Calibration Table for Schiotz Tonometry in Dogs*

	Schiotz Scale Reading	IOP (mm Hg) 5.5 g wt	IOP (mm Hg) 7.5 g wt	IOP (mm Hg) 10.0 g wt
	0.5	52.6	71.2	93.6
	1.0	49.3	67.0	88.3
	1.5	46.3	63.1	83.3
	2.0	43.4	59.4	78.6
	2.5	40.8	55.9	74.1
Normal range with 5.5 g wt	3.0	38.3	52.6	69.9
	3.5	36.0	49.6	66.0
	4.0	33.9	46.7	62.2
	4.5	31.9	44.0	58.7
	5.0	30.1	41.6	55.4
	5.5	28.4	39.2	52.3
	6.0	26.9	37.1	49.4
	6.5	25.5	35.1	46.7
	7.0	24.2	33.2	44.2
	7.5	23.0	31.5	41.8
	8.0	21.9	29.9	39.6
	8.5	21.0	28.5	37.5
	9.0	20.1	27.1	35.6
	9.5	19.3	25.9	33.8
	10.0	18.6	24.8	32.1
	10.5	18.0	23.8	30.6
	11.0	17.4	22.8	29.1
	11.5	17.0	22.0	27.8
	12.0	16.6	21.3	26.6
	12.5	16.3	20.6	25.5
	13.0	16.0	20.0	24.5
	13.5	15.8	19.5	23.6
	14.0	15.7	19.1	22.8
	14.5	15.7	18.8	22.0
	15.0	15.7	18.5	21.4
	15.5	15.8	18.3	20.8
	16.0	15.9	18.1	20.3
	16.5	16.1	18.0	19.9
	17.0	16.4	18.0	19.5
	17.5	16.8	18.1	19.2
	18.0	17.2	18.2	19.0
	18.5	17.7	18.4	18.8
	19.0	18.3	18.7	18.7
	19.5	19.0	19.0	18.6
	20.0	19.7	19.4	18.7

*From Peiffer, R.L., et al. (1976): Proc. Am. Coll. Vet. Ophthalmol., 7:47.

Magrane's
CANINE OPHTHALMOLOGY

Magrane's
CANINE OPHTHALMOLOGY

Lloyd C. Helper, D.V.M., M.S.

Charter Diplomate American College of Veterinary Ophthalmologists;
Professor, Clinical Medicine (Ophthalmology);
Associate Dean of Academic Affairs,
College of Veterinary Medicine,
University of Illinois at Urbana-Champaign.

FOURTH EDITION

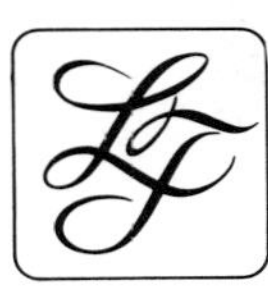

Lea & Febiger Philadelphia • London 1989

Lea & Febiger
600 Washington Square
Philadelphia, PA 19106-4198
U.S.A.
(215) 922-1330

Lea & Febiger (UK) Ltd.
145a Croydon Road
Beckenham, Kent BR3 3RB
U.K.

Library of Congress Cataloging in Publication Data

Magrane, William G.
Magrane's canine ophthalmology.

Rev. ed. of: Canine ophthalmology. 3rd ed. 1977.
Includes bibliographical references and index.
1. Dogs–Diseases. 2. Veterinary ophthalmology.
I. Helper, Lloyd C. II. Title. III. Title: Canine ophthalmology. [DNLM: 1. Dog Diseases. 2. Eye Diseases–veterinary. SF 991 M212c]
SF992.E92M28 1989 636.7'08977 88-9389
ISBN 0-8121-1173-7

PRINTED IN THE UNITED STATES OF AMERICA

Print number: 5 4 3 2 1

Dedicated to my wife Jean
whose skill and help made this work possible,
and to our children,
Debra, Mark, David, and Patti
who have brought so much joy and satisfaction to our lives.

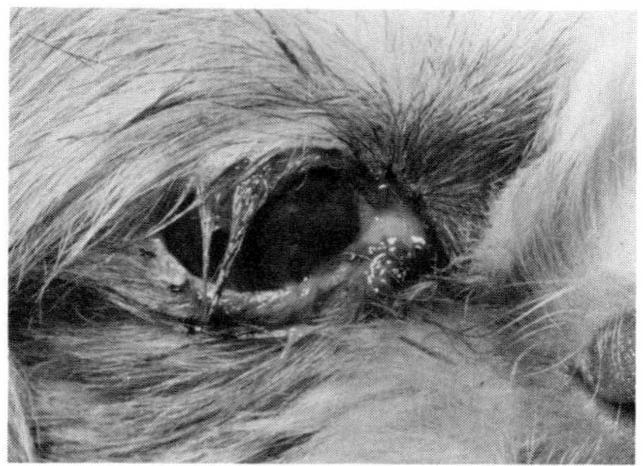

Fig. 4–16. Trichiasis. Some of the regular eyelashes have assumed an abnormal, inferior deviation.

nictitating membrane or palpebra tertia, and by dog breeders and fanciers, the "Haw." The term third eyelid seems most appropriate in the dog and other animals in which it is a thick, more complex structure; and the term membrana nictitans, or other terms implying a membranous structure is more appropriate for birds and other species in which the structure is more like a membrane. It is composed of a T-shaped cartilage covered on both surfaces by conjunctiva. The conjunctiva in the inner surface is continuous with the bulbar conjunctiva and that on the outer surface with the palpebral conjunctiva (Fig. 1–10). A seromucinous gland, similar histologically to the lacrimal gland, envelops the base of the T-shaped cartilage and extends well up on its inner and outer surfaces. A small cluster of lymphocyte follicles is located on the bulbar surface of the membrana nictitans superior to the glandular tissue. Figure 4–19 illustrates the relationship between the cartilage, gland,

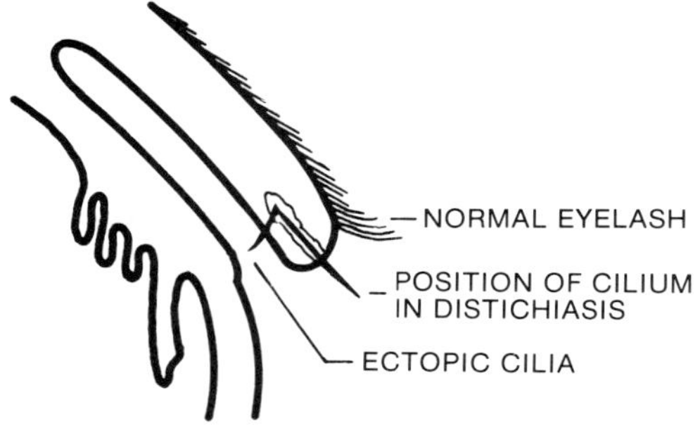

Fig. 4–17. Contrast of lid cilia.

and the follicle area. There is no muscle in the membrana nictitans in the dog, or in the tissue connecting it to the globe and to the lower eyelid. Severin[30] suggests that there is a connective tissue band anchoring the base of the gland to the orbital tissue. The relative position of the free edge of the membrana nictitans on the globe is controlled by the position of the eyeball. Retraction of the globe by the retractor oculi muscles causes the third eyelid to elevate, and relaxation of the retractors allows it to recede to normal position. Conditions that produce enophthalmos generally cause elevation and increased visibility of the membrana nictitans while conditions that produce exophthalmos generally cause the membrana nictitans to recede and become less visible. Space-occupying lesions or marked inflammation or edema in the orbit below or behind the globe are exceptions, in that they tend to produce exophthalmos while concurrently forcing the membrana nictitans out of the orbit and up on the globe. The third eyelid acts to protect the cornea when the eye is retracted and to aid in distribution of the precorneal film. This latter function is especially important in dogs with poor cornea-eyelid apposition or lid function. Most dogs with obicularis oculi muscle paralysis due to injury or a long-acting nerve block of the palpebral branches of the auriculo-palpebral nerve maintain normal distribution of the precorneal film by action of the third eyelid. The gland of the third eyelid produces part of the watery layer of the precorneal film. The percentage produced by the lacrimal gland and the gland of the third eyelid seems to vary from dog to dog.[18] One should be aware that removal of the gland reduces tear production and, because the percent reduction is variable and unpredictable, such treatment may lead to keratoconjunctivitis sicca, immediately or later, if remaining tear production is compromised by other factors.

4:46 In the past the third eyelid has been surgically removed by many clinicians for a variety of reasons, few of which have had any validity. Hypertrophy elevation or eversion/

PREFACE TO THE FIRST EDITION

In this book I have endeavored to present a concise, practical, and systematic review of the diseases and surgical procedures of the canine eye. The text is intended for the student and general practitioner in veterinary medicine and includes principles of ophthalmology applicable to any of the species.

To remain within the scope of a manual, excessive detail, extensive discussion, theories and rare conditions are allotted minimal space. It is hoped that the reader will seek further knowledge in the subject by references to the more exhaustive and comprehensive textbooks of human ophthalmology. However, since some important differences do exist between the canine and human eye, a comparison will be made as deemed necessary.

There has been no attempt to categorize all of the preparations and drugs or surgical procedures, nor to describe all methods of treatment or operative techniques. Only those with which I am most familiar are included.

Illustrations and photographs have been used when it seemed that they would be of value in clarifying the text. I am indebted to many colleagues in human and veterinary medicine for permission to use illustrative material and for their inspiration and help.

I wish to express my special appreciation to Denyes Studio of South Bend, Indiana, and Mr. James Sprunger in particular, illustrators for this book; and to my daughter-in-law Barbara, who typed and helped to edit the complete manuscript. I am deeply grateful to the many practitioners throughout the country who have provided me with the cases that have made this specialized study and this book possible.

William G. Magrane

PREFACE

In this, my first revision of *Canine Ophthalmology*, I have attempted to continue Dr. William Magrane's original intent to provide a concise text for the student or general practitioner that includes the principles of ophthalmology applicable to any species.

The rapid expansion of knowledge in veterinary ophthalmology makes it impossible to include, or even cite, all of the new information that has evolved since the last edition and maintain a concise text of reasonable length.

Obsolete material has been deleted, and those new diagnostic methods, medical treatments, and surgical techniques that we have found most useful have been added.

Those interested in further study are referred to more comprehensive texts in veterinary ophthalmology that have been published since the last edition of this book, such as Gelatt's *Veterinary Ophthalmology*, Lea & Febiger, 1981, 788 pages; the numerous human texts; as well as the journal articles cited herein and elsewhere.

Urbana, Illinois Lloyd C. Helper

CONTENTS

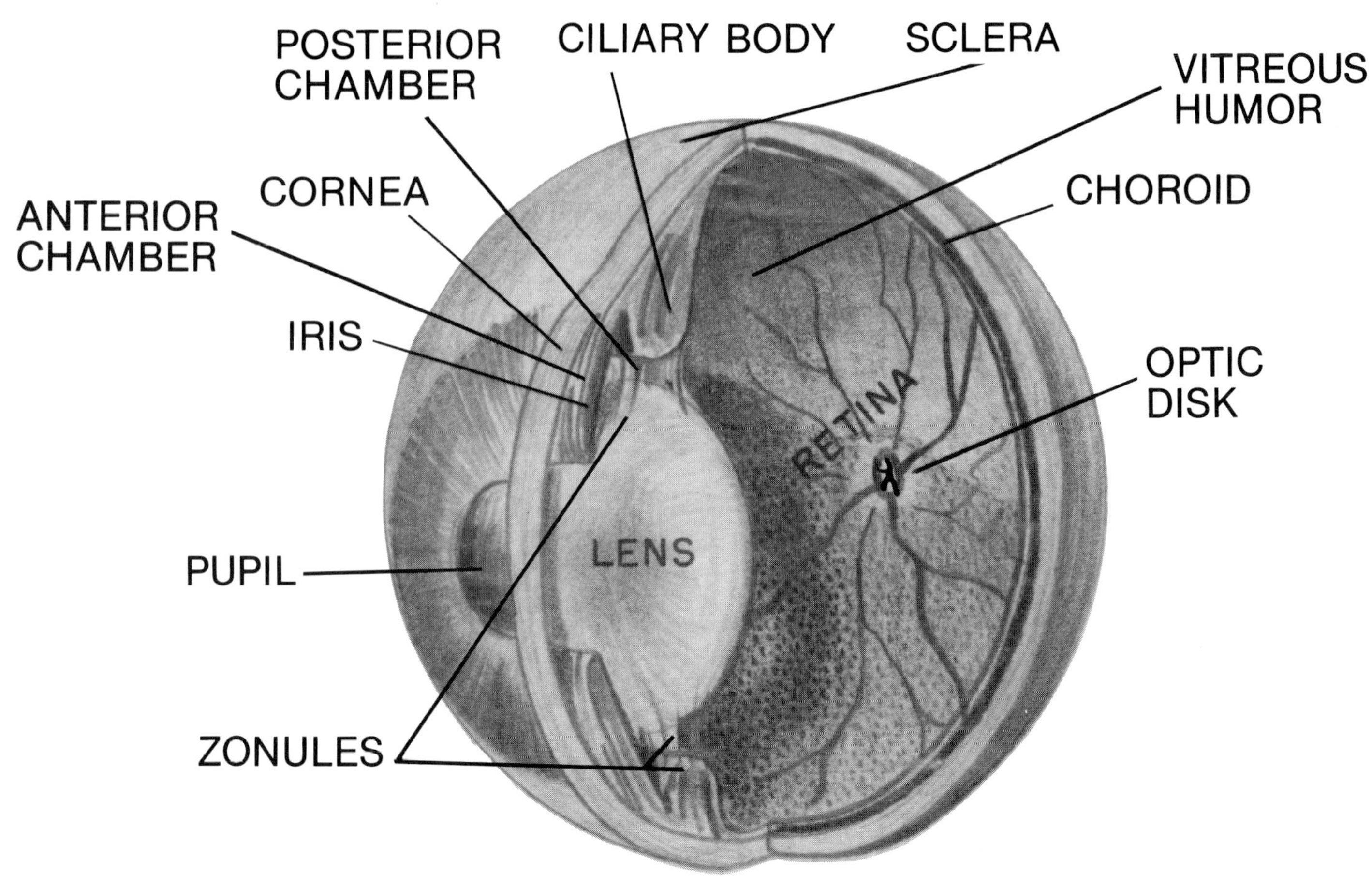

Fig. 1–1. The eye with section removed.

1 THE NORMAL EYE

Vision

1:1 It is generally agreed that the domestic dog is myopic (near sighted), astigmatic (uneven cornea), color blind, and accommodates poorly. Roberts[6] concludes that the selection process which has produced dog breeds of greatly varying anatomical types has produced haphazard combinations of the various genetic factors that account for the optical system, the corneal size and shape, lens curvature, and anteroposterior measurements resulting in the poor visual apparatus of the dog breeds we know today. The dog has sharpened his other senses because his vision is so poor, at least when we compare it to man.

1:2 Although the ophthalmoscope gives the examiner a rough idea of the refractive error, retinoscopy is a much more accurate means for making such determinations. Wyman,[8] examining 52 dogs of various breeds with an ophthalmoscope, found that −2D to +2D produced the clearest focus. When refracting 9 dogs with a hand retinoscope, he found the refractive error ranged from 0 to −1.75 diopters, indicating dogs are normal-sighted to somewhat myopic (Fig. 1–2). We have noted variances in myopia of 1 to 8 diopters, as determined by the minus settings on the ophthalmoscope, and commonly use a −3.0 setting to initiate examinations of the fundus. The apparent disparity in these two observations may be due, in part at least, to inadvertent accommodation of the lens of the observer, which could require a compensation of up to −4.0 diopters in the ophthalmoscope. Although one should attempt to relax accommodation as if looking off into the distance when looking through the direct ophthalmoscope and then adjust the diopters setting of the ophthalmoscope, the student or infrequent user will find it advantageous to *start* with a slightly exaggerated minus (red) diopter setting. The observer can compensate for the exaggerated minus setting by making his own lens more *plus* (accommodation), thus bringing the fundus into focus; whereas, such compensation is not possible if the ophthalmoscope is initially set without enough minus (red) diopters.

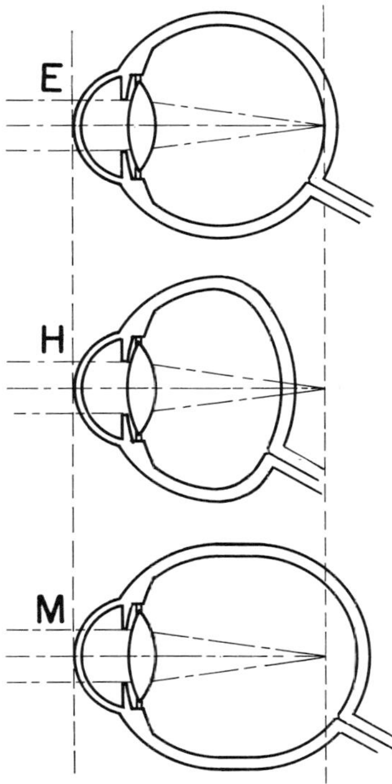

Fig. 1–2. E. Emmetropia (normal sight). H. Hyperopia (far sighted). M. Myopia (near sighted).

1:3 The poor accommodation (ability to

focus) is the result of a weak ciliary muscle and a firm lens. This anatomic difference (*i.e.* from man) produces a naturally presbyopic eye (old sight) in the dog.

1:4 For academic interest, investigations[7] into the color vision of the dog have been undertaken. The investigators have concluded: for the dog, it is form and (to a less extent) brightness which are important qualities of visual stimuli. It is doubtful if the animal experiences color at all. Whatever weakly chromatic sensations his cones may afford are further unsaturated and greatly diluted by his superabundant rods. For example, he sees shades of grey when looking at and comparing red and pink blankets.

1:5 Fortunately for the dog other factors play a role in providing satisfactory vision. He has a larger pupil and larger visual field than man, with a better peripheral vision. With the aid of the tapetum lucidum and abundant rods, the dog can see better in semi-darkened to darkened areas (Par. 11:18). He has a fair degree of binocular vision (depth perception), but when one eye is lost the other takes over in remarkable fashion, using a sense of perspective and parallactic displacement to compensate in part. On the whole, as is the case with all the species, the dog is supplied with the type of vision most suited to its needs, and is most adept in following moving objects.

1:6 The question is often asked: how long does it take after the eyes are open until the new puppy can see. Anatomically, the developmental processes of the eye itself are complete at birth, even though the lid junction does not disappear until approximately 10 days postpartum. The time of lid opening, however, coincides closely with that at which the rods and cones of the retina have finished their differentiation. Retinal maturation takes place in the early postnatal period and proceeds from the central to the peripheral regions. Slender rod and cone inner and outer segments are present in the central retina by 16 days after birth and in the peripheral retina after 35 days.[1] We can only postulate when single binocular vision, with depth perception and fusion occurs. Based on an age comparison with man, this would be at about 6 weeks in the puppy.

Anatomy of Vision

1:7 The eye may be considered as an optical instrument comparable to the camera, in which by means of a refracting (dioptric) system a small and inverted image of external objects is formed on the retina.[2]

1:8 In passing through the eyeball, rays of light traverse the cornea, aqueous, lens, and vitreous. These light rays are refracted (bent) to converge on or near the retina. The refracting surfaces of the eye are the cornea, and the anterior and posterior surfaces of the lens. If the canine eye is about 20 mm from cornea to retina (Par. 1:22), it represents an optical system of about 50 diopters refracting power. (One diopter brings parallel light rays into focus at 1 meter.) Fifty diopters will bring parallel rays into focus at 20 mm. The cornea provides most of the refraction of light. Since the lens contributes only about 10 diopters of refraction, removal of the lens tends to make the eye quite hyperopic (far-sighted) and causes a blurred image, but does not alter the inversion of the image, as some clients commonly conclude.

1:9 The amount of light that enters the eye is regulated by the eyelids and the pupillary action of the iris. Light reaching the retina is absorbed by its deeper layers and a photochemical reaction converts this light into electrical impulses. Electrical impulses arising here are transmitted in the reverse direction to the innermost retinal nerve fiber layer, and then to the optic nerve. Impulses continue along the optic nerve, optic chiasm (where a partial decussation of fibers takes place), optic tract, and into the lateral geniculate body. From the lateral geniculate body, optic radiations travel to the calcarine area (visual cortex) of the occipital lobe of the cerebrum. It is here that impulses are recorded and interpreted (Fig. 1–3).

1:10 The eye, then, must not be considered

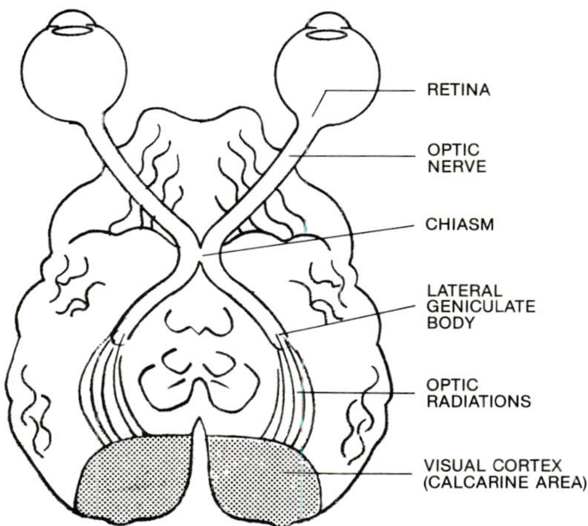

Fig. 1–3. The anatomy of vision.

an isolated organ, for the retina and all the refractive media are useless if the nerve connections to the cerebral cortex of the occipital lobe are diseased or cut off.[4]

THE EYEBALL

Anatomy

General Considerations

1:11 The anatomic parts with which ophthalmology is concerned are the eyeball proper, the appendages of the eye, *i.e.* the cavity which contains the eye, the eyelids which protect it, the muscles which move it, the lacrimal apparatus which constantly moistens its transparent portion, and the visual pathways just described (Par. 1:9).

1:12 This chapter concerns itself only with a view of the eyeball as a whole. The anatomy and physiology of each of the parts constituting the visual apparatus are more precisely discussed at the beginning of the chapters dealing with the diseases and surgery of these parts.

1:13 Prince[5] describes the eye (Fig. 1–1) simply as a layer of neural light-sensitive tissue (the retina) held in shape by surrounding coats which protect it (sclera) and nourish it (choroid), and served by an optical system of a lens of modified transparent epithelium behind a transparent anterior extension of the sclera (cornea), all of which combine to focus light on the retina.

1:14 The eyeball proper consists of three layers or tunics:

1. *External fibrous tunic.* The outer protective layer which, with the intraocular pressure gives the globe its definite semi-rigid shape. This layer can be likened to the box of a camera.
   a. Anterior portion: *Cornea*
   b. Posterior portion: *Sclera*
   Both of these parts are covered by conjunctiva which is represented by epithelium only over the transparent cornea.
2. *Vascular tunic* (Uvea). This layer provides for the nourishment of the eyeball and is composed of:

   a. Iris } (Anterior uvea)
   b. Ciliary body }
   c. Choroid (Posterior uvea)

3. *Inner layer: Retina.* A thin, delicate membrane which is really an extension of the brain. All parts of the eye serve the purpose of protecting and maintaining the retina.

1:15 Within the eyeball are the principal structures referred to as:

1. The *anterior chamber* containing *aqueous* humor.
2. *Pupil*—formed by the margin of the iris.
3. *Posterior chamber*—containing aqueous humor.
4. *Lens* and its *zonular* attachments.
5. *Vitreous humor*—a jelly-like mass occupying the greater part of the ocular cavity and lying between the posterior surface of the lens and the retina. Its outer surface presents a thin, structureless condensation, the *hyaloid membrane,* which, in turn, is firmly attached to the posterior capsule of the lens.

1:16 Structures and areas include:

Bulbar conjunctiva—covers the globe proper.

Palpebral conjunctiva—lines the upper and lower lids.

Limbus—the area 1 mm wide which forms a transition zone between the cornea and the conjunctiva-sclera. It is rich in blood vessels and nerve endings. The conjunctiva, Tenon's capsule and sclera are firmly adherent one to another in this area and not easily separated by dissection.

Tenon's capsule—a dense connective tissue membrane that lies between the conjunctiva and sclera from the limbus back to the attachment of the extraocular muscles. From the area of muscle attachment, Tenon's capsule extends posteriorly along the muscles and does not cover the sclera from the area of muscle attachment to the posterior pole of the eye (Fig. 1–4).

Episclera—a thin, spongy, vascular, elastic membrane whose purpose is to provide nutrition to the outer parts of the almost avascular sclera. It is contained by Tenon's capsule and loosely attached to the globe by fibrous connective tissue.

Fornix (retrotarsal fold)—the transition portion of bulbar to palpebral conjunctiva, forming a fold between lid and globe.

Cul-de-sac—the fold (pouch) formed by the junction of the palpebral and bulbar conjunctivae.

1:17 *Extraocular muscles* (Figs. 1–5, 1–9, and 1–10) are seven in number. There are four recti, two obliques and a retractor oculi (absent in man). The recti and obliques are poorly developed as compared to those of man.

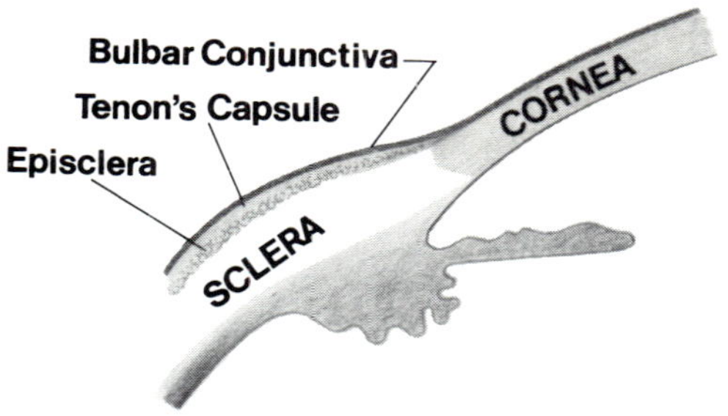

Fig. 1–4. Relationship of external structures.

1:18 All four recti muscles are flat, have their origins around the optic foramen and orbital fissure and insert into the globe with aponeurotic tendons between 6 and 8 mm from the limbus.

1:19 The inferior and superior oblique muscles which serve as rotators of the eye in the dog are attached near the insertions of the recti in the anterior portion of the eye. This is in sharp contrast to man in whom these muscles insert posterior to the equator.

1:20 The retractor oculi may be either a complete cone of muscle, the apex at the orbital fissure and the base at its insertions into the globe, or it may be divided into four parts, two inserting on either side of the superior rectus and the other two on either side of the inferior rectus. The retractor oculi serves a useful purpose in providing a protective mechanism for the eye. Since there is no complete bony orbit in the dog, it is important that the eye can be retracted in impending danger.

Measurements (Fig. 1–6)

1:21 The eye is almost spherical and is relatively large for the size of the animal. The geometrical center of the cornea is known as the *anterior pole* of the eye and the *posterior pole* is exactly opposite and is usually dorsal and medial to the nerve head. The *geometric axis* connects the anterior and posterior poles.

1:22 There are three diameters which are commonly referred to as: the *sagittal* (anteroposterior), the *transverse* and the *vertical*. The length of these varies among the different breeds with a dimensional range of:

20 to 25 mm in the anteroposterior direction
19.7 to 25 mm in the transverse direction
18.7 to 25 mm in the vertical direction

1:23 The total absolute volume of the eyeball is from 4.5 to 5 ml and the weight from 4 to 8 g.

The Vascular System (Fig. 1–7).

1:24 The main blood supply to the orbit is derived from the internal maxillary artery,

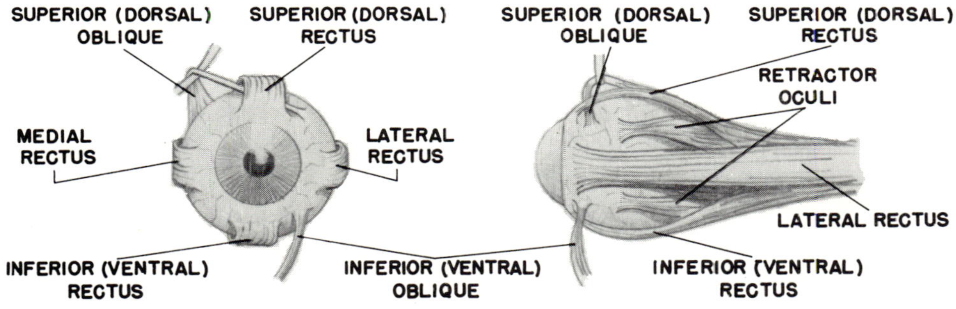

Fig. 1–5. The extraocular muscles.

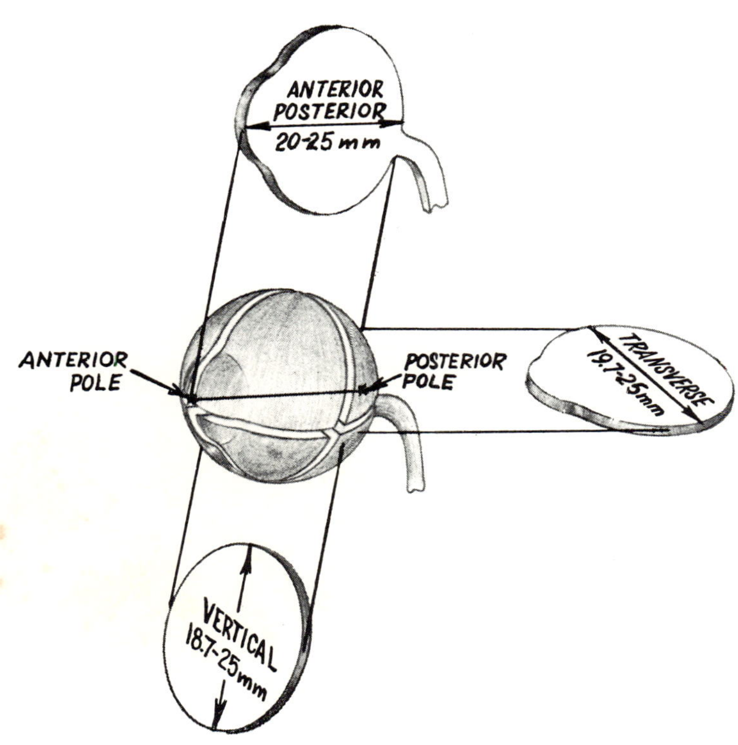

Fig. 1–6. Measurements of the canine eye.

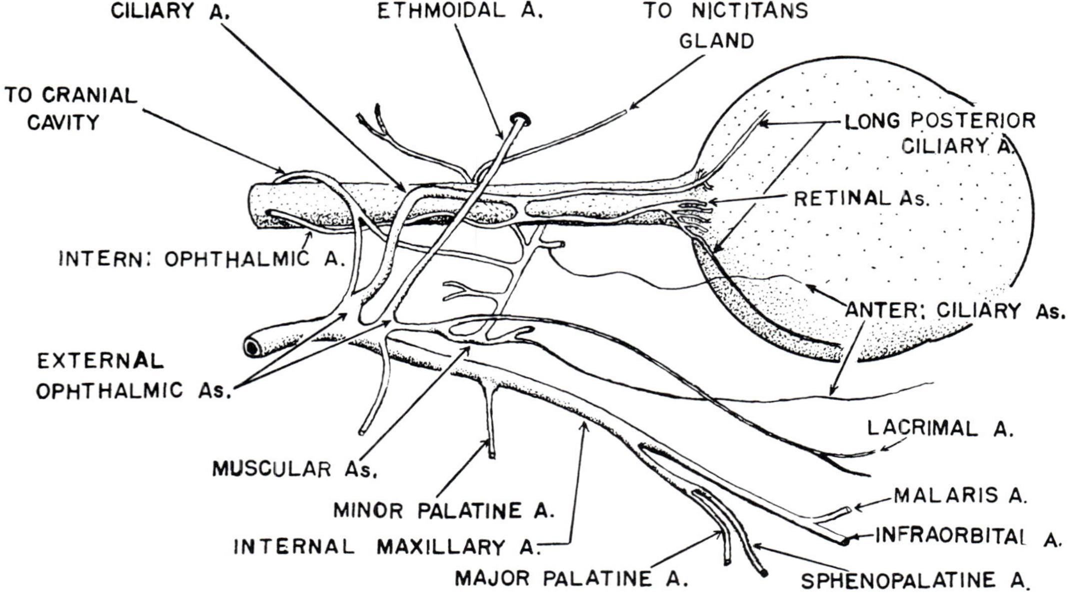

Fig. 1–7. The orbital arterial system. (Prince, Diesem, Eglitis and Ruskell, *Anatomy and Histology of the Eye and Orbit in Domestic Animals,* courtesy of Charles C Thomas.)

which is a continuation of the external carotid artery. Two branches of the internal maxillary artery penetrate the periorbita and represent the external ophthalmic artery.

1:25 In contrast to man, in which the main blood supply to the eye is derived from the internal carotid, the ciliary system in the dog is derived from the external ophthalmic artery, a branch of the maxillary artery which anastomoses with the *external* carotid. It is distributed to the vascular tunic (the uvea) and the sclera by:

(1) Four to six short posterior ciliary arteries which ramify within the choroid.
(2) Two long posterior ciliary arteries which run between the sclera and choroid and give off branches to the ciliary muscle, ciliary processes, and the iris.
(3) The anterior ciliary arteries which supply branches to the conjunctiva, sclera, ciliary muscles, and limbal region.[5]

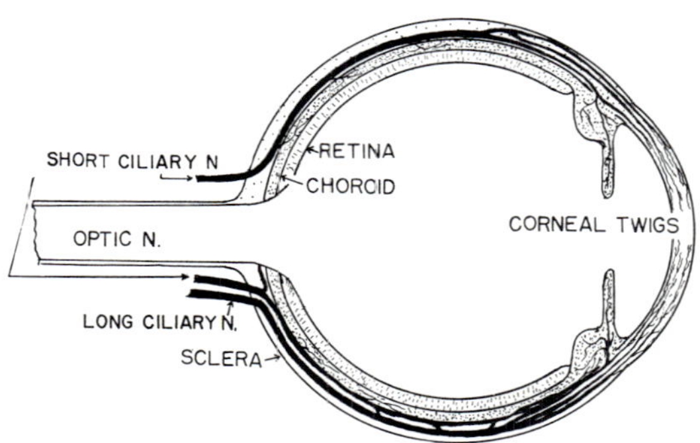

Fig. 1–8. The paths by which the various ciliary nerves enter the eye, anastomose, and travel to their destinations. (Prince, Diesem, Eglitis and Ruskell, *Anatomy and Histology of the Eye and Orbit in Domestic Animals,* courtesy of Charles C Thomas.)

1:26 The venous tributaries converge toward the equator, perforate the sclera and pass into the ophthalmic vein. The anterior branches unite into an annular plexus which receives the veins of the ciliary body and iris. The anterior ciliary veins communicate with the *plexus venosus sclerae* (drainage system).

Nerve Supply (Fig. 1–8)

1:27 The nerves of the eyeball course toward the cornea between the sclera and choroid and form a plexus in the choroid and then the plexus gangliosus ciliaris on the ciliary

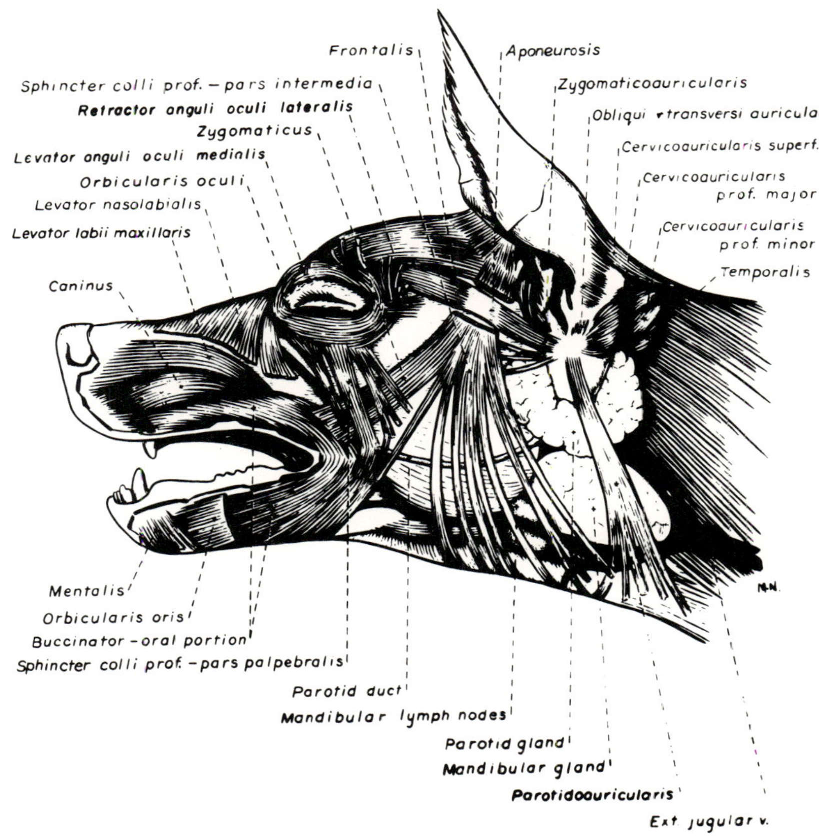

Fig. 1–9. Lateral view of the face, illustrating the position and relationships of the orbicularis oculi and retractor oculi muscles. Also note the position of the parotid salivary gland and duct. (Platysma and sphincter colli superficialis muscles have been removed) (Evans and Christiansen, *Miller's Anatomy of the Dog,* courtesy of W.B. Saunders Co.)

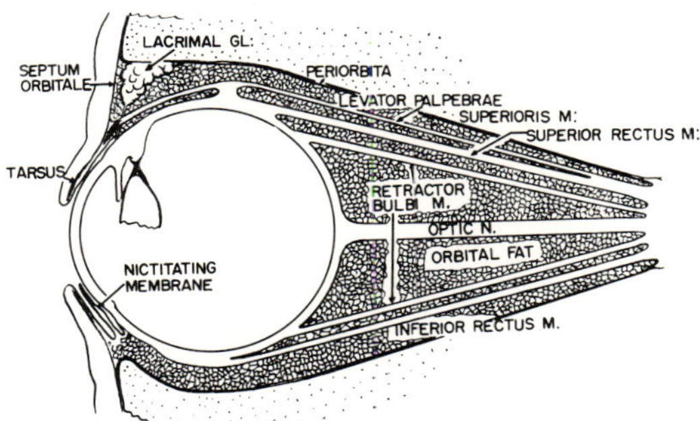

Fig. 1–10. Diagrammatic cross-section of the orbit, illustrating the relationships of the eyelids, orbital septum and lacrimal gland and the extraocular muscles. Note the relationship between the levator muscle, which raises the upper lid, and the superior rectus muscle. (Prince, Diesem, Eglitis and Ruskell, *Anatomy and Histology of the Eye and Orbit in Domestic Animals,* courtesy of Charles C Thomas.)

body, which gives rise to the nerves for the ciliary muscle, the iris, and the cornea.

General Nerve Supply

1:28 Third (Oculomotor) supplies motor fibers to: superior, inferior and medial recti muscles, portion of the retractor oculi, inferior oblique, levator, sphincter of iris, ciliary muscle.

Fourth (Trochlear) supplies the superior oblique.

Fifth (Ophthalmic branch of trigeminal) supplies: lids, conjunctiva, cornea, dilators of the iris.

Sixth (Abducens) supplies the lateral rectus and portions of the retractor oculi.

Seventh (Facial) supplies the orbicularis muscle.

For a more comprehensive study of the neurology the reader is referred to the texts mentioned in the references.

REFERENCES

1. Aguirre, G.D., et al.: Development of the Canine Eye, Am. J. Vet. Res., 33:2399, 1972.
2. Allen, J.H.: *May's Diseases of the Eye*, 23rd ed., Baltimore, The Williams & Wilkins Co., 1963.
3. Evans, H.E., Christiansen, G.C.: *Miller's Anatomy of the Dog*, 2nd Ed., Philadelphia, W.B. Saunders Co., p. 668, 1979.
4. Leinfelder, P.J.: Outline of Neuro-ophthalmology, Home Study Course, Am. Ac. Ophth. & Otolar.
5. Prince, J.H., Diesem, C.D., Eglitis, I. and Ruskell, G.L.: *Anatomy and Histology of the Eye and Orbit in Domestic Animals*, Springfield, Charles C Thomas, 1960.
6. Roberts, S.R.: Animal Vision, J.A.V.M.A., *127*:236, 1955.
7. Walls, G.L.: *The Vertebrate Eye*, Bloomfield Hills, Cranbrook Institute of Science, p. 506, 1942.
8. Wyman, M. and Donovan, E.F.: The Ocular Fundus of the Normal dog, J.A.V.M.A., *147*:17, 1965.

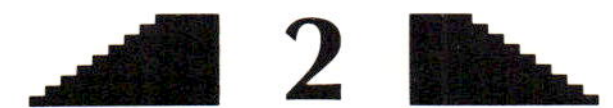

EXAMINATION OF THE EYE AND ITS ADNEXA

External Examination

2:1 The clinician must ever remember that ophthalmology is a branch of medicine and surgery. Examination of an eye (Fig. 2–1) or eyes does not mean merely that an isolated organ is being studied, rather, that the animal is being examined with special reference to that organ and its functions. It is often imperative that an accurate case history, thorough physical examination, and laboratory studies are necessary before an evaluation of the ocular lesion is possible. The value of the history depends on how observant the owner is and the ability of the clinician to elicit information. Questions should include: (1) owner's description of signs and which eye is involved. If both, which eye was involved first?, (2) what is vision like at night, daytime, for stationary and moving objects?, (3) duration of signs and previous medications? The breed and age should always be considered. Certain breeds exhibit a predisposition to ocular disease within an age group. This knowledge is most helpful in establishing a firm diagnosis (Appendix 1).

2:2 Every examination should include a systematic plan, a routine that will enable the examiner mentally to catalogue his findings in orderly fashion and instill in him the concept of thinking of the eyeball and adnexa as a whole. Unless this principle is adhered to, an obvious lesion of one part of the globe will often distract the examiner so that either the real cause of that lesion or an associated pathologic condition is completely overlooked. It is very important that the history and findings during examination be recorded in a manner, such that the examiner or another veterinarian can, at a later date, understand what was said and what was found.

2:3 Examination of the eye may be divided into: *objective* and *subjective* (functional).

2:4 The objective examination consists first of a naked eye examination of the dog. This procedure is applicable primarily to the orbit and eyelids. It is conducted with *minimal restraint* being used and is for the purpose of ascertaining obvious abnormalities such as swellings, comparing size of the eyes, nystagmus, strabismus, position of the nictitating membrane, discharges, size of the palpebral aperture, and especially the position of the lids in relation to the globe. It may be necessary to withhold all restraint or even examine the patient on the floor in order to determine accurately the lid relationship (*e.g.* entropion, ectropion) to the globe. Further evaluation of the orbit may necessitate examination of the mouth or special techniques, *e.g.* radiography of the skull, ultrasonography (Par. 2:71) and surgical exploration.

2:5 The remainder of the objective examination should be conducted in a quiet, semidarkened to dark room with the aid of proper equipment and a suitable, focal light source. For convenience and maneuverability, the examiner should be seated on an adjustable caster-equipped stool. The seated position places the examiner at eye level with the animal which facilitates examination, and provides stability to hold the instruments being used. A binocular loupe of 2.5× magnifica-

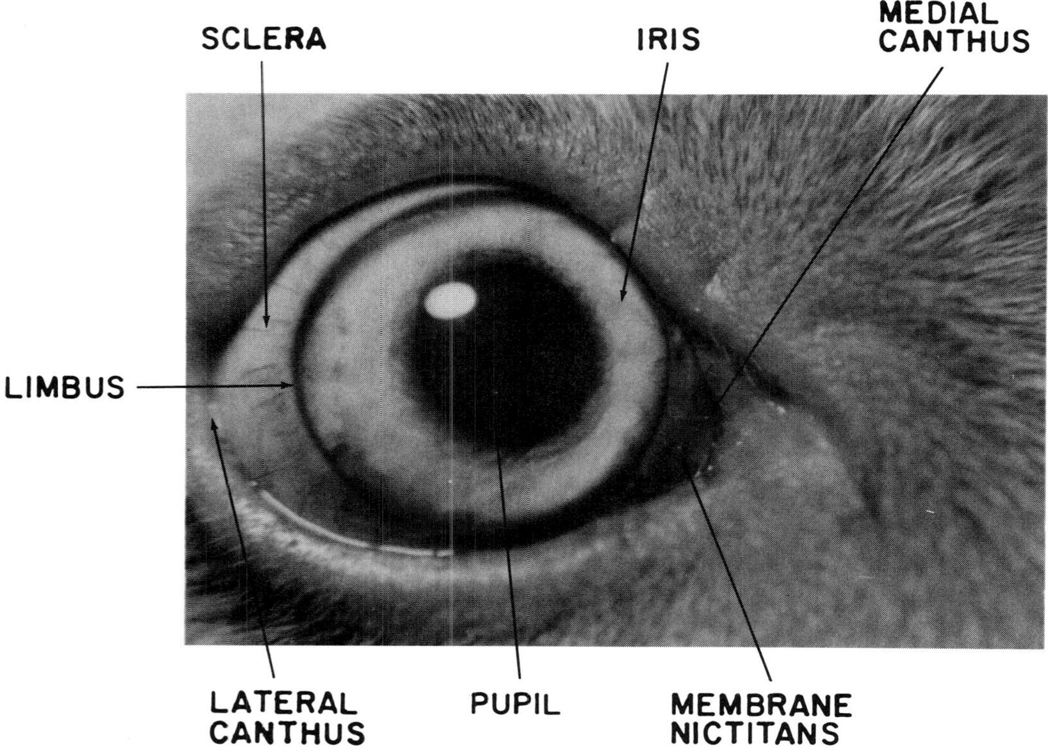

Fig. 2–1. The external eye.

tion, and a focal light source, *e.g.* a pen light, or ideally, a transilluminator (Figs. 2–2 and 2–3) is usually adequate to examine properly all structures from the lids back to the face of the vitreous. The fiber optic Finoff transilluminator with a Halogen bulb (Fig. 2–2) is an ideal focal light source and can also be used for conducting the pupillary light reflex tests, as well as for limited use in transillumination of the eye. (Par. 2:8) A hand-held monocular slit lamp (Fig. 2–4) that is relatively inexpensive provides a magnification and the spatial relationship of ocular structures seen by slit illumination. It should, however, not be confused with the hand-held binocular slit lamp-biomicroscope (Fig. 2–5) that provides up to 20× magnification and binocular viewing, or the larger table or stand-mounted binocular slit lamp-biomicroscope that provides up to 60× magnification (Fig. 2–6).

2:6 Überreiter[30] pioneered in the use of *biomicroscopy* for examination of the eye in animals. The combination of the corneal microscope with illumination by a slit-lamp for the examination of the anterior portion of the eye offers a magnification of 10 to 60 diameters and enables the viewer to observe finer structures and localize the depth of pathologic processes. This piece of equipment is essential to the human or veterinary ophthalmologist, but because of the cost and need for special training in its use, is not practical for general use. Various slit-lamp models may be modified for use by the veterinary ophthalmologist. The external and anterior segment of the eyes can usually be examined with the slit lamp biomicroscope without the need for drug restraint. For prolonged, or an examination of deeper structures, a combination of Rompun (xylazine)† at the rate of 1.0 mg per

†Rompun, Chemagro Corp., Kansas City, Mo.

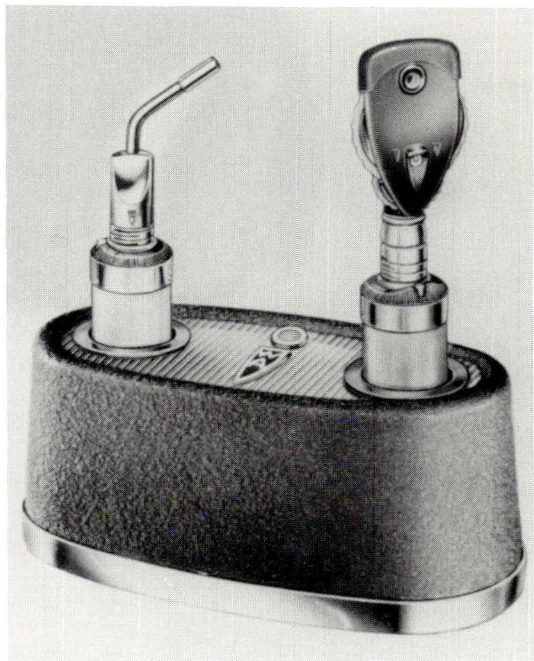

Fig. 2–2. Finoff transilluminator and ophthalmoscope battery set (Welch Allyn). Handles are automatically charged when placed in unit.

pound intramuscularly and atropine 0.01 mg per pound, followed in seven minutes by 5 mg per pound of ketamine hydrochloride‡ intramuscularly has proven most efficacious.[13] The eye stays forward and open thus eliminating the disadvantage of general anesthesia and tranquilizers which often cause the eye to recede and the nictitating membrane to elevate. On occasion the use of biomicroscopy has proven to be the *only* means of arriving at a correct diagnosis with subsequent correction of a chronic condition. Martin[19] conducted an exhaustive study in slit lamp biomicroscopy of the normal eye of the dog. The ocular structures are described and illustrated in exquisite detail and the significant differences from the human eye noted.

2:7 Each year there is an increase in the use of the slit-lamp as veterinarians complete residencies and graduate training in ophthalmology. This development is imperative if we are to solve a myriad of ocular diseases and surgical problems.

2:8 *Transillumination* is useful when corneal edema or flocculent debris in the anterior chamber precludes examination of the iris and pupillary area.[2] Often even the lens and vitreal cavity can be visualized by this means. This method of examination uses the passage of a beam of light through the sclera. The light source is applied directly to the globe at different aspects of the sclera, usually near the limbus. Good results can only be obtained when the examining room is absolutely dark. The development of ultrasonography (Par. 2:72) has diminished the use of transillumination; however, it remains a valuable inexpensive diagnostic aid in certain cases.

2:9 Various types of transilluminators are used. Diagnostic equipment with an intense focal light source, such as the Finoff transilluminator, will also serve the purpose (Fig. 2–2). However, the best results will be obtained with a specially designed transilluminator (Fig. 2–7).

2:10 *Gonioscopy*—The angle of the anterior chamber (irido-corneal angle) is hidden from view in man and animals by the forward projection of the opaque edge of the scleral limbus. None of the ordinary methods of examination of the iris and chamber allows access to this recess. Gonioscopy involves the observation of this angle of the anterior chamber of the living eye.

2:11 Whereas visualization of the chamber angle is desirable for other reasons, *e.g.* tumors, cysts, congenital anomalies, foreign bodies, the most important aspect of gonioscopy is in the study of glaucoma (Par. 9:47). Since the angle area is important in returning the aqueous humor to the blood stream, narrowing, closure or changes in the tissues can cause inhibition of outflow and give rise to an increase in intraocular pressure (Chapter 9). Study of the angle may reveal both cause and effect of glaucoma, and by so doing may furnish clues for medical or surgical treatment.

‡Ketamine, Parke Davis Co., Detroit, Mich.

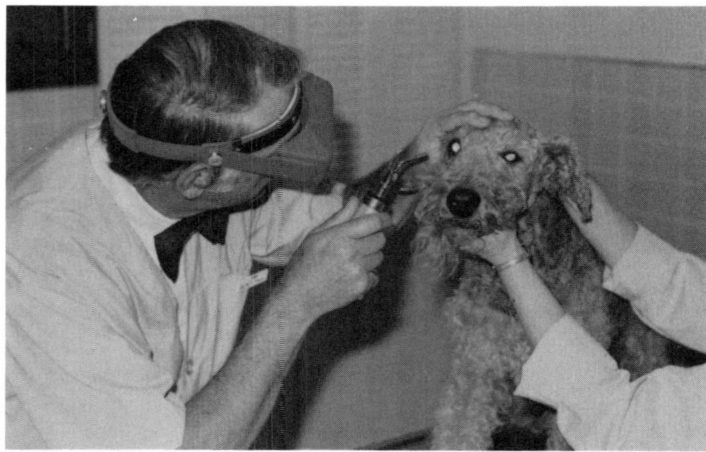

Fig. 2–3. Examination of the eye using a binocular loupe and focal light source (darkened room essential).

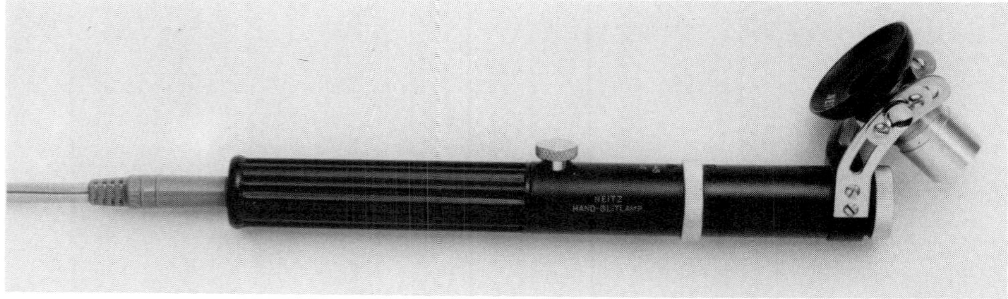

Fig. 2–4. A hand slit-lamp (Neitz). (Neitz, Western Optical, 1200 Mercer St., Seattle, Washington 98109)

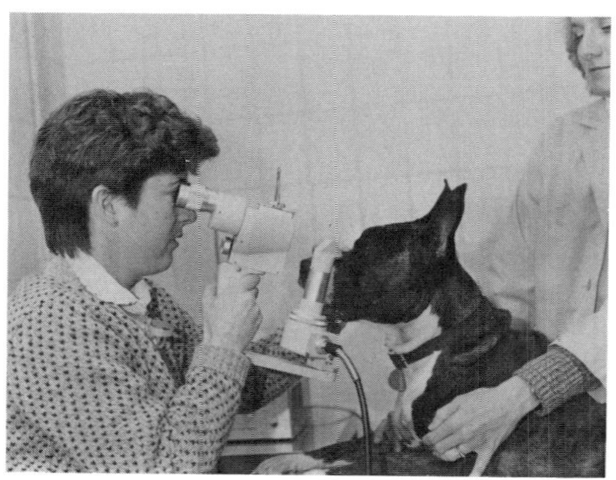

Fig. 2–5. Kowa hand-held, fiber optic slit lamp and biomicroscope, capable of up to 20× magnification.

Examination of the not yet glaucomatous fellow eye may also be of some prognostic value.

2:12 Gonioscopy in the dog is not particularly difficult to perform and has proven to be a most practical clinical procedure, although, admittedly its use is limited to the clinician who tends towards specialization.

2:13 Troncoso[29] gives a splendid word picture and color drawing of the canine chamber angle. Lescure[16] has described his technique, choice of instruments, and method of photographing the angle. Martin[18,19] correlated the gonioscopic appearance with specially prepared gross dissections, histology and scanning electron microscopy, in an attempt to better understand the anatomy and physiology of aqueous circulation. One of the several contact gonioscopic lenses designed for

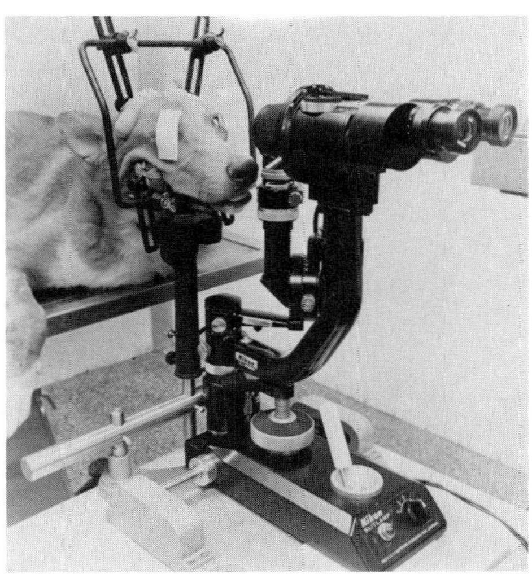

Fig. 2–6. The slit-lamp and corneal microscope *(biomicroscopy)* modified for use in the dog.

use in man is satisfactory. The silicone flange type* (Fig. 2–8) is favored by most veterinary ophthalmologists. The lens is filled with 1 percent methylcellulose or similar gonioscopic solution and placed on the cornea. Air bubbles are to be avoided. When securely in place the prism bends light rays so that the angle and pectinate ligaments may be examined. It is necessary to have good focal

*Franklin Optical, 1624 Franklin St., Oakland, Calif.

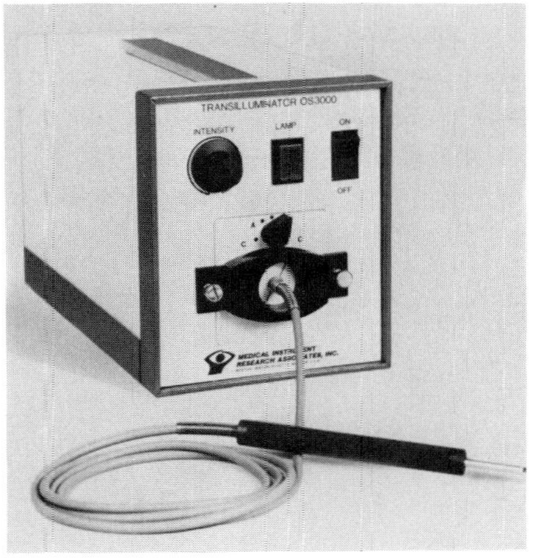

Fig. 2–7. Commercial type of transilluminator. (Model OS 3000 Medical Instrument Research Associates, 150 Causeway, Boston, Mass. 02114)

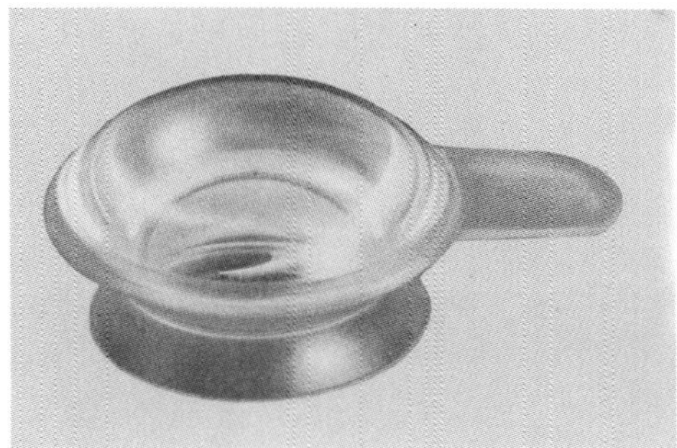

Fig. 2–8. Plastic gonioscopic lens (Franklin). The rubber scleral flange adjusts to the curvature of the sclera.

illumination in combination with magnification (loupe, otoscope head, ophthalmoscope, gonioscope [Fig. 2–9], or slit-lamp head).[17] Practical methods and uses for gonioscopy are elaborated on by Gelatt[9] and Bedford.[4]

Specific Structures

2:14 To begin the gross examination it is necessary that the eye be cleaned when secretions obscure the globe and membranes (Par. 3:9). However, since it is often advantageous to take material for bacteriological and sensitivity studies, these tests should be anticipated before the irrigation and cleaning process is initiated. The Schirmer Tear Test (Par. 2:19) should also be conducted prior to irrigation of the eyes. The nature and duration of these discharges should be noted as well as whether one or both eyes are involved. This, and the character of the secretion, whether mucoid, purulent, or stringy and tenacious, may be of significance in eliciting the cause.

2:15 *Lids:* Note their thickness and position (entropion, ectropion); condition of their margin, whether swollen, crusted or ulcerated; presence of neoplasms; size of the opening; ability to open and close; openings for the lacrimal drainage system; presence of misdirected or a second row of cilia. A structure (caruncle) in the medial canthus should also be noted for the possible presence of hair follicles protruding from it. The conjunctival

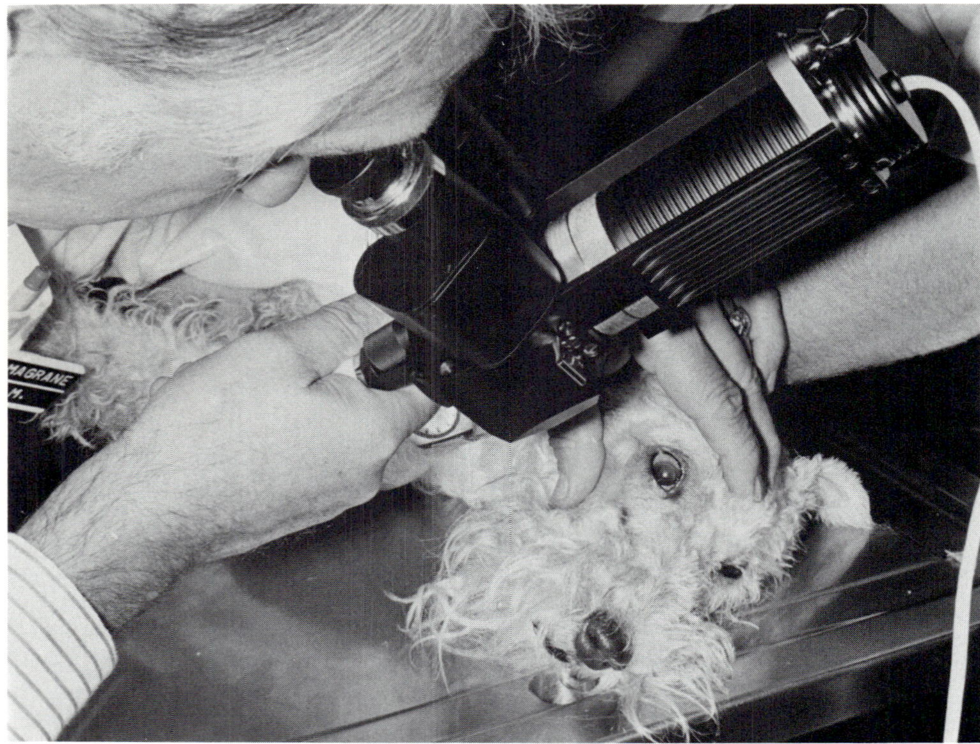

Fig. 2–9. Gonioscopy using the hand-held gonioscope.

surface (palpebral conjunctiva) is next inspected, especially if the presence of a foreign body is suspected. Exposure of the conjunctiva of the lower lid is easily accomplished by placing a finger near the margin of the lid and pressing downward. Eversion of the upper lid for viewing of the inner surface is more difficult but can be accomplished by grasping the center, pulling away from the globe and then back and upward. A topical anesthetic (Par. 3:37) may be necessary for the proper examination of this structure, the bulbar conjunctiva, and the cornea.

2:16 *Globe* proper: Note its situation in the orbit (exophthalmos, enophthalmos), mobility as compared to the companion eye and the presence of nystagmus, or strabismus, or periorbital swelling. Observe the size of both eyes in relation to the orbit and compare one with the other. Microphthalmia is not an infrequent finding and is often associated with other ocular anomalies (Par. 8–12).

2:17 *Conjunctiva*—bulbar: observe whether there is any edema (chemosis), signs of anemia, jaundice, hemorrhage, congestion, follicles, hyperplasia, growths, rents, or unusual amount of pigment deposition. Check whether the conjunctiva is smooth and dry or excessively moist. Additional tests may be required. These include the Schirmer Tear Test (Par. 2:19), culture, cytologic examination or the use of stains. Note possible presence of any foreign bodies, especially in the area of the *fornix* (upper transition of palpebral to bulbar conjunctiva), or in the *cul-de-sac* (lower transition of palpebral to bulbar conjunctiva).

2:18 *Membrana Nictitans, Nictitating Membrane or Third Eyelid:* All of these terms are used to describe the structure that lies between the lower lid and the globe and can be elevated to cover the globe. The term Third Eyelid, however, seems more appropriate for the dog and other species in which the structure is thick. Membrana nictitans is more appropriate for the structure in birds and other species in which it is truly a thin membrane that moves across the cornea. Observe its relationship to the globe and whether there is elevation, hypertrophy, eversion or inversion. This structure is best examined under topical anesthesia. The superior border is grasped with smooth thumb forceps (Fig. 2–10), pulled up and out for a good view of the inner surface and straight up to best see the external surface and conjunctival cul-de-sac. Note possible presence of lymphoid follicles on either surface and especially for foreign bodies (*e.g.* weed seeds, etc.) between the inner surface and the globe.

2:19 *Lacrimal Apparatus:* Examination encompasses evaluation of the tear production and the patency of the nasolacrimal duct. (1) *Secretion.* Hyposecretion of the lacrimal glands is either a temporary or permanent problem. There may be partial or complete hyposecretion. The Schirmer Tear Test* is easily performed and offers an accurate means of assaying the amount of lubrication being produced for the conjunctival and corneal surfaces. This test should be performed before any eyewash or anesthetic is instilled. Stringy secretions can be removed with cotton applicators before introducing the test strip into the cul-de-sac area (Fig. 2–11). Based on my own observations and those of others who routinely use this test, most dogs secrete enough tears to wet 15 mm or more of the test paper in one minute. A reading of under 10 mm should arouse suspicion and a reading of 0 to 5 mm indicates significant hyposecretion (Par. 6:66). If irrigation of the conjunctival sac has been accomplished prior to deciding to conduct the Schirmer test, the lid margins and conjunctiva can be dried with cotton balls and the test conducted. The results will be similar to those that would have been obtained prior to irrigating the eye. Topical anesthesia, however, reduces the Schirmer values considerably. In one study, the mean Schirmer value, without topical anesthesia (Schirmer I) was 22 mm/min, while following topical anesthesia (Schirmer II), it was 11 mm/min.[12] (2) *Drainage.* It is often necessary to determine the patency of the tear conducting channels to their nasal termination. This is easily accomplished under

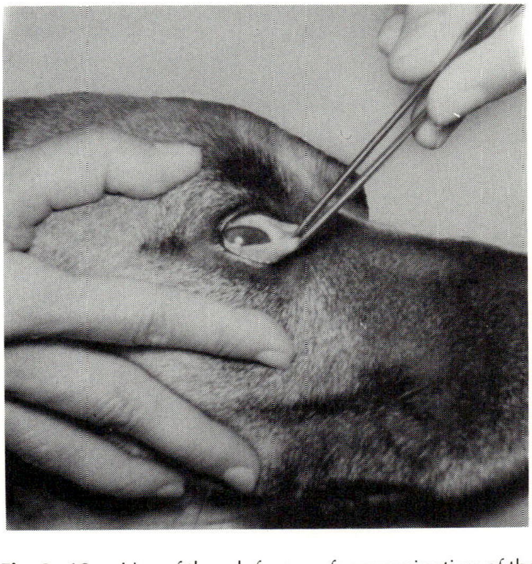

Fig. 2–10. Use of thumb forceps for examination of the membrane nictitans.

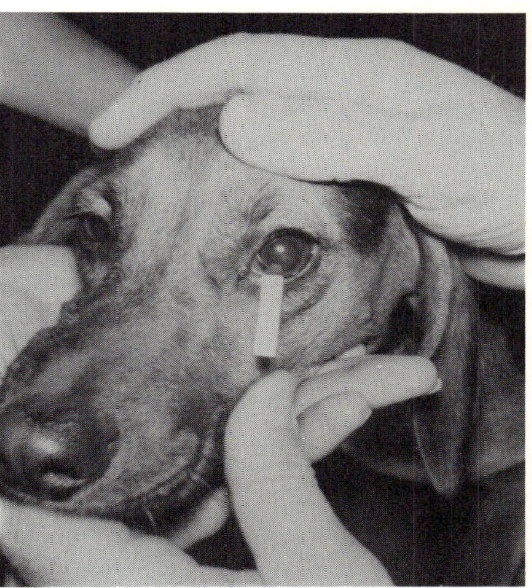

Fig. 2–11. Schirmer Tear Test strip in place in lower conjunctival cul-de-sac.

*Schirmer Tear Test. Cooper Labs, Wayne, N.J.

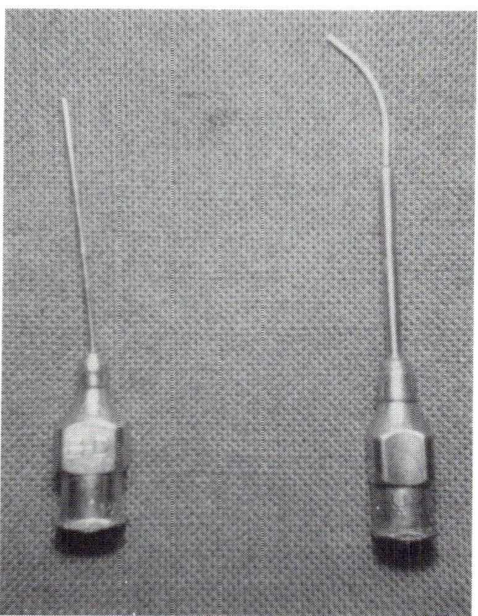

Fig. 2–12. Lacrimal cannulae.

topical anesthesia or tranquilizers by introducing a blunt lacrimal cannula (Fig. 2–12) into the upper opening (punctum) of the lacrimal canal and infusing saline solution (Fig. 2–13). When the drainage system is functioning properly, the solution will escape freely through the lower punctum and through the nostril. If the upper punctum cannot be found, location may be assisted by flushing the lower punctum. Whereas flushing the nasolacrimal duct will detect patency or obstruction of the duct, the primary dye test can be used to detect tear flow through the duct. To conduct this test, apply fluorescein liberally to the cornea or conjunctiva and then apply eye wash carefully to keep the lacrimal lake at the medial canthus filled, preferably without overflow onto the face. Hold the dog's head with the nose down below the eye level and watch for fluorescein stain in the nostril. It should appear within 2 minutes if flow is normal. In cases of unilateral epiphora, the test should be conducted on both eyes to compare results. For probing the ducts, various whalebone or metal bougies may be employed (Fig. 2–14); however probes are seldom needed, and use may traumatize or puncture the ducts. Nasolacrimal abnormalities associated with obstructions, deviations, congenital defects, infection, and neoplastic involvement can be further evaluated by means of dacryocystorhinography.[10,32]

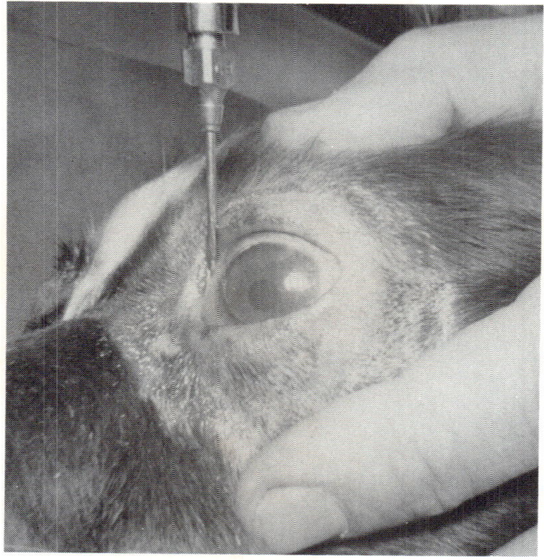

Fig. 2–13. Infusion of saline through the upper canaliculi to determine patency of the lacrimal drainage apparatus.

2:20 *Cornea:* The cornea is normally clear, transparent and there should be no visible blood vessels. Inspect for presence of dullness, opacities, vascularization, foreign bodies, growths, conjunctival encroachment, pigmentation, and whether the surface is smooth and curved properly. Minute changes may be seen by directing the light through the cornea at an angle to the line of sight. The layer or layers of the cornea involved should be noted and recorded, by drawing, for further reference. To bring an abrasion or ulceration into view, a moistened fluorescein impregnated paper† is inserted in the lower cul-de-sac long enough to transfer the stain to the anterior aspect of the globe (Fig. 2–15). The excess is rinsed away with the wash bottle. Or, the wash bottle may be used to moisten the strip with a clinging drop of stain applied to the cornea before the rinsing begins. These strips are sterile and eliminate the danger of using

†Fluores-Strip. Ayerst Laboratories, New York, New York 10017.

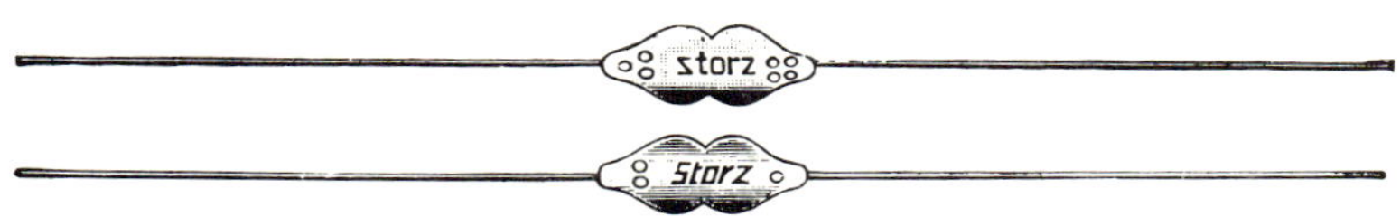

Fig. 2–14. Metal probes (Bowman) used for probing the lacrimal ducts.

fluorescein solutions which are known to be good culture media for *Pseudomonas*. Eyes have inadvertently been inoculated with contaminated solutions with disastrous results.[7,15] Vital staining of the cornea and conjunctiva with rose bengal[11] and a combination of fluorescein-rose bengal and alcian blue[27] are adjuncts for demonstrating the mucous thread and for differentiating mucus and cellular debris.

2:21 The sensitiveness of the cornea may be noted by touching it with a wisp of cotton, thread, or glass rod. The head of the dog should be held in such a position as to eliminate squinting caused by discomfort.

2:22 If deep ulceration and an impending prolapse are evident, the examination is stopped immediately and adequate sedation administered. At the appropriate time following sedation, a general intravenous anesthesia is administered, the examination concluded, and, if possible, corrective measures are taken, thus eliminating the danger of anterior chamber rupture caused by undue restraint and activity on the part of the patient.

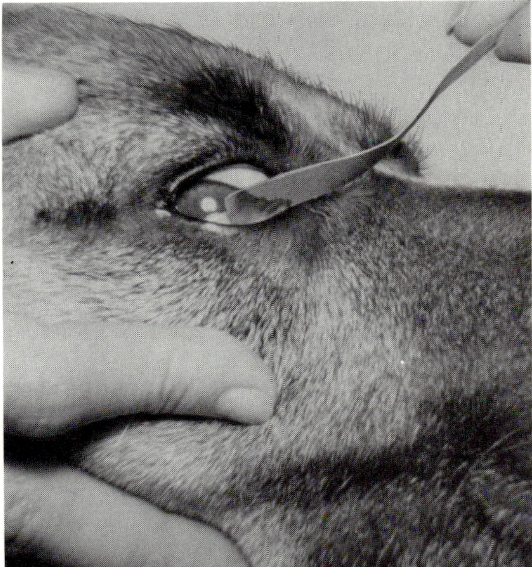

Fig. 2–15. Use of sterile fluorescein impregnated papers.

2:23 The sclera is best examined by opening the palpebral fissure as widely as possible with the fingers and by changing the head position. This structure should be white and glistening underneath its covering of bulbar conjunctiva. Note the possible presence of subconjunctival hemorrhage (ecchymosis), episcleral injection and congestion, growths, embedded foreign bodies or the site of their entry into the globe, and jaundiced discoloration.

2:24 *Anterior Chamber:* Note its depth, whether normal, shallow, or increased, comparing it with the other eye when possible. The depth is apt to be shallow in glaucoma, or deep if the lens is thinned by partial absorption or is luxated. The aqueous humor should be clear. If altered, observe whether there is a diffuse cloudiness (aqueous flare) or exudates consisting of pus (hypopyon) or blood (hyphema). Both direct and lateral illumination should be used. Directing a slit beam of light from the ophthalmoscope held at the lateral aspect, while viewing the eye through the binocular loupe, is helpful in determining the characteristics of the aqueous. Any opacities of the aqueous will appear as dust particles in a beam of light in a darkened room. Nearly complete darkness is essential. The angle of the anterior chamber can only be accurately evaluated by gonioscopy (Par. 2:10).

2:25 *Iris:* The iris should be examined with both direct and lateral illumination. Observe its mobility, color, smoothness and texture, and whether it is steady or tremulous during movements of the eyeball (iridodenesis). The latter condition is seen when the iris is not properly supported by the anterior aspect of the lens, *e.g.* in absence (aphakia), subluxation, or luxation of the lens (Par. 9:72). Note especially whether there are adhesions to the cornea (anterior synechia) or to the anterior capsule of the lens (posterior synechia) and for atrophic changes of the pupillary border in particular. Remnants of persistent pupillary membranes are not infrequently seen (Par. 7:26).

2:26 *Pupil* (Par. 7:14–7:24) Note its size, shape, position. Compare its size with that in the other eye, and especially its reaction to light (the pupillary light reflex-PLR). The PLR is helpful in determining optic nerve and retinal function, if conducted in a standard manner. Since the PLR is reduced in apprehensive dogs and in dogs that are not dark-adapted, it should be evaluated after the dog has been in a darkened quiet room for 10 minutes or more and is at ease. The same bright focal light source should be used each time . . . a Finoff transilluminator is ideal. To observe the direct light reflex, the examiner should sit in front of the dog, hold the dog's head by the muzzle with one hand and with the other, direct the focal light source above the eye to be tested, then bring it quickly down to approximately 2 inches in front of the cornea, and hold it there until the pupil constriction is complete. Now quickly direct the light to the other eye to see if that pupil is constricted (indirect reflex). For a closer observation of the indirect reflex, the iris can be illuminated from the lateral aspect with an ophthalmoscope or other light source, just bright enough to allow visualization of the pupil, and an assistant should direct the transilluminator into the other eye upon command, while the examiner observes the indirect reflex. The examination should be repeated for the other eye after the pupils have been allowed to dilate again in the darkened room. The direct and indirect reflexes can be recorded as 'normal,' 'sluggish,' 'incomplete,' 'sluggish and incomplete,' or 'absent.' Although the PLR is a rather inexact test, it can be quite helpful in determining the cause of blindness, and in diagnosis and prognosis of retinal and optic nerve disease if one becomes familiar with the test by including it as a part of all routine eye examinations.

2:27 *Lens:* Dilation of the pupil (Par. 3:28) is essential for complete evaluation of the lens. Pupil dilation should be avoided in eyes with luxated or subluxated lenses, or if glaucoma from any other cause is suspected or might be induced. If, after dilation, a predisposition to glaucoma is found, one should conduct an examination of the eye and then instill a miotic such as 4% Pilocarpine and monitor the intraocular pressure (Par. 3:32–3:33) until the pupil is constricted. Although lens opacities can be visualized with the ophthalmoscope using the proper settings (Fig. 2–23), the examiner only sees an out-of-focus view of the retina when attempting to examine a normal lens with an ophthalmoscope. Most all abnormalities of the lens can be seen with a focal light source and a binocular loupe. Inspect for lenticular opacities, size, dislocation and uveal pigment deposits on the anterior capsule and for iris adhesions (posterior synechia). The inverted Y of the posterior suture lines is usually visible. In some instances, a white dot (Mittendorf's dot) is visible with a remnant of the hyaloid artery extending from it and swinging in the vitreous. In older dogs, a blue-gray reflection from the nucleus of the lens (nuclear sclerosis) is normal and should not be confused with a cataract. A slit-lamp-biomicroscope (Par. 2:6) is ideal for detecting small or developing lens lesions and determining exact location of lens lesions.

Palpation and Intraocular Pressure Determination

2:28 To complete the external examination, palpation is helpful in determining the presence or absence of pain in the ciliary region and in determining the existence of tumors and swellings in and around the orbit. Retropulsing the globe, *i.e.* gently pushing the globe back into the orbit with the thumb or index finger, is helpful in detecting space-occupying lesions of the orbit. The degree and ease of retropulsion can be compared to the normal eye.

2:29 With practice, a fairly accurate approximation of intraocular pressure can also be achieved by digital palpation. With the two index fingers placed upon the upper lid, the globe is palpated by an alternating rolling motion of the fingers (Fig. 2–16). Some idea of the degree of pressure may then be determined by comparison with the other eye, if normal, or with another healthy eye. However, tonometry should be used to more accurately assess the intraocular pressure (IOP) in dogs with ocular inflammation or episcleral congestion in order to detect developing glaucoma (elevated pressure) or anterior uveitis (decreased pressure). Subtle changes in pressure associated with developing glaucoma would probably be missed with digital palpation alone, and sight lost before institution of proper therapy.

2:30 Two general types of tonometers are: (1) applanation tonometers, which detect the amount of pressure needed to flatten a small area of the cornea. Measurements are influenced very little by scleral rigidity and more accurately correlate with actual intraocular pressure, but are impractical for the practicing veterinarian, at present, because all are priced in the thousands of dollars. (2) Indentation tonometers, which detect the indentation that a given weight can cause on the cornea. The Schiötz tonometer (Fig. 2–17) is the commonly used tonometer which functions on the latter principle.

2:31 Tonometry has been found especially useful (1) in the early diagnosis of glaucoma, (2) following surgical procedures or medicinal treatment for the correction of glaucoma, and (3) for keeping a "check" on the unaffected eye in glaucoma patients.[17]

2:32 In cooperative animals, readings can be made following an instillation of a topical anesthetic. An assistant holds the animal's head so that the eyes are directed upward, the lids are separated, and the tonometer is allowed to rest by its own weight upon the near center of the up-turned cornea (Fig. 2–18). If difficulty is encountered in recording pressure by this method, the animal can be rolled over on its back. Again, the nose and head should be held so as to direct the center of the eye toward the ceiling. In a cooperative patient, the examiner should be

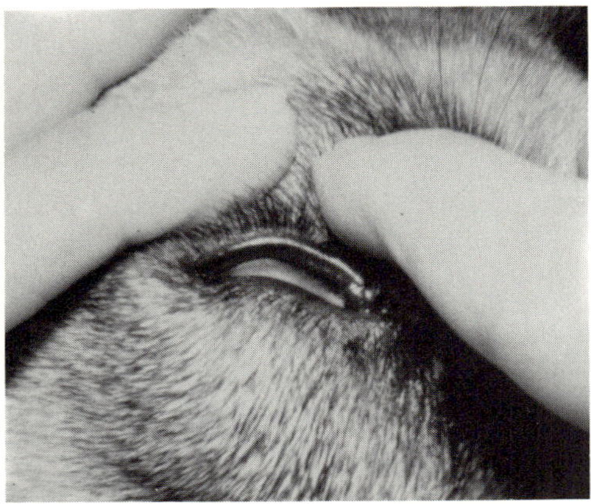

Fig. 2–16. Testing the tension of the eyeball by digital tonometry.

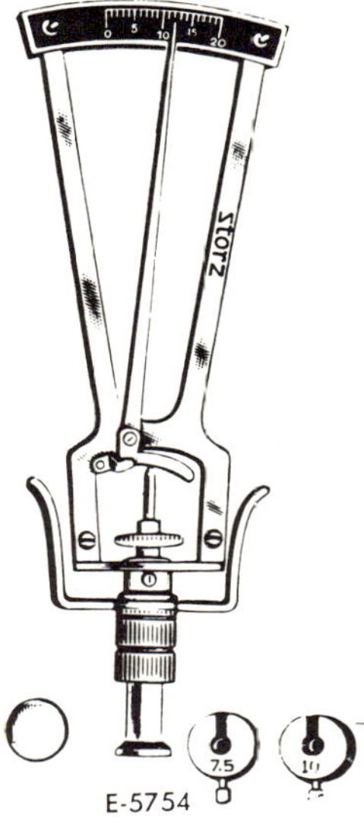

Fig. 2–17. Schiötz tonometer.

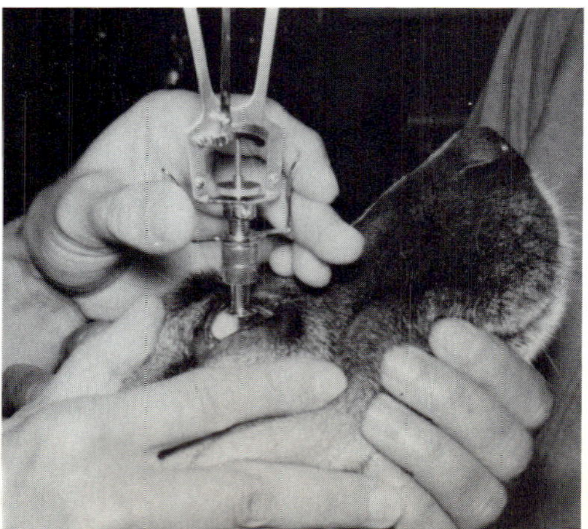

Fig. 2–18. Testing the intraocular pressure by Schiötz tonometry.

able to accomplish accuracy with three consecutive readings that agree to within one scale reading. One should be careful to hold the tonometer vertical, place the footplate evenly on the cornea, and make certain no pressure is being applied to the eyeball elsewhere by the examiner's fingers or the dog's eyelids. The results of tonometry should be recorded in scale readings indicating the weight used. A convenient way of recording, for example, is $5.5 = \frac{\text{R reading}}{\text{L reading}}$. This method allows comparison on subsequent measurements.

2:33 Scale readings between 3 and 7 on the Schiötz tonometer with a 5.5 g weight indicate normal intraocular pressure in the dog. This converts to 24.4 to 12.2 mm Hg when using the conversion chart for humans (inside front cover), which is supplied with the tonometer. Tonometer scale values below 3 generally imply elevated pressure, and, for a more accurate evaluation, a heavier weight, preferably the 10 g should be used, and the scale reading recorded for future comparison. The conversion of scale readings to mm Hg with the various weights does not usually agree, if the human conversion table is used, primarily because of the difference in scleral rigidity between dogs and humans. Generally, the heavier weights convert to lower mm Hg than lighter weights, if both are used on the same eye. Peiffer[22] reported that the normal true intraocular pressure in the dog is considerably higher than in man. He prepared a Schiötz conversion table (inside front cover) for the dog indicating that a 3 to 7 scale reading implies normal range of 24.2 to 38.3 mm Hg. While this revelation is important in the study of aqueous dynamics, it should not confuse the fact that Schiötz values between 3 and 7 are normal for the dog.

Subjective Examination and Assessment of Visual Function

2:34 Subjective or functional examination of the eye is, of course, difficult in animals. A true evaluation of pain, light and dark adaptation, field of vision, and percentage of vision is impossible. Veterinary clinicians then should not be guilty of assuring the client that his pet has, let us say, 25% vision in the right eye and 75% in the left. Regardless of cause, in evaluating blindness from the subjective aspect, an animal that was born blind or has gone blind gradually adapts well to its environment. A change in environment prompts confusion and more accurately reveals the extent of vision loss. Loss of vision in only one eye will probably go unnoticed by the owner.

2:35 Much can be learned by eliciting a good history regarding movement of the dog throughout the house, up and down lighted and unlighted stairs, out of doors on dark versus sunlit days, reaction to large versus small objects, reaction to changes in furniture placement, ability to jump on sofas and beds, follow rolling balls, and find tidbits held up or thrown. Animals that go blind quickly usually move with caution and sniff their way around; however, animals that go blind slowly and have minimal or no vision often act normal in familiar surroundings. Pain is demonstrated by squinting the affected eye, especially in bright light (photophobia), tearing, and often, by a change in disposition and eating habits and by general lethargy. Rubbing the affected side may be a sign of pain, but it is much more often a sign of itching, such as is seen with conjunctivitis or blepharitis.

2:36 Patching of the unaffected eye (Fig. 2–19) and subjecting the dog to an obstacle course around the examining room will also be of value in vision determination. The clinician and owner should remain stationary while this test is being conducted. A cotton ball or similar lightweight object may be dropped a few feet ahead of the animal and the reaction observed. The visual behavior should be tested under normal room illumination as well as in semi-darkness. Testing in this environment evaluates the function of the receptors responsible for vision under subdued illumination (rods), but is best performed after a five- to ten-minute period of dark adaptation. Minimal vision (light perception and projection) can often be determined by opening the door of a darkened examining room just enough to allow a beam of bright light to enter. A dog with any remaining vision will generally find the beam of light and follow it to the door.

2:37 Finally, the clinician is cautioned about using the "hand waving technique" for vision determination. Air currents created by this motion cause lid blinking and globe reaction which are not indications of sight.

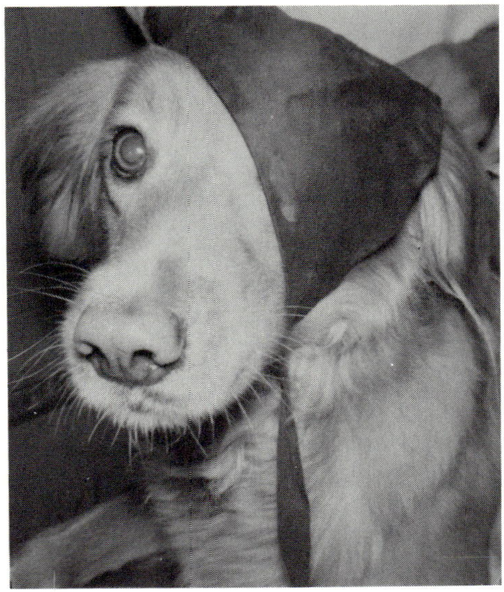

Fig. 2–19. Black patch with ties used to test the vision of the fellow eye.

Internal Examination (Ophthalmoscopy)

2:38 When the ocular media is sufficiently clear, the deeper internal structure, *i.e.* vitreous humor and fundus, are examined with an ophthalmoscope. Ophthalmoscopy has been recognized as a valuable addition to medical diagnostic procedures for over a hundred years. Its use in veterinary medicine has been limited primarily because of insufficient training and lack of emphasis of its importance. The ophthalmoscope, when used properly and frequently, becomes a most useful diagnostic tool for the determination of ocular fundic degenerations and lesions, injuries, congenital anomalies, growths, and even certain systemic diseases (Chaper 12). In addition, by utilizing the plus lens system, lesions of all parts of the eye from the cornea through the vitreous can be studied with this instrument (Fig. 2–20). The +40D lens gives a magnification of about 4×. Although the focal distance is quite critical, this setting is useful for close examination if other sources of magnification are not available.

2:39 There are two general methods of ophthalmoscopic examination: direct and indirect. The *indirect* method utilizes a condensing lens between the patient's eye and the ophthalmoscope (Fig. 2–21). This lens projects a virtual image of the retina that the examiner views (Fig. 2–21). The image presented is much smaller (2 to 4½× vs. 14× of the direct ophthalmoscope) and is inverted, but is of a much greater area of the retina. Although the instruments are expensive, indirect ophthalmoscopy does offer many advantages to the clinician willing to pursue its potential. It is of great value when the eyes of many patients must be "screened." It permits visualization of a larger field at one time and provides stereoscopic vision. This enables the examiner to more readily recognize such lesions as fundic depressions and retinal detachments. In addition, the fundus can or-

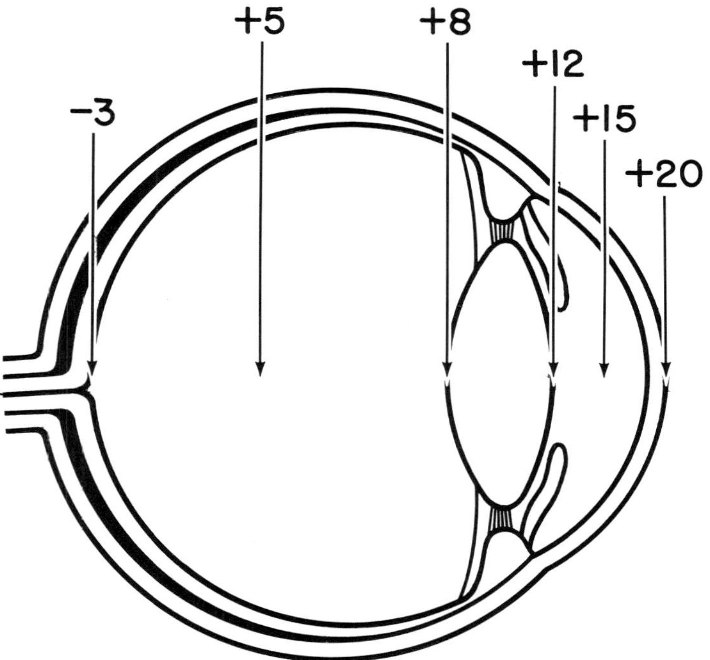

Fig. 2–20. With the ophthalmoscope 1 inch in front of the eye, the lenses in the rotating wheel produce clear view of lesions at points indicated in the diagrammatic eye.

dinarily be examined through a more hazy lens than it is possible to penetrate by direct means. Since the examination is made from a distance, the animal is often less apprehensive and close contact is avoided. For teaching purposes an accessory prism on the instrument enables the observer to see the same image viewed by the clinician. A monocular indirect ophthalmoscope is also available (Fig. 2–22). It contains a lens system that allows the examiner to see an upright image of about 2.5× magnification. Its advantage is ease in use; disadvantages are high price and lack of the stereoscopic view provided by the binocular instrument. Monocular indirect ophthalmoscopy can also be performed by the examiner holding a focal light source, such as a Finoff transilluminator, just below his/her eye at about 18 to 24 inches from the patient's eye and directing the beam of light through a 20 diopter lens held about 4 inches in front of the patient's eye. An inverted image is observed.

2:40 In the *direct* method a beam of light is projected into the interior of the patient's eye by a reflector or prism, while the aperture in the lens-disc, which opening is situated above the level of the reflector, allows a portion of this light, after returning from the patient's eye, to pass into the eye of the observer. This method utilizes the common electric ophthalmoscope.[6] A magnification of about 14× is obtained. Other advantages over indirect ophthalmoscopy include the obtaining of a direct image, expense, and comparable ease in mastering the technique.

2:41 In initiating the examination with the ophthalmoscope, it is often useful to hold the instrument at a distance of about 2 feet. At this distance and with the 0 setting, one is better able to detect lesions, especially of the lens, that may be missed when the instrument is held close to the eye.

2:42 The clinician with a refractive error of his own may choose to wear his glasses or not when using the ophthalmoscope. If, how-

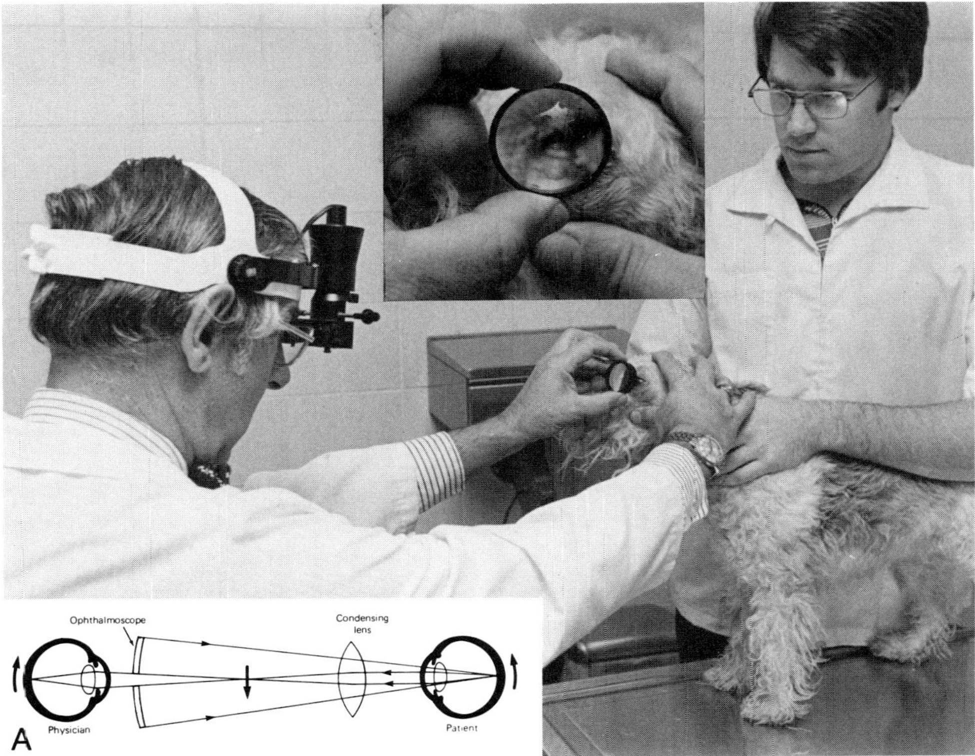

Fig. 2–21. Binocular indirect ophthalmoscopy.

ever, this refractive error is marked and he chooses not to wear glasses for the examination, the difference should be taken into consideration. For example, hyperopia of one's eye will tend to neutralize myopia of the patient's (Par. 1:2).

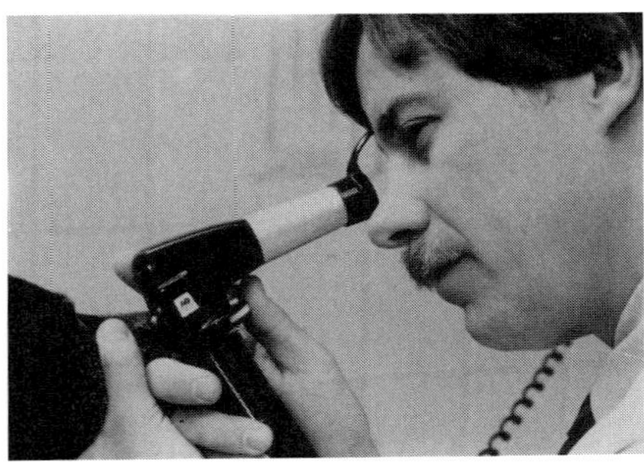

Fig. 2–22. Monocular indirect ophthalmoscope.

Suggestions for Using the Ophthalmoscope

2:43 1. The examination should be performed in a semi-darkened room, and where distracting influences are minimal. One of the deterrents to the successful use of this instrument is the lack of cooperation of the patient. This is seldom a problem if the dog is restrained comfortably in a quiet room with only the owner, assistant and observer present. It is well to have the owner stand where the dog can see and be reassured of his presence.

2:44 2. Dilation of the pupil is not always necessary, but it is helpful to the novice, and is advisable for complete examination of the fundus. In pathological dilatation (Par. 11:54) this, of course, will not be necessary. Agents which may be used for dilatation include Mydriacyl (tropicamide), Neosynephrine, or Cyclogyl (Par. 3:28). Mydriacyl is preferable.

One or two instillations made 20″–30″ prior to examination provide good dilation. These mydriatrics lose their effect within a few hours. Atropine should not be used because of its long action.

2:45 3. The owner or assistant may satisfactorily restrain the animal's head. Obviously, however, a trained assistant is preferred for this purpose.

2:46 4. The head of the ophthalmoscope should be held as close to the examiner's eye as possible and about 1 inch away from the patient's cornea. Both eyes should be examined. When examining the right eye, the observer uses his right eye from the right side. When examining the left eye, the observer should be to the left and use his left eye. If, however, the habit of using only one eye for the examination has already been established, it is not important that this routine be changed.

2:47 5. The ophthalmoscope is held vertically (Fig. 2–23) in front of the observer's eye with the light beam directed toward the patient, and the right index finger is placed on the serrated edge of the dial in order to change lenses as necessary. The observer will soon learn to follow the natural movement of the dog's eye or, it may be advantageous to remain fixed, thus allowing the movements to bring the different aspects of the fundus into view. I find it an advantage to mentally divide the retina into 4 quadrants with the optic disc at the intersection, and systematically examine each quadrant.

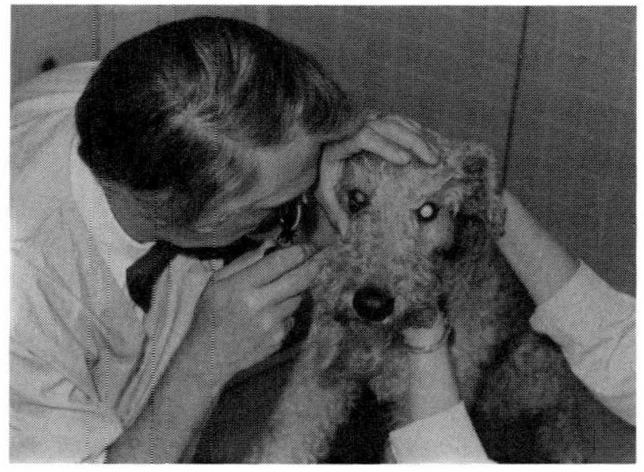

Fig. 2–23. Direct method of ophthalmoscopic examination.

2:48 6. In looking through the ophthalmoscope the observer should relax his accommodation and gaze through the eye, not at the eye, *i.e.* across the fields into the distant horizon. The observer's other eye may be suppressed without closing, in the manner of using a monocular microscope.

2:49 7. Since most dogs are myopic (Par. 1:2), and there is a tendency for the examiner to accommodate the lens, the minus 3 lens is first used to focus on the optic disc and retina. By changing the lens to more or less minus, the fundus is brought into the clearest view for the observer. Ophthalmoscopy is also a means of determining the approximate degree of myopia, or hyperopia (if the plus lens system must be used). Then by rotation from the minus through the plus lens the structures anterior to the fundus may be brought into view (Fig. 2–20). Vitreous opacities may be picked up between 0 and plus 6–8, opacities of the lens between plus 6–8 and plus 12, then through the plus lens to the iris, anterior chamber, and the cornea itself, which is in focus at about plus 20. Those ophthalmoscopes equipped with a plus 40 lens provide still more magnification but the instrument must be held very close to the cornea.

2:50 8. Patience and precise observations are necessary for obtaining diagnostic information, and thorough familiarity with the normal structure of the eye is necessary before disease processes can be recognized. This is especially true of the dog's eye in which there are many variations of the normal.

2:51 Familiarity with the normal can only be achieved by using the ophthalmoscope at every opportunity. Its routine use in the general physical examination of a patient will soon result in a surprising acumen and will, in addition, often prove of value in assaying systemic diseases (Chapter 12).

Fundus and Retina of the Adult Dog (after H. B. Parry)[21]

2:52 The fundus of the dog differs from that of man in the presence of a tapetum lucidum and a heavily pigmented choroid, as well as in the absence of a true macula or fovea. This area in the dog is known as the *area centralis*.

2:53 The fundus can be divided conveniently into two portions (Plate 1A):

1. The tapetal fundus in the dorsal quadrants backed by the brightly reflecting tapetum lucidum.
2. The non-tapetal fundus (tapetum nigrum) dark with choroidal pigment in the ventral quadrants.

The tapetal fundus is half-moon shaped, occupying most of the dorsal quadrants, but *not* extending to the periphery of the fundus, where it is surrounded by a narrow zone of non-tapetal fundus.

2:54 The color of the tapetum lucidum varies from a light lemon yellow through orange to a deep apple green, dependent upon the breed and the individual. In some breeds, such as pointers, the color of the reflection appears to be inherited with certain coat colors (*e.g.* liver coat color and a light orange brown tapetum), but in most breeds this association is not very distinct.

2:55 Over the tapetal fundus, the retina appears to be fully translucent without refractive distortion and its surface is flat, but the substance of the fundus appears to have a definite texture of fine granular beading, which becomes slightly coarser toward the periphery. Between the beading is a very fine reticulum of dark triangular spaces, the stellulae of Winslow. The granular beading is most marked in adolescent dogs; in some animals over two years old the texture of the granular beading is so fine that it appears to be even.

2:56 In the retinal vascular pattern, three main divisions of vessels exist: (1) primary veins (2) secondary veins (3) arterioles. The primary veins are most visible and vary only in number. They cross the disc dorsally, ventrotemporally, ventrally, and ventronasally and join within the disc. The secondary veins are smaller and join the primary veins within the disc to form the venous ring. The arterioles will be recognized by their bright red color, tortuous arrangement and origin at the periphery of the disc. They are much smaller in diameter. The venous circle or ring may pulsate, thus appearing and disappearing during the examination. This is especially obvious if one places slight pressure on the sclera during examination.[23] See Pars. 1:25 and 11:17 for further information on the blood supply.

2:57 The non-tapetal fundus varies from bright red to deep brown in color, depending on the amount of choroidal pigment. If dark brown, there often appears to be slight gray over-wash. The granular texture is not so well marked in this region. The blood vessels arising from the two main medial and lateral horizontal retinal vessels are more numerous over the ventral nontapetal fundus than over the tapetal fundus and the larger vessels reflect the light from their surface, producing a thin regular "silver-wire" reflection, which is not seen with the tapetal vessels.

2:58 The optic papilla (disc) usually lies just within the ventral border of the tapetal fundus not infrequently surrounded by a narrow zone of nontapetal fundus. It is situated nasally from the center and is round to oval. Its margins are well demarcated in some dogs and ragged in others. This irregular shape is due to myelin in the nerve fiber layer of the retina, which appears cream to white in color, and extends varying distances away from the disc. Usually the papilla (disc) is flat with its periphery level with the inner surface of the retina. The papilla is usually pinkish white with a dark or grayish physiologic pit or cup near the center. (Plate 1, B, C, D.) Additional variations in the optic disc include: Deep physiologic cupping; pigmentation; increased myelination and micropapilla.

2:59 Observation of the choroid, other than the tapetum, is restricted to the dense brown pigment in its inner layers over the non-tapetal fundus. The pigment completely obscures the choroidal blood vessels in many dogs, although it is often possible to view the choroidal circulation in light-coated dogs (Plate 19H).

2:60 Szutter[28] has described the development of eye-background coloring in the puppy two weeks until the fourth month of age. The colors most often seen in the tapetum lucidum were greenish yellow, yellow gold, and bright green. During the development of the colors the most consistent intermediate color was lilac. In the tapetum nigrum (non-tapetal fundus) the commonly seen colors were: rust red, yellowish brown, greenish brown, and brownish-black. From the time the eyelids opened until the thirtieth day, the overall color of the eye background appeared bluish-grey.

2:61 Wyman and Donovan[31] conducted a study of the fundus in 52 dogs of various breeds and concluded: (1) there is a refractive error of 0 to -1.75 diopters; (2) the color of the tapetum lucidum varies greatly and cannot be correlated directly with coat color; (3) the tapetum lucidum comprises approximately one-third of the fundus; (4) tapetal beadiness increases with the age of the dog; (5) coloring of the nigrum is dependent upon the degree of pigmentation of the choroidal layers and can be correlated to the degree of pigment in the iris; (6) the retinal vascular pattern generally displays four primary veins and several secondary veins; (7) the arterioles are more tortuous and brighter red; (8) the tapetum lucidum is located just behind the pigmented epithelium of the retina and is penetrated intermittently by the small choroidal vessels; (9) no central retinal artery or veins are demonstrable in the dog's eye; (10) the retinal arteries are cilioretinal in origin.

2:62 In several other detailed studies[8,20] the authors describe some areas of the fundus somewhat differently from each other and from the Wyman and Donovan study. Presumably, the breeds studied by these observers differed. There remains no doubt that there are many variations of the normal fundus and these must be taken into consideration during the examination.[3] For a thorough and pictorial description the reader is referred to Rubin's text.[25] The words *tapetal fundus* and *tapetum lucidum* are used interchangeably by various authors, as are the terms *non-tapetal* and *tapetum nigrum.* Whereas the terms *tapetal* and *tapetum lucidum* are appropriate, the term *tapetum nigrum* does not seem to be appropriate, as there is no actual tapetal structure present in that area of the fundus. The term *non-tapetal* seems much more appropriate to identify the part of the fundus (or an entire fundus) in which there is no tapetum behind the retina. The tapetum is evident on histologic examination as a layer of modified choroid just behind the pigment epithelium of the retina.

Other Means of Internal Examination

2:63 Beyond the scope and economic practicability of the practitioner, but within the realm of veterinary ophthalmology, several important diagnostic aids are being utilized.

2:64 *Electroretinography* (ERG). As with other nervous tissue, the retina generates electrical currents. The electroretinogram is a measurement of retinal function obtained by placing electrodes on the cornea and adjacent to the eye and measuring the response of the retina to a strobe light via the corneal electrode attached to a specialized electroencephalograph. Studies[1,14,19] indicate that there are instances in which the ERG can be used to provide the clinician with a clear-cut estimate of the functional integrity of the retinal photoreceptors when such evaluation would not otherwise be possible, *i.e.* when the retina cannot be visualized ophthalmoscopically because of corneal, lens or vitreal opacities, hypopyon or hyphema.

2:65 The chief clinical diagnostic problem which the ERG will solve is the evaluation of dogs presented for cataract extraction. Cataract secondary to retinopathies occurs frequently in, for example, the middle age Poodle and Cocker spaniel (Par. 11:64). When visualization of the fundus is precluded by the presence of opaque lenses, when the pupil response to light stimuli is questionable, and the history of vision loss is inconclusive, the ERG is essential to the determination of retinal viability. A normal ERG answers the question as to whether a dog's vision can be restored.

2:66 In *progressive retinal atrophy* (PRA), changes in the ERG are seen before ophthalmoscopic changes, and more subtle changes in the ERG provide evidence that puppies as young as 9 weeks of age will develop clinical signs of PRA when they get older. Testing of puppies and other ERG diagnosis depending on subtle changes requires considerable experience and instrument calibration and standardization. However, this diagnostic service is available at only a few places in the country.

2:67 Electroretinography is also useful in determining whether blindness is of central or of ocular origin.

2:68 In retinal dysplasia with or without retinal detachment, a congenital cataract is sometimes an accompanying feature, making visualization of the fundus difficult. Although the ERG cannot tell the clinician the extent of a congenital retinal anomaly except at the extremes, it will indicate whether photoreceptor function is present.

2:69 *Ultrasonography.* Rubin and Koch[16] have shown that time amplitude ultrasonography (A-scan) is a useful adjunct to the diagnosis of ocular diseases. While a specific diagnosis may not be obtained by ultrasonography, the added evidence can strengthen a clinical judgment. The technique requires a time amplitude portable ultrasound machine with attached transducer. The examination is made by placing the transducer on the corneal surface in various positions along the horizontal and vertical axes.

2:70 When corneal opacification obscures observation of the intraocular structures the unsuspected presence of anatomic abnormalities may alter the prognosis, or suggest and alter the course of treatment. A determination of subluxation or luxation of the lens is possible by this means.

2:71 Ultrasonography is valuable in detecting retinal detachment in eyes in which the fundus is not visible. By applying the probe in various directions, a map of the detachment can be constructed. In those animals affected with complete hyphema it is of value in ascertaining whether intravitreal hemorrhage, intraocular tumor or other complications are concurrent.

2:72 Ultrasonographic diagnosis in the presence of cataract is useful in determining the presence of clotted blood in the vitreous, retinal detachment, and neoplastic masses. The ultrasonogram also aids in the assaying of lenticular thickness. Another application is in diseases in which the axial length of the eye may be increased, and in which an increase may influence the prognosis. B-scan is also useful. It is helpful in detecting lesions of the orbit.

2:73 *Fluorescein Angiography.* In this diagnostic procedure, a series of photographs of the fundus are used to record the progress of fluorescein through the retina, optic nerve and choroidal vasculature following intravenous injection. It is used extensively in man to study ocular vascular disease, but it is just beginning to be explored in veterinary medicine.[5,23]

REFERENCES

1. Aguirre, G.D., et al.: Electroretinography in Veterinary Ophthalmology, J.A.A.H.A., 9:234–237, 1973.
2. Allen, J.H.: *May's Diseases of the Eye*, 23rd ed., Baltimore, The Williams & Wilkins Co., 1963.
3. Barnett, K.C.: *Variations of the Normal Ocular Fundus of the Dog*, A.A.H.A. Publication, South Bend, Ind., 1972.
4. Bedford, P.G.: A Practical Method of Gonioscopy and Goniophotography in the Dog and Cat, J.S.A.P., *14*:601–606, 1973.
5. Bellhorn, R.W.: Fluorescein Fundus Photography in Veterinary Ophthalmology, J.A.A.H.A., 9:227–232, 1973.
6. Catcott, E.J.: Ophthalmoscopy in Canine Practice, J.A.V.M.A., *121*:35, 1952.
7. Cello, R.M. and Lasmanis, J.: Pseudomonas Infection of the Eye of the Dog Resulting from the Use

of Contaminated Fluorescein Solution, J.A.V.M.A., *132*:297, 1958.

8. De Carvalho, C.M.F.: Fundo de Olho normal do Cao (Canis familiaris) e alteracoes que nele ocorrem em algumas doencas, Arquivos da Escola Veterinaria Universidade de Minas Gerais, Belo Horizonte, Brasil. *15*:205–260, 1963.
9. Gelatt, K.N., and Ladds, P.W.: Gonioscopy in Dogs and Cats with Glaucoma and Ocular Tumors, J.S.A.P., *12*:105–117, 1971.
10. Gelatt, K.N., et al.: Dacryocystorhinography in the Dog and Cat, J.S.A.P., *13*:381–397, 1972.
11. Gelatt, K.N.: Vital Staining of the Canine Cornea and Conjunctiva with Rose Bengal, J.A.A.H.A., *8*:17–21, 1972.
12. Gelatt, K.N.: Evaluation of Tears Formation in the Dog, Using a Modification of the Schirmer Tear Test, JAVMA, *166*:368, 1975.
13. Helper, L.: Diagnostic Techniques in Conjunctivitis and Keratitis, Vet. Clin. No. Am., *3*:357–365, 1973.
14. Howard, D.R., et al.: Clinical Electroretinography, J.A.A.H.A., *9*:219–226, 1973.
15. Kimura, S.J.: Fluorescein Paper, Am. J. Ophthal., *34*:446, 1951.
16. Lescure, F.: L'Angle Camerulaire du Chien Étude Goniophotographique. *Proceedings XVIIth World Veterinary Congress*, Hanover, Germany, *2*:1001–1004, 1963.
17. Magrane, W.G.: Thesis—Canine Glaucoma, University of Pennsylvania Graduate School of Medicine, Philadelphia, 1956.
18. Martin, C.L.: Gonioscopy and Anatomical Correlations of the Drainage Angle of the Dog, J.S.A.P., *10*:171–184, 1969.
19. Martin, C.L.: Slit Lamp Examination of the Normal Canine Anterior Ocular Segment, J.S.A.P., *10*:143–169, 1969.
20. Monti, F.: L'Esame Clinico del Fondo Dell'Occhio Nel Cane, La Nuova Veterinaria, *4*:262–279, 1967.
21. Parry, H.B.: Structure and Development of the Retina of the Normal Dog, Brit. J. Ophthal., *37*:385, 1953.
22. Peiffer, R.L.: Calibration of the Schiötz Tonometer for the Normal Canine Eye, Am. J. Vet. Res., *38*:1881–1889, 1977.
23. Peruccio, C., Helper, L.C., Monte, F., and Brightman, A.H.: Fundus Fluorangiography in the Cat, J.A.A.H.A., *18*:939–945, 1982.
24. Rubin, L.F. and Koch, S.A.: Ocular Diagnostic Ultrasonography, J.A.V.M.A., *153*:1706–1716, 1968.
25. Rubin, L.F.: *Atlas of Veterinary Ophthalmoscopy*, Philadelphia, Lea & Febiger, 1974.
26. Rubin, L.F.: Clinical Electroretinography in Dogs, J.A.V.M.A., *151*:1456–1470, 1967.
27. Slatter, D.H.: Differential Vital Staining of the Canine Cornea and Conjunctiva with Fluorescein-rose bengal and Alcian Blue, J.S.A.P., *14*:291–296, 1973.
28. Szutter, I.: *Ophthalmoskopische und Lupenspielgeluntersuchungen an Neugeborenen.* Haustieren. 1., Acta Veterinaria Academiae, Scientiarum Hungaricae, Vol. 2, Issue 2, 1961.
29. Troncoso, M.U.: *Gonioscoy*, Philadelphia, F.A. Davis Co., 1948.
30. Überreiter, Von Otto: Examination of the Eye and Eye Operations in Animals, *Advances in Veterinary Science*, Vol. 5, New York, Academic Press, Inc., 1959.
31. Wyman, M. and Donovan, E.F.: The Ocular Fundus of the Normal Dog, J.A.V.M.A., *147*:17, 1965.
32. Yakely, W.L. and Alexander, J.E.: Dacryocystorhinography in the Dog, J.A.V.M.A., *159*:1417–1421, 1971.

3

OCULAR THERAPEUTICS

3:1 The eye is a delicate and sensitive organ and in applying various therapeutic preparations care must be exercised to limit the strength of applications and the manner in which they are applied. Generally, almost anything used on the cornea will interfere with corneal healing. Ointments retard more than solutions, and powders more than ointments.

3:2 Remedies employed in the treatment of diseases of the eye may be divided into: (1) systemic, and (2) local.

3:3 *Systemic:* Many systemic disorders present ocular manifestations (Chapter 12), and an important part of the treatment of the latter consists in general medication intended to correct the constitutional disturbance. Several good examples of this in canine practice are: distemper, systemic mycotic infections, especially blastomycosis and a variety of other infectious diseases. Heavy internal parasite infestation, and nutritional deficiencies may also cause ocular manifestations. It is evident that, in cases of this sort unless the systemic condition is corrected, the ocular manifestation will not respond satisfactorily.

3:4 *Local Remedies:* Drugs intended for local use are dissolved in aqueous solutions or used in oily, ointment, or powder forms. In recent years a tremendous improvement in the preparation and packaging of eye preparations has been realized. Isotonic and buffered solutions now being generally used are stable, nonirritating, sterile, and possess optimum activity. Ointment base vehicles of today are far superior to those of the past. The use of methylcellulose and related compounds as the vehicle for solutions is largely responsible for this improvement. Methylcellulose is nonirritating to ocular tissue and its incorporation in ophthalmic solutions results in the medication remaining in contact for a longer time. Polyvinyl alcohol is another suitable vehicle for various ophthalmic preparations and compares favorably with methylcellulose.

3:5 Generally, for the long term effect solutions need to be instilled more frequently than ointments. Thus, ointment preparations have usually been more popular for use by veterinarians. Solutions, however, exert a quicker effect and are often to be preferred in, for example, acute ulceration. The use of powders in the eye is to be condemned.

3:6 In applying an aqueous solution to the eye, it is best to raise the upper lid and instill the drops just above the limbus at 12 o'clock, allowing it to flow over the cornea. If the solution is instilled into the lower cul-de-sac, it is diluted immediately with tears and passes readily into the lacrimal passages, thus a full therapeutic effect to the cornea is not obtained.

3:7 Oily solutions and ointments may be instilled on the cornea or into the lower cul-de-sac where they are not diluted with tears and tend to remain longer in contact with the eye structures.

3:8 Any extended discussion of eye therapy is beyond the scope of this chapter. Only the drugs and therapeutic measures proved to be of value by our extensive clinical use are included.

Cleansing Solutions

3:9 Cleansing solutions are used for flushing the conjunctival sac and removing secretions to facilitate examination (Par. 2:14) and *always* prior to the topical instillation of drugs. They should be bland and used warm or at room temperature. Instillation is accomplished most often by soft-rubber bulb syringe, or plastic irrigating bottle (Fig. 3–1). Saturated cotton balls can be used to clean debris and discharge from the conjunctiva and lids.

3:10 Cleansing solutions recommended for home preparation and use include: (1) boric acid (1 teaspoonful in a cup of water), and (2) saline solution (1 teaspoonful NaCl in a pint of water).

3:11 An excellent cleansing, comforting solution for clinic use is:

Sodium bicarbonate ½ oz
Boric acid or Borax ½ oz
Sodium chloride ½ oz
Glycerine 2 oz
Water q.s. 1 gal. Filter or use the supernatant fluid.

3:12 To this preparation may be added 4 ml of 10% Roccal or a similar quaternary ammonium chloride solution. This then becomes a 1 to 10,000 solution. Quaternary ammonium solutions of this strength are nonirritating, do not inhibit regeneration of corneal epithelium, provide a good vehicle for drugs (low surface tension), are compatible with antibiotics, and are bacteriostatic. When compared with other commonly used antiseptic-germicides, the quaternary ammonium compounds exert the best relative disinfectant action and a good persistency of action.

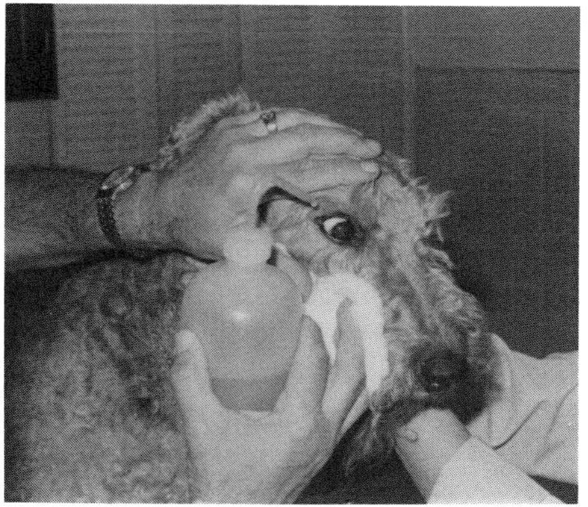

Fig. 3–1. Removal of secretions with plastic irrigating bottle.

3:13 The use of plain tap water for removing secretions from the eye is not condoned, especially in view of the ease with which the above soothing preparation can be prepared.

Stimulating and Astringent Remedies

3:14 These are drugs which are used locally to contract tissue and which produce a precipitate action on proteins. They are used chiefly in various forms of conjunctivitis but have been replaced in many instances by antibiotic and other chemotherapeutic preparations.

3:15 Zinc sulfate, silver nitrate, copper sulfate and yellow oxide of mercury have all been used primarily to treat chronic conjunctivitis. "Painting" the conjunctival surfaces with a copper sulfate crystal, held in a thumb forceps has been used to treat follicular conjunctivitis. Such treatment is effective in destroying the follicles, but is often much more severe than needed, even when done carefully. Mechanical debridement (Par. 5:33) is preferred. A silver nitrate stick should not be used. These agents, especially silver nitrate and copper sulfate, can cause corneal damage if not neutralized with saline or other chloride-containing eye wash and flushed from the conjunctival sac.

Disinfectants-Cauterants

3:16 Three preparations in common use as disinfectant-cauterants are:

1. Pure carbolic acid
2. Trichloroacetic acid (25% to pure).
3. Tincture of iodine (mild to strong)

3:17 Disinfectant-cauterants are principally used for cauterization of corneal ulcers. (Par. 6:114)

3:18 Acids, such as carbolic have been used for producing corneal sloughs because the corneal proteins are immediately precipitated by the acid.[14] This precipitate in turn acts as a barrier to the further penetration of the acid into the deeper structures of the cornea (Fig. 6–5). In contrast, alkalies do not form a precipitate with the proteins of the cornea, but rather pass through and in many instances cause irreparable damage.

3:19 Strong tincture of iodine (7%) is much less damaging to the cornea than the acids mentioned above. It is the preferred mild disinfectant-cauterant for infected corneal ulcers or corneal epithelial erosions (Boxer indolent ulcers). Stromal staining, that has been mentioned as a contraindication in man, does not appear to be a problem to the dog.

Mydriatics and Cycloplegics

3:20 Mydriatics are agents that produce dilatation of the pupil; cycloplegics are agents that cause paralysis of the iris, sphincter, and ciliary body with a resultant dilatation of the pupil and loss of accommodation. Thus, a cycloplegic always acts as a mydriatic, but a mydriatic does not necessarily cause cycloplegia. These topically applied autonomic drugs are among the most useful pharmacologic agents in ophthalmic practice. They comprise two groups of drugs: (1) Parasympatholytics and (2) sympathomimetics.

3:21 *Parasympatholytic* drugs produce dilatation and cycloplegia by rendering the pupillary sphincter and ciliary muscle insensitive to acetylcholine. The most commonly used cycloplegics in veterinary ophthalmology are atropine, scopolamine, and tropicamide. The duration of action of atropine may be a week or more. A noted side effect is salivation and drooling which occurs immediately following instillation but persists for a short time only. This effect is the response to the bitter taste the dog senses after the drug reaches the mouth via the nasolacrimal duct.

3:22 Atropine sulfate in solution or ointment form (1 to 4%) is one of the most *important* and *useful* drugs in canine ophthalmology. There are few contraindications to its use, *e.g.* glaucoma not associated with uveitis, and its value in the following conditions cannot be overemphasized:

3:23 1. In iritis and uveitis, to dilate the pupil, prevent adhesions, and to relieve pain by paralyzing the ciliary body. Ciliary spasm is an important source of pain.

3:24 2. In various diseases of the cornea, from ulceration to interstitial (deep) keratitis. Its effect in these conditions is superior to that of topical anesthetics. In corneal inflammation the iris and ciliary body are usually affected to some degree. These structures share a common innervation (Fig. 1–8) and the ensuing iris-ciliary spasm adds to the pain which is reduced by the atropine.

3:25 3. After certain operations, *e.g.* extracapsular cataract extraction.

3:26 4. As a mydriatic for ophthalmoscopy, although short-acting preparations (Par. 3:27) are preferred.

3:27 Scopolamine is used in combination with phenylephrine* to achieve mydriasis prior to intraocular surgery and in an attempt to break down iris adhesions.

3:28 Tropicamide,† 1% has proved to be the most useful mydriatic for use in canine ophthalmoscopy. A maximum mydriasis can be obtained within 20 to 30 minutes and the pupil will return to normal within several hours. Rubin's[19] investigation discloses that some of the more common preparations advocated for use in man failed to achieve the same effect in the dog.

3:29 *Sympathomimetic* agents imitate or potentiate the action of adrenalin, and their effect is upon the dilator muscle of the iris. Those in common use are epinephrine and phenylephrine. They do not cause cycloplegia. Adrenalin (epinephrine) is considered a mydriatic although its rapid destruction precludes its clinical use for this purpose. As a vasoconstrictor it is useful in the control of hemorrhage both from the smaller arterioles

*Murocoll #2. (Muro Pharmaceuticals, Inc., Tewksbury, MA, 01876).

†Mydriacyl. (Alcon Laboratories, Inc., Ft. Worth, Texas 76101).

and the capillaries of the conjunctiva, and for the relief of congested mucous membranes. It has been injected subconjunctivally in an attempt to release recent iris adhesions and dilate the pupil, but with questionable effect. Its use is in conjunction with cocaine for the diagnosis of Horner's syndrome. Its use for this purpose has been superseded by paradrine (Par. 12:25). Epinephrine 2% has been used for its ocular hypotensive effect in certain types of glaucoma in man even though its mode of action is not well established. It is thought that the aqueous outflow facility is enhanced by its action. I have found epitrate (2% epinephrine) of greatest value in treating low-grade glaucoma associated with iris atrophy in old dogs, especially poodles.

3:30 Phenylephrine HCl alone, 10% (viscous sol.)* or in conjunction with scopolamine,** is used for ophthalmoscopy and pre- and postoperatively. Weaker solutions (0.12 to 0.2%) are used as decongestants in combination with other drugs.

Miotics

3:31 These drugs diminish the size of the pupil, producing tonic contraction of the sphincter of the iris and of the ciliary muscle, and hence, enhance aqueous outflow. They are employed chiefly in glaucoma. These parasympathomimetic drugs are either *cholinergic* (*i.e.*, simulate the effect of acetylcholine at autonomic synapses or the neuroeffector junctions of the parasympathetic system), or *anticholinesterases* (prevent the hydrolysis of acetylcholine by the enzyme cholinesterase).

3:32 The most commonly used cholinergic drug is pilocarpine (1 to 4%). Its duration of miotic action is but three to four hours. Therein lies its disadvantage.

3:33 Miotics that have proved most useful for control of glaucoma in the dog are in the anticholinesterase group. These include Echothiophate iodide,* and Demacarium bromide.† Either of these preparations requires fewer instillations and exerts a more dramatic effect (Par. 9:91).

3:34 Phospholine is prepared in four strengths (0.03, 0.06, 0.125, and 0.25%). The reconstituted solution is stable for several months if kept refrigerated. Systemic toxic effects caused by the use of these drops can occur, especially at the higher concentration and in small dogs. They include vomiting, diarrhea, and muscle rigidity.

3:35 Demacarium bromide (Humorsol) is supplied in two strengths: 0.125% and 0.25%. Systemic toxic effects approximate those of phospholine iodide. An advantage is its stability. It is in solution when received and does not need refrigeration.

Anesthetic Agents

3:36 Topical anesthetics play an almost indispensable role in the proper examination and treatment of the eye. These agents permit the clinician to perform ocular procedures such as tonometry, removal of superficial foreign bodies, and lacrimal canalicular irrigation. Most work within several minutes and their duration of action is between 10 to 20 minutes. Preparations in common use include phenacaine hydrochloride (Holocaine), butacaine sulfate (Butyn), tetracaine hydrochloride (Tetracaine, Pontocaine). These drugs are effective in producing topical anesthesia, but disadvantages include a stinging sensation following instillation and occasionally chemosis, thought to be an allergic reaction.

3:37 Proparacaine hydrochloride¶ solution has proved of real value because of its quick, efficient manner in producing topical anesthesia with freedom from undesirable side ef-

*Neo-Synephrine (Winthrop Laboratories, New York, N.Y., 10017)

**Muracoll (Muro Pharmaceuticals, Inc., Tewksbury, MA, 01876)

*Phospholine Iodide (Ayerst Labs., New York, N.Y. 10017).

†Humorsol (Merck Sharp and Dohme, West Point, Pa. 19486).

¶Ophthaine (E.R. Squibb and Sons, New York, N.Y. 10022) or Ophthetic (Allergan Pharmaceuticals, Santa Ana, Calif. 92705).

fects.[13] A disadvantage is in its relatively short shelf life and need for refrigeration after opening.

3:38 They have the additional undesirable effect of making the cornea insensitive, and thereby making it more vulnerable to further damage by the dog abrading it with a paw or rubbing it on the floor or furniture. The safest rule is to use topical anesthetics to facilitate examination of the eye, but refrain from using them in treatment.

3:39 Procaine, 2 to 4% solution, or xylocaine are the anesthetics of choice for hypodermic use in lid growth operations.

Antibiotics and Chemotherapy

3:40 Antibiotics and the sulfonamides have an important place in the treatment and prevention of ocular infections. In order to achieve optimum results, however, one must know: (1) the penetrating properties into the eye through the cornea and through the blood aqueous barrier, (2) the sensitivities and (3) the spectrum they encompass. Studies as regards toxicities or effectiveness elsewhere in the body mean little, *e.g.* penicillin may be effective in a streptococcic infection of the throat, but that same organism in the eye will not be affected by penicillin since this particular antibiotic penetrates the blood aqueous barrier of the eye very poorly.

3:41 An appreciation of the importance and a knowledge of the function of the blood aqueous barrier of the eye is essential. This barrier differs from the blood tissue barriers in the rest of the body, except for perhaps the brain, because of the low concentration of protein in the aqueous as opposed to its much higher concentration in all other tissues.

3:42 In diseases of the eye, then, there are additional problems because of the peculiarities of the blood aqueous barrier. The presence of adequate blood concentrations in the body does not guarantee adequate concentrations in the aqueous and vitreous that may be involved in the infectious process. In other words, we must be concerned not only with whether or not the organism responsible for the infection in the ocular tissue is susceptible to the drug chosen, but also whether the drug will penetrate into the involved ocular tissues in sufficient concentration to bring about the desired result. (Par. 7:10)

3:43 Most of the commonly used antibiotics, *e.g.* penicillin, streptomycin, aureomycin, and terramycin, must be given in massive doses and by injection to feebly penetrate the blood aqueous barrier. Neither do they penetrate an intact corneal epithelium. They do, however, penetrate an abraded epithelium.

3:44 Chloramphenicol, on the other hand, is absorbed rapidly, secreted slowly and penetrates the blood aqueous barrier readily when given orally.[15] It also penetrates an intact epithelium when applied topically. When used orally, the dosage should be 75–100 mg/pound/day in divided doses.

3:45 Neomycin, bacitracin, and polymyxin, in addition to the aforementioned antibiotics, are all used topically to treat infections caused by sensitive organisms. Medications containing these 3 antibiotics are preferred over chloramphenicol for routine use because of the danger of chloramphenicol to the person treating the dog. However, if the infection is severe or intraocular in nature, systemic treatment with chloramphenicol is imperative.

3:46 Gentamicin sulfate is effective against gram-positive and gram-negative bacteria, including some strains of *Staphylococcus* which are penicillin resistant, and many strains of *Pseudomonas, Escherichia coli* and *Proteus*. However, many strains of B hemolytic streptococcus are resistant. It is well tolerated when administered as a topical solution or as a subconjunctival injection and is capable of penetrating both normal and inflamed eyes. Gentamicin penetrates the aqueous humor of human eyes in therapeutic levels when injected subconjunctivally (10 mg).[7] My own experience with its use in this manner has been most gratifying. To initiate therapy in severe ulcerative keratitis where *Pseudo-*

monas is suspected or proven, 5 to 10 mg* is injected subconjunctivally. This is followed by the topical preparation.

3:47 Sulfonamides have largely been supplanted by the antibiotics, but they are still very useful and more of their mode of action is understood. In the local use of sulfonamides, these points must be kept in mind.

3:48 (1) Their efficacy is impeded by the presence of pus and other secretions containing large amounts of para-aminobenzoic acid, and irrigation of the conjunctival sac should be employed before instillation. High concentrations should be used, *e.g.* sulfacetamide sodium (30% solution or 10% ointment).

3:49 (2) Sulfonamides have been incriminated for delaying the regeneration of corneal epithelium; however, newer preparations with smaller particle size have essentially eliminated the disadvantage.

3:50 Sodium sulfacetamide appears to possess the best power of penetrating the intact corneal epithelium, but when the cornea is infected, its permeability is altered and all sulfonamides pass through readily. When used systemically, the sulfonamides penetrate the blood aqueous barrier and diffuse readily into all ocular tissue.

3:51 *Collagenase Inhibitors* are often combined with antibiotics to treat melting corneal ulcers. Collagenase, produced by bacteria such as *Pseudomonas* sp., epithelial cells and white blood cells, is responsible, in part, for the collagen break down that occurs in melting corneal ulcers. Collagenase inhibitors include acetylcysteine, EDTA, fresh serum and iodine compounds. Acetylcysteine, available as Mucomyst† (20%), is most commonly used. The formula for preparation of ophthalmic solutions is given in the following table:[21]

Amount Needed to Prepare 24 ml	Final Conc. in Ulcer Sol.
1. 1.2 ml 20% Chloramphenicol succinate	1 %
or	or
1.5 ml 5% Gentamicin solution	0.3%
2. 6 ml 20% Acetylcysteine	5 %
3. 6 ml 1% Atropine ophthalmic solution	0.25%
4. 10.8 or 10.5 ml Artificial tear (*e.g.* Adsorbotear)	to q.s. to 24 ml

3:52 Mucomyst deteriorates in about 2 days at room temperature, but will keep for 6 weeks if refrigerated; so, the prepared solution with exception of a 24- to 48-hour supply should be kept refrigerated. Drops should be applied hourly the first day, every 2 hours the second day, and then 4 times a day.

Anti-Fungal Agents

3:53 Diseases in which the fungi have assumed an important role are on the increase. The one clinical denominator in these cases has been the use of antibiotics and steroids. Antibiotics enhance fungus growth by inhibition of the normal bacterial flora, while steroids facilitate fungus proliferation through interference with the host's anti-inflammatory and immune responses.

3:54 Natamycin, a new polyene antibiotic, is the least irritating and least toxic drug in this group. It is effective against Candida, Fusarium, Aspergillus, and other ocular fungi.[9] Natamycin recently has been approved for use in the eye, and is available in 5% suspension or a 1% ointment. It is currently a drug of choice for topical treatment of superficial fungal corneal diseases. As with other polyenes, it penetrates the cornea poorly, and is not effective against deeper infection of the cornea. Its antifungal activity seems to be a result of its ability to cause lysis of cell membranes of susceptible fungi.[2]

3:55 Amphotericin B has a broad antifungal activity. It is the drug of choice in therapy for systemic infections caused by Blastomyces, Coccidioides, Histoplasma, and Cryptococcus. In vitro testing has shown it also to be fairly effective against Candida and Aspergillus infections of the cornea. It does not pen-

*Gentocin (50 mg per ml) (Shering, Kenilworth, N.J. 07033).

†Mucomyst (Mead Johnson Laboratories, Evansville, Indiana 47721)

etrate the blood-aqueous barrier well when given systemically nor does it penetrate the normal cornea when administered topically. A solution of 1 to 5 mg/ml is recommended for topical use. In humans, intraocular doses of up to 25 micrograms have been used for Candida endophthalmitis. Its inability to penetrate the cornea and high degree of corneal irritation have limited its use topically.[2]

Anti-Viral Agents

3:56 Antiviral drugs have been infrequently prescribed in veterinary ophthalmology because the role of ophthalmic virus infection has not been well established, except for feline viral rhinotracheitis-induced keratoconjunctivitis in the cat. Idoxuridine, Vidarabine and Trifluridine are used in man and in the cat. These agents act by inhibiting DNA replication, and hence inhibit viral replication, rather than being viracidal. To be effective, they must be used 5 to 6 times a day, or more frequently if drops are used.

Anti-Inflammatory Agents—Steroids

3:57 Perhaps the greatest usefulness of the corticosteroids in veterinary medicine lies in the field of ophthalmology.[12] This importance has become manifest primarily because good therapeutic results depend upon sufficient amounts of the steroids reaching the sites where needed. Since the eye is readily accessible, optimum results can be expected.

3:58 However, enthusiasm must be tempered with the realization that there are definite contraindications to their use.[16] Steroids do not affect the causative agents but rather the tissue response to those agents. They *do not* have antibiotic or chemotherapeutic effect, but, even when combined with a suitable antibiotic, there still are contraindications to their use, *e.g.* acute ulceration (Par. 6:119).

3:59 The ocular effects of steroid therapy are to:

1. Suppress hypersensitivity reactions
2. Suppress ocular reactions to irritants
3. Suppress inflammatory processes that result from infections
4. Suppress neovascularization of the cornea
5. Reduce fibroblastic activity in the cornea
6. Interfere with effective immunological reactions.

3:60 The anti-inflammatory effects of steroids are nonspecific, occurring whether the cause is allergic, traumatic or infectious. One of the best means of combatting vascular invasion of the cornea and of inducing regression of existing vessels is to administer a repository form by the subconjunctival method. In addition, when used properly, steroids will markedly reduce the amount of permanent scarring. Whereas formation of collagen and fibroblastic activity are inhibited by steroids, some clinicians have been reluctant to use them until a week or more following surgery. However, if care is exercised to assure good wound closure and the sutures are allowed to remain intact for 12 or more days, good healing will result and many postoperative complications will be avoided. A study[1] showed that the administration of topical corticosteroid ointment twice daily, even when started immediately postoperatively, did not affect the tensile strength of corneal wounds in rabbits tested 21 days after surgery.

3:61 Steroids reduce resistance to many types of invading microorganisms and should *never* be used in the presence of such infections except concurrently with an effective antibiotic. There is also general agreement that the topical use of steroids increases ocular susceptibility to fungus infection. Fungus induced ulceration, if unrecognized, can lead to the loss of an eye. Not only viral and fungal, but bacterial corneal infections may be worsened by the use of steroids. When used over a long period of time progressive gray-white corneal infiltrates may appear and coalesce to produce a form of dystrophy. Glaucoma and posterior subcapsular cataract formation have been reported in the human as a complication of long-term, high-dosage systemic corticosteroid therapy. I have not encountered this side effect in the dog. The cause of degenerative disease is not influenced by the administration of steroids. Havener[8] sums it up by stating, "the greatest contraindication to corticosteroid therapy, however, holds for both systemic and topical routes of administration; it is *the lack of a specific indication for steroid use.*"

Uses

3:62 As with all medications, it is important to delineate specific fields of action. Medications administered topically or subconjunctivally can provide adequate drug levels in extra-ocular tissues and the anterior segment (back through the iris and ciliary body), but not in the posterior segment (vitreous, retina, or choroid). Systemic administration can provide adequate levels in the posterior segment, but generally does not provide as high a level in the extraocular tissue and anterior segment as can be obtained by the topical or subconjunctival routes.

3:63 Topical instillation and/or subconjunctival injections:

(1) lid and conjunctival allergies and diseases
(2) superficial keratitis (vascularization, pannus, exuberant granulation tissue)
(3) episcleritis
(4) iridocyclitis (anterior uveitis)
(5) postoperative.

3:64 Systemic

(1) Iritis (anterior uveitis)
(2) Posterior segment disease (chorioretinitis, optic neuritis, retinal detachment [serous-inflammatory]).

3:65 Routes of administration and dosage

1. Drops. Topical agents mainly used in conjunction with anti-infective agents include: hydrocortisone; prednisolone; dexamethasone; flumethasone; and betamethasone. Frequency of application is more effective than use of a stronger concentration. Instillation every hour or two is made until a response is obtained and thereafter 4 × a day.

2. Ointments containing most of the same combinations as the drops are instilled 2–4 × a day.

3. Subconjunctival injection. The repositol form of methylprednisolone* or triamcinolone† provides a constant source of corticosteroid, lasting for 2 to 4 weeks. Depending upon weight, a 2.5 to 10 mg injection is made. Technique: Adequate topical anesthesia is first obtained by applying the agent 2–3 × at 2–3-minute intervals. Then, using a 26 gauge needle mounted on a disposable 1 ml syringe, the injection is made underneath the bulbar conjunctiva at any accessible area (Fig. 3–2). A bleb results which usually subsides within a few hours. A residue of the suspension may remain indefinitely. If only a short action is required or there is some doubt as to whether a steroid should be continued beyond a prescribed time, the nonrepositol type of preparation should be considered, *e.g.* Flucort (.125 to .25 mg).‡ These preparations afford adequate steroid concentration for approximately forty-eight hours. The same anti-inflammatory effect could be obtained with topically applied drops, as outlined above; however, the frequent instillation of drops needed makes subconjunctival injection a desirable method of gaining control of inflammatory diseases prior to using drops or ointments for maintenance.

4. Systemic. This administration may be either by intramuscular injection or per os.

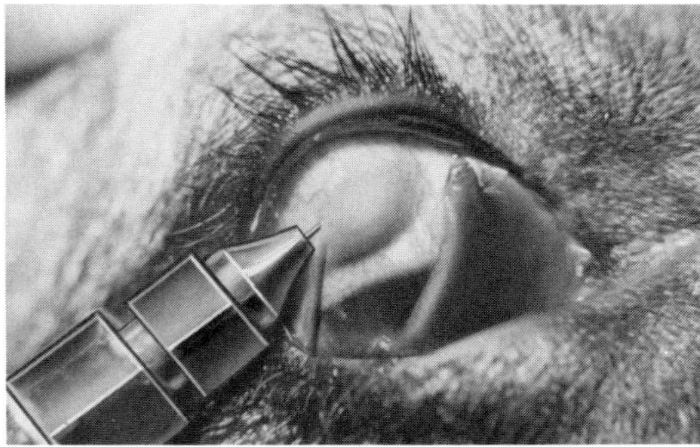

Fig. 3–2. Bleb arising from a subconjunctival injection.

*Depo-medrol (Upjohn).
†Kenalog (Squibb).
‡Flucort (Syntex Labs., Palo Alto, Calif. 94304).

Dosage depends upon the preparation used and the condition to be treated. Specific recommendations are made as these diseases are discussed throughout the book.

3:66 *Non-Steroidal Anti-Inflammatory Agents—Prostaglandin Inhibitors.* Since prostaglandins, primarily PGE, are important mediators of inflammation in the uveal tract,[6] prostaglandin inhibitors are potent agents in preventing inflammation. The two agents most commonly used in the dog are aspirin 10 mg/pound given orally, 4 to 6 hours prior to surgery,[3] and flunixin meglumine,* 0.25 to 0.5 mg/pound given IV, 30 minutes prior to surgery. Banamine is not approved for use in small animals, but is widely used by veterinary ophthalmologists, and appears to be more effective than aspirin. It can, however, cause severe side effects, including hemorrhagic diarrhea, and even kidney failure in some dogs when given in conjunction with deep general anesthesia, so must be used with caution. Aspirin can cause vomiting which is quite undesirable in a dog being prepared for cataract extraction.

Antihistamines

3:67 These preparations, as histamine antagonists, will relieve the seasonal allergic symptoms of ocular itching, redness and tearing. They must be given systemically, rather than topically, to produce the desired effect. The corticosteroids, however, generally achieve a more sustained and dramatic response and are, in addition, effective when instilled topically.

Vitamins

3:68 In ophthalmology we are concerned with vitamin therapy, especially in those avitaminoses caused by the absence of an insufficient amount of vitamins A, C, and riboflavin and niacin of the B complex.

3:69 Vitamin A assumes an extremely important role in the physiology of vision.[22] In vitamin A deficiency, various tissues all over the body begin to deteriorate, the retina included. The rods in the retina exhibit marked changes and, as the deficiency progresses, other layers of the retina become involved. Fortunately, however, even rods which have ceased to function appear to regain function within 2 to 4 months of vitamin A administration.

3:70 Vitamin A is also thought necessary and essential for the normal life of the epithelial cell. In the absence of this vitamin, these cells degenerate and atrophy, followed by a proliferation on the part of the basal cells, resulting in keratinization and keratomalacia (Par. 6:110).

3:71 Vitamin C (ascorbic acid) is essential for the proper maintenance of intercellular cement substances. In vitamin C deficiency the characteristic lesion is the occurrence of capillary hemorrhages due to the failure of the endothelial cells to produce cement substance and thus allowing the capillaries to rupture. This vitamin is also important to the regeneration of corneal epithelium and is useful in ulcerative keratitis.

3:72 Riboflavin (B_2) deficiency is characterized by superficial vascularization with a possible ulceration and subsequent opacity of the cornea.

3:73 Niacin is believed to enhance the regeneration of corneal epithelium and, thus, is also useful in the therapy of ulcerative keratitis.

3:74 *Dosage*

Vitamin A	10,000 to 25,000 units daily
Vitamin C	50 to 150 mg daily
Riboflavin	5 to 15 mg daily
Niacin	50 to 150 mg daily

3:75 Daily administration of a therapeutic capsule containing approximate amounts of the above vitamins constitutes good adjunctive therapy in cases of corneal ulceration or ocular manifestations resulting from improper nutrition or debilitating disease.

*Banamine (Schering, Kenilworth, N.J. 07033)

Other Therapeutic Measures

3:76 *Carbonic anhydrase inhibitors** have proved to be a most useful addition in the treatment of glaucoma as they lower intraocular pressure by inhibiting secretion of the aqueous (Par. 9:96). They have the advantage of being effective in the oral form. I prefer Daranide at 0.5 mg to 1.0 mg/pound of body weight, twice a day. Diamox at 2.5 mg to 5.0 mg per pound, twice a day is second choice; however, side effects of labored breathing and gastrointestinal disorders seem to be more common. Dividing the doses and giving them 4× a day is even better, but owner compliance is often a problem. Reduction of tension can be expected within a few hours of oral administration. Ordinarily carbonic anhydrase inhibitors are reserved for short-term therapy of glaucoma.

3:77 *Osmotic agents* have also proved useful as an emergency measure to gain control of acute glaucoma. Glycerol and mannitol effectively reduce increased intraocular pressure within an hour of administration. They reduce aqueous production and also dehydrate the vitreous, thereby allowing the lens and iris to move back and open the iridocorneal angle. Their main use is to bring tension under control in those cases which have not responded to miotic and carbonic anhydrase inhibitor therapy (Par. 9:91) Once the tension is brought under control, the miotic may effectively maintain that control.

3:78 Mannitol is administered intravenously as a 20% solution. It can be given at the rate of 2.5 to 5 ml per pound body weight over a 5- to 10-minute period. The hypotensive effect lasts for several hours. Mannitol is especially useful for softening an eye before removal of a subluxated or luxated lens. Mannitol powder can be purchased and the solution prepared and autoclaved at considerable savings to the clinician.

3:79 Glycerol has the advantage of being effective when taken orally and is relatively nontoxic, although it may produce gastrointestinal upset in dogs. It is administered at the rate of 1 ml per pound body weight, preferably diluted with a syrup base to render it more palatable. This dose may be repeated at 8- to 12-hour intervals.

3:80 *Enzymes.* Trypsin and Chymotrypsin† in combination have been used to promote the absorption of intraocular debris (hypopyon, hyphema); however, the benefit is questionable. Alpha-chymotrypsin is a proteolytic enzyme useful in human ophthalmology because of its selective lytic action upon zonular fibers. This facilitates cataract extraction by the intracapsular method. However, this enzyme exerts no appreciable effect on the normal vitreolenticular attachment of the dog, thus limiting its usefulness.

3:81 *Nonspecific Protein Therapy.* Foreign proteins supposedly stimulate or increase the antibodies thus increasing the natural resistance against the invading bacteria. The indications for foreign protein therapy are: infected corneal ulcers, uveitis and some cases of purulent conjunctivitis. Prior to the advent of the corticosteroids, sterile milk and typhoid-paratyphoid vaccine were routinely used. It is now generally agreed, however, that steroids create a therapeutic response superior to that obtained with foreign protein injections and, therefore, they are seldom used anymore.

3:82 *Heat.* Hot, moist compresses are prescribed in infections of the cornea, iris, ciliary body, sclera and orbit as a whole. Hot cloths are usually applied on the closed lids and renewed every few minutes for fifteen minutes several times a day. Heat is a vasodilator producing an active hyperemia with an increase of leukocytes and antibodies and thus aiding in the absorption of inflammatory products.

3:83 *Cold.* Moist, cold compresses are of distinct benefit to those injuries of the eyelids, eyes and surrounding tissues that produce swelling and pain and are sometimes

*Ethoxzolamide (Cardrase—Upjohn Co.) Dichlorphenamide (Daranide—Merck Sharp & Dohme) Acetazolamide (Diamox—Lederle).

†Chymar, Chymoral (Armour).

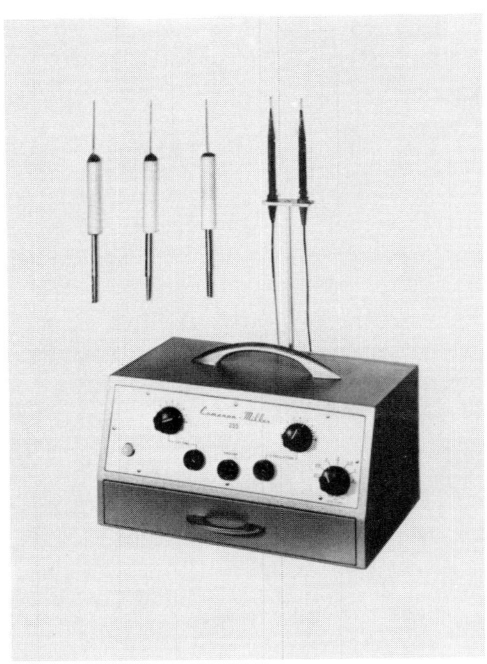

Fig. 3–3. The Cameron-Miller electrosurgical unit Model 255 and epilation needles used in distichiasis and trichiasis.

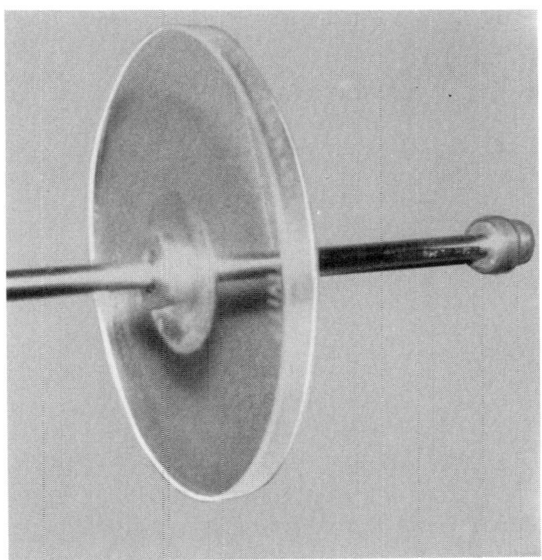

Fig. 3–4. The beta-ray applicator.

accompanied by hemorrhage. As a vasoconstrictor it produces an ischemia in tissues that are swollen, chemotic or edematous, thereby hastening recovery. I use cold compresses if treating within 4 hours of injury and hot compresses after 4 hours.

3:84 *Electrosurgery* (Fig. 3–3). Electrosurgery and coagulation are most useful for: (1) removal of distorted or unwanted cilia causing distichiasis, trichiasis (Par. 4:34), (2) removal of lid tumors (Par. 4:86), (3) scleral incision (Par. 9:140), and (4) cautery in intraocular surgical procedures, including iridectomy (Par. 7:98).

3:85 *Radiation.* X-ray or beta-ray therapy has been well investigated and utilized in canine ophthalmology.[11,17,18] Although radiation is sometimes useful adjunct therapy, its importance has been lessened considerably with the development and use of the newer steroid preparations.

3:86 X ray and other forms of deep radiation are occasionally used for lid and orbital tumors not amenable to surgical excision; however, cataract formation and even brain injury are potential complications.

3:87 Beta-ray therapy (Fig. 3–4) has an advantage over other forms of radiation in the treatment of superficial corneal or conjunctival lesions, because Beta rays do not penetrate the cornea or sclera.

3:88 I use Beta-ray therapy infrequently after removal of corneal and scleral neoplasms (primarily in horses and cattle) to further reduce the chance of regrowth. Four thousand to six thousand R.E.P. should be delivered to each area and repeated to cover all of the area of tumor removal.

3:89 Beta-ray irradiation has also been advocated for treatment of vascular lesions of the cornea and to reduce neovascularization of the cornea by application to the limbus following keratectomy (Fig. 3–5). It is somewhat effective, but, in my estimation, is not as effective as steroids.

3:90 *Cryotherapy.* The destruction of tissue by the application of substances or instruments to freeze tissue (diagram p. 40). The most important use in canine ophthalmology

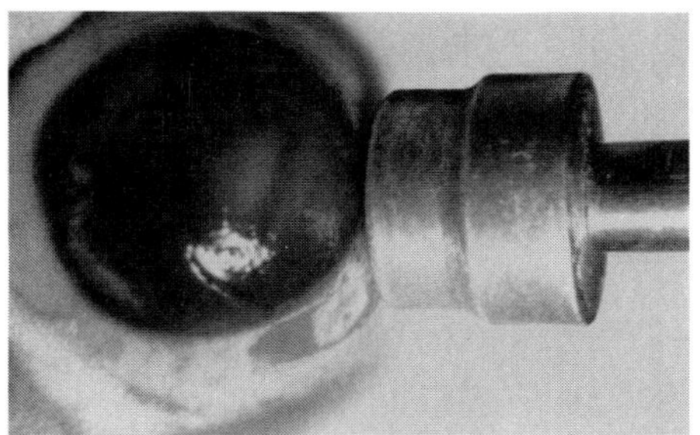

Fig. 3–5. The beta-ray source in position at the limbus following a superficial keratectomy.

is the treatment of glaucoma[4,20] (Par. 9:129–132).

Theory of Cryosurgery

Rapid Freeze
↓
Intracellular Ice Crystals
↓
Slow Thaw
↓
Cell Destruction
Capillary Disturbance
Combination of Both
↓
Aseptic Necrosis

In cyclocryotherapy, a cold probe is applied to the bulbar conjunctival surface over the ciliary body (Fig. 3–19). Rapid freezing and slow thawing causes destruction of ciliary epithelial cells without seriously damaging the conjunctiva and sclera, because of the difference in cellular susceptibility. Cryotherapy is also used for destruction of lid tumors (Par. 4:93) and treatment of distichiasis (Par. 4:38). The cryogens most often used are (1) liquid nitrogen (Fig. 3–17), −196° C, which can be applied directly as a spray or indirectly through a cold probe, and (2) nitrous oxide, −89° C, which is applied through a cold probe (Fig. 3–18). Freon, −40° C, is used in some cryoprobes for lens extraction (Par. 10:114), but not for cryosurgery.

3:91 *Bandaging.* With an ordinary amount of patience and practice, the eye or eyes of most breeds can be easily bandaged. A comfortable bandage will be well tolerated and offers three important advantages: (1) protection of the globe, (2) extra warmth (conducive to healing), and (3) prevention of contamination.

3:92 A sterile piece of combined roll or fracture padding can be held in place by an elastic type adhesive* or stockinette (Fig. 3–6). Eyes are routinely bandaged following intraocular surgery, including intraocular prosthesis and, often, enucleation.

3:93 *Castor Oil and Cod Liver Oil* are soothing preparations which can be recommended for first aid use. They are useful for protection prior to bathing and can be used following minor abrasions of the cornea and conjunctiva.

3:94 *Artificial Tears.* Methylcellulose† is commonly used in from 0.5 to 1% solution as artificial tears and as a soothing base for many ophthalmic preparations. It has a minimum effect on regeneration of corneal epithelium and has the important feature of increasing corneal contact time by a considerable margin over non-methylcellulose solutions. In one study[10] the ideal ophthalmic vehicle for ocular absorption of active ingredients appeared to be hydroxpropyl methylcellulose 1%; a 0.5% solution of the same substance was next most suitable. Solutions of polyvinyl alcohol are also used as an ophthalmic vehicle and lubricant.

3:95 Artificial tears can be purchased under several different trade names. The bulk powder may also be purchased and a stock solution made for use as artificial tears or as a vehicle for numerous ophthalmic preparations the clinician may want to prepare.

*Elasticon (Johnson and Johnson).

†Methocel 4000 CPS USP (Dow Chemical Co.)

GENERAL CONSIDERATIONS FOR EYE SURGERY

3:96 Ocular surgery can be divided into two parts: extraocular and intraocular. Essentially, extraocular surgery involves procedures of the lids, conjunctiva and cornea which are easily performed by the veterinarian possessing the qualifications essential to general surgery. Intraocular surgery (*e.g.* cataract, glaucoma procedures), on the other hand, demands the skills of a person willing to devote an unusual amount of time to the study of a specific specialty.

3:97 The intraocular surgeon must be temperamentally suited and have patience. It is not sufficient to simply be an accomplished surgeon. To achieve any degree of success he must be well versed in medical ophthalmology, and have an intimate knowledge and a thorough understanding of the surgical anatomy of the eye. A distance of 1 mm may not be critical in performing an incision elsewhere in the body, but it can mean the difference between success or failure in an eye operation. In addition, a knowledge of ophthalmic pathology is a most important aid in the proper selection of cases. For example, some cataract extractions, even though properly executed, are doomed to failure without this knowledge (Par. 10:37).

3:98 Other considerations which are important to the degree of success are: adequate practice surgery, a sufficient number of cases for perfection of a technique, and religiously adhering to the time-proved procedures of preoperative care, surgical techniques, and postoperative care practiced by the qualified ophthalmologists of both human and veterinary medicine.

3:99 The rules of asepsis and antisepsis which govern general surgery are also valid in ophthalmic operations. This is especially true in consideration of intraocular procedures where introduction of infection, a cilia, lint, glove powder, etc., will nullify the best effort. By following a rigid aseptic routine and utilizing the aid of a well-trained assistant, many complications leading to failure can be avoided.

3:100 It is most important that the area about the eye is prepared properly and that the eye is draped in such a manner that skin and lid exposure is minimized. A small sheet of rubber dental dam with a slit cut for insertion of the eye speculum is included in the pack for this purpose, and is used to envelop the lids and skin area left exposed by the head and body drape (Fig. 3–7).

Preparation of the Patient

3:101 Intraocular surgery is usually elective surgery, and should be done under ideal circumstances. In a preoperative evaluation and preparation, any discharge other than normal tearing should be noted by the surgeon. Intraocular surgery should not be performed in the presence of infection. The preparation of the patient is begun at least 24 hours prior to surgery, so that no clipped hair is present in the conjunctival sac at the time of surgery.

1. Instill an antibiotic ointment in the lower cul-de-sac, allowing a film of the ointment to form over the cornea for protective purposes prior to steps 2, 3, and 4.
2. Clip the hair with surgical blade approximately 1½ to 2 inches back from the upper and lower lids, as well as the lateral commissure of the lids. Brush or vacuum loose hair away.
3. With blunt point scissors, the blades of which have been anointed either with water or mineral oil, cut the lashes of the upper lid. Lashes will cling to the scissors.
4. With a cotton ball, rub undiluted surgical soap into the clipped areas around the lids. Wet a ball of cotton, squeeze out excess water, work up a lather, and with succeeding balls of wet cotton remove all dirt and soap.
5. Remove any remaining hair or lashes by irrigating eye and lids.

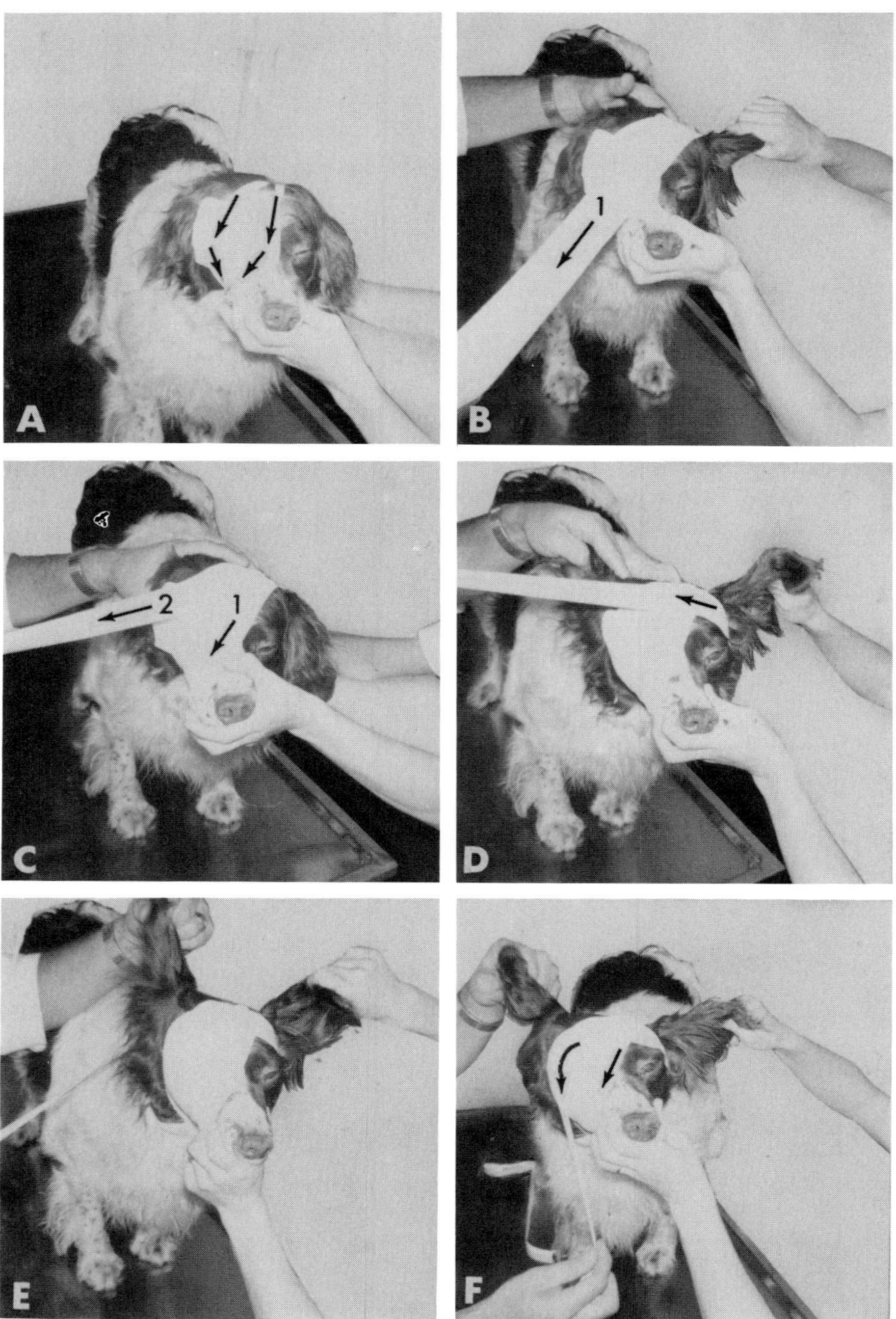

Fig. 3–6. Method of bandaging with pad and elastic adhesive. *A*. The pad is held in place by a continuous strip of adhesive, starting at the base of the opposite ear, to include the medial and lateral aspects of the pad. *B*. Depending upon head size, 1 or 2 inch Elasticon is started at the base of the opposite ear. The assistant holds a corner of the eye pad at all times. The first roll of the bandage (1) should just miss the commissure of the mouth. C. A second roll (2) around the head is made to encompass the lateral aspect of the pad. Then the roll is brought under the jaw to and around the temple in front of the ear on the opposite side. *D*. The roll is continued to the opposite temple and in front of the ear on the bandaged side. *E*. The roll is then continued around the neck back of the ears. This roll, then, is parallel with the support encircling the head in front of the ears. *F*. A final strip of adhesive is used to "nail down" the medial aspect of the bandage. Inclusion of some hair along this border helps to prevent slippage. The strip is continued around the lateral aspect of the bandage.

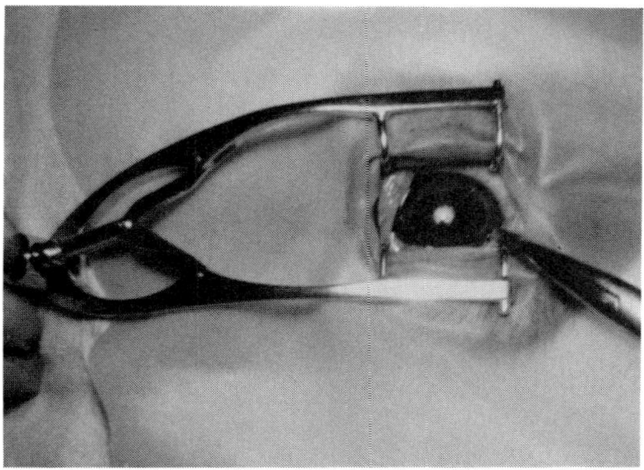

Fig. 3–7. The use of rubber dental dam and the eye speculum for draping.

6. Dry lids with cotton, apply betadine solution carefully with a cotton ball and instill into the cul-de-sac the previously used antibiotic ophthalmic ointment, also massaging same into the clipped area around the eye.

7. If surgery is for cataract extraction, use a mydriatic (Par. 10:91) prior to step 6.

8. Several times before surgery the ointment application and mydriatic (if cataract) are repeated as in step 6.

If the surgery is for relief of glaucoma, removal of the lens, or an intraocular tumor, 20% mannitol is given IV at 3 ml per pound of body weight at the time of induction of anesthesia. If an IV prostaglandin inhibitor such as Banamine (Par. 3:66) is being used, it is given at this time also.

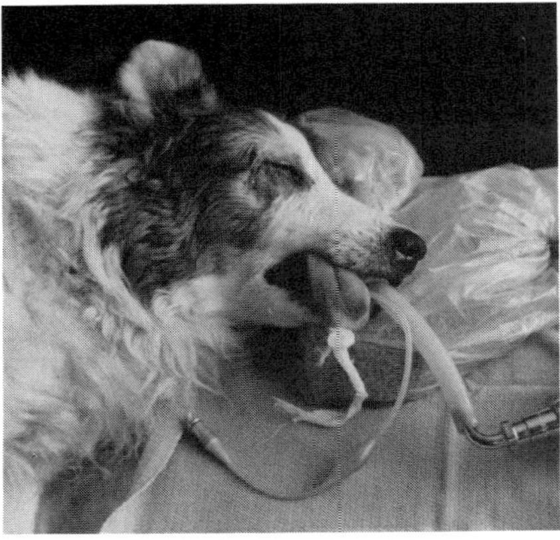

Fig. 3–8. The head positioned for eye surgery using plastic bags filled with "Kitty Litter."

Positioning of the Patient

3:102 Position depends somewhat on the procedure to be performed. Basically, however, the dog is placed on its side with the eye to be operated uppermost. Its head should be at the end of the table and supported in the desired position by sand bags (Fig. 3–8). One sand bag is placed under the ear and back of the head to raise and stabilize the head. The second sand bag is placed under the nose to raise the nose to the desired height. Elevation of the nose is often sufficient. With the head at the end of the table, the instrument stand is within easy reach of the surgeon and assistant (Fig. 3–9).

The Operating Room

3:103 The design of an ophthalmic operating room need not be different from that of a general surgery but the lighting requirements are different. Intraocular surgery cannot be satisfactorily performed in a brilliantly lighted room since this type of light tends to produce a reflection from the cornea, and reduce the apparent brightness of the focal illumination, making it impossible to see details within the anterior chamber. Artificial focal illumination in a darkened room is essential. A combination operating loupe with an attached, adjustable and concentrated light source (Fig. 3–10) has proved to be ideal for performing both intra- and extraocular procedures. For exacting procedures in which additional magnification is needed, the operating microscope (Fig. 3–11) has proven very helpful to the veterinary ophthalmologist. The cost of this equipment and infrequent need precludes its use for the general practitioner.

Instruments

3:104 The instruments used in eye surgery are similar to those used in general surgery, but are much smaller to allow for greater precision in their manipulation.

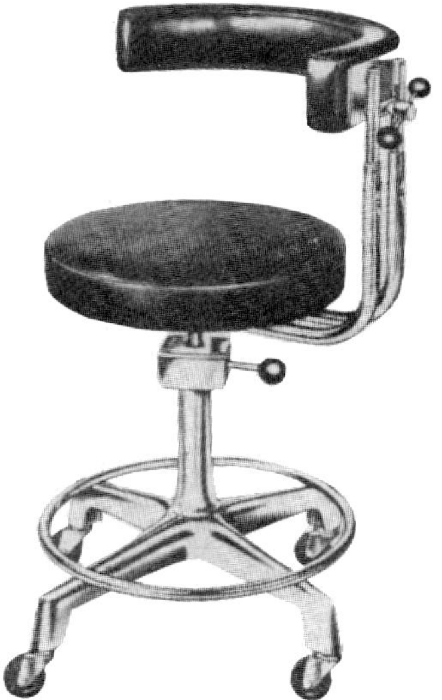

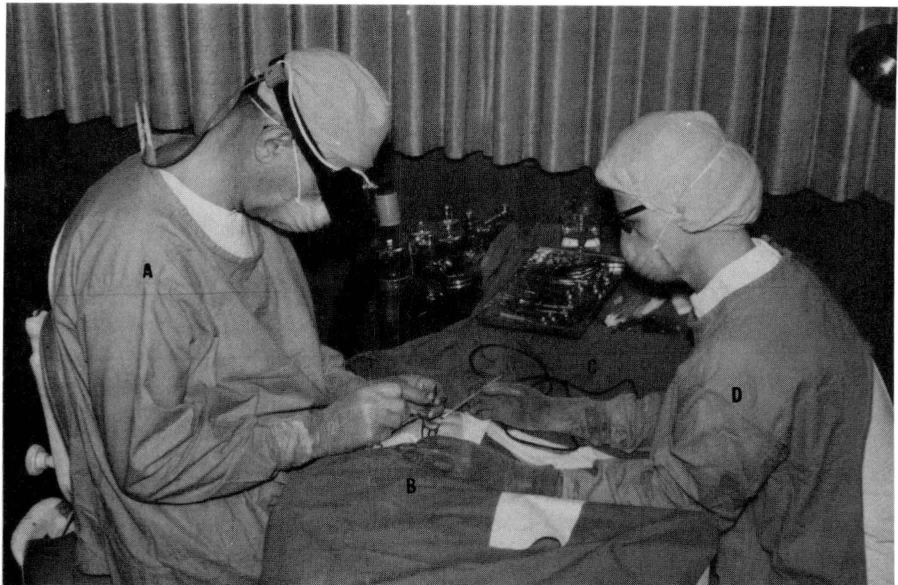

Fig. 3–9. *Above.* Commercial operating stool. *Below.* Position assumed for surgery on the right eye. *A.* Surgeon sitting in operating chair with arms supported. *B.* Dog's head under the drape. *C.* Instrument stand accessible to surgeon and assistant. *D.* Assistant.

3:105 Most eye surgical instruments are very delicate and utmost care must be exercised in their handling and sterilization. The cutting edges, grasping teeth and other functional parts must not strike other objects. Sterilization can be accomplished in the usual way, but dry heat (Fig. 3–12) or gas (Fig. 3–13) has proved to be the best, especially as regards preservation of cutting edges. After use, instruments should be thoroughly cleaned as soon as practical, removing all residue with hot water, soap or a noncorrosive solvent. Cleaning of sharp instruments and forceps with delicate teeth should be done with as little wiping as possible. Storage in cases is recommended, especially when infrequent use is anticipated. We have found that an ultrasonic cleaner (Fig. 3–14) is the most efficient way to clean ophthalmic instruments and keep them "looking like new."

3:106 Ophthalmic instruments are many

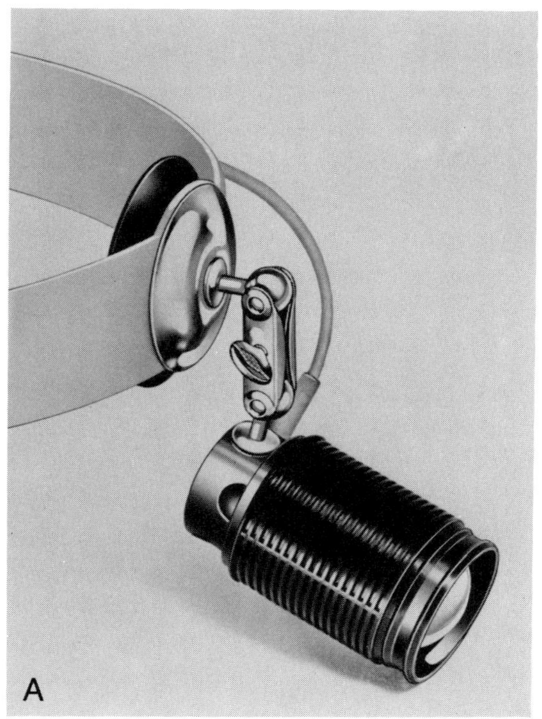

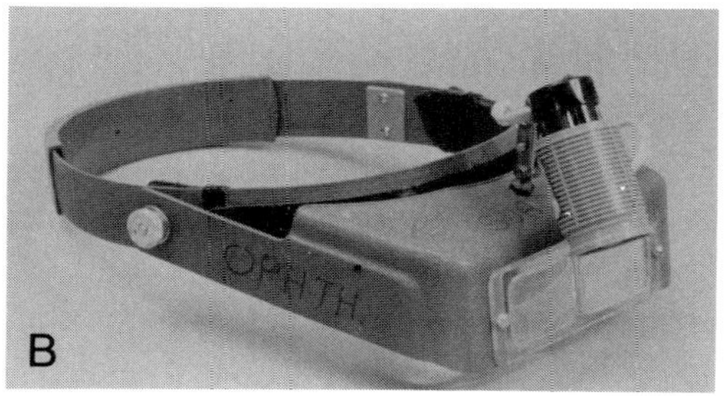

Fig. 3–10. Welch Allyn focusing spot light (left) attached to binocular loupe (right) for eye surgery.

and varied but a good basic set (Fig. 3–15) includes: Castroviejo eye speculum (medium), straight blunt strabismus or tenotomy scissors, dull iris hook, 2 rat tooth curved mosquito forceps, several lacrimal cannulas, McGuire corneal scissors, Graefe strabismus hook (medium), eye dressing forceps (straight serrated), tissue forceps (1 and 2 teeth), fixation forceps with catch, eye needle holder,

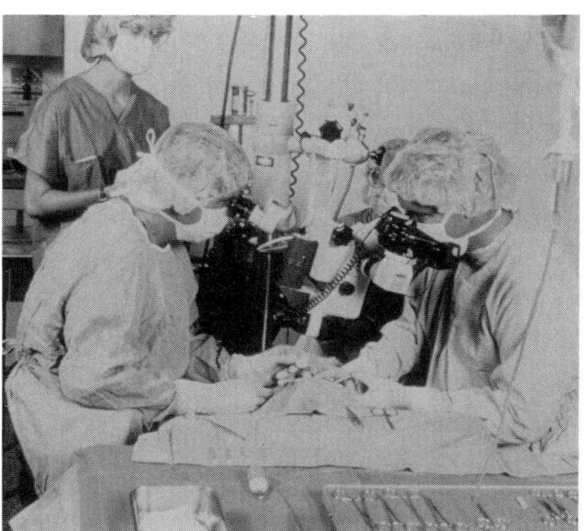

Fig. 3–11. Zeiss opmi 6 operating microscope with urban quadrascope adaptation allowing face-to-face seating of surgeon and assistant. (Carl Zeiss Inc., 444 5th Avenue, NY, NY 10018)

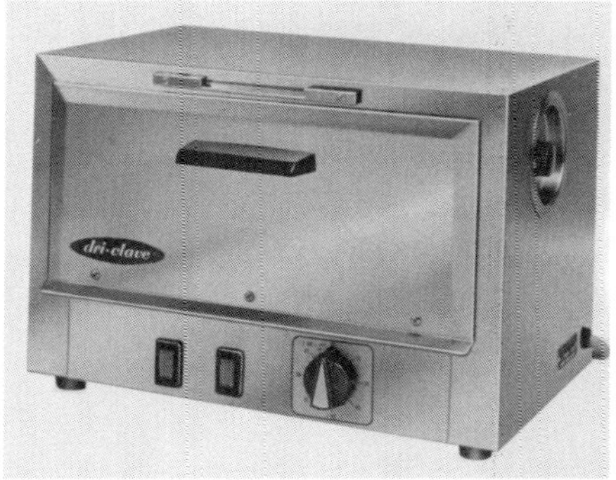

Fig. 3–12. Dry heat sterilizer. (Dri-Clave (Model 75), 54 Kinkel St., Westbury, L.I., N.Y. 11590)

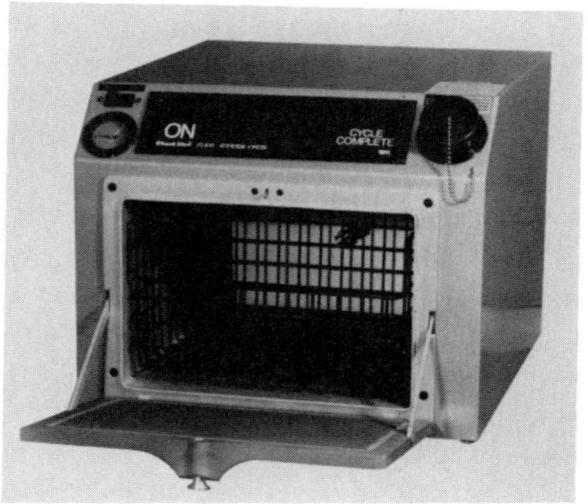

Fig. 3–13. Gas sterilizer. (3M (Model 100 Steri-vac), 3M Co., Saint Paul, Minn. 55101)

Beaver blades #64 and 65 and handles* (Fig. 3–16). Finally, suitable magnification (Fig. 2–3) must be used by the surgeon. It is impossible to work within millimeters without this aid.

3:107 In addition to the instruments required for a specific operation a pack usually also includes:

- cotton applicators
- irrigation jar and bulbs
- eye pad
- a piece of bed sheet or similar cloth 8 to 10 inches square, to be cut as an eye drape at the time of surgery, if a regular surgical drape with a large hole is being used
- rubber dam

*Beaver, 480 Trapelo Rd., Belmont, Mass, 02179.

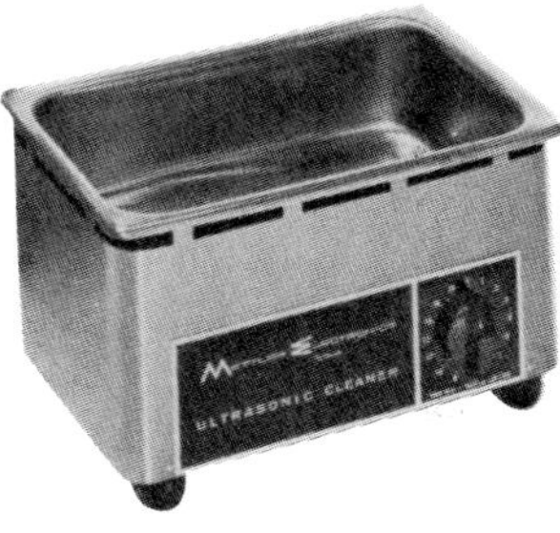

Fig. 3–14. Ultrasonic instrument cleaner. (Mettler 2.1 qt.)

3:108 6–0 to 8–0 silk, nylon or mersilene† have been commonly used for closure in intraocular procedures. These sutures are available with fine atraumatic needle attachments. In recent years synthetic absorbable sutures, *i.e.* collagen and polyglycolic acid (Dexon‡), have become available. They have good tensile strength, an adequate but not prolonged absorption time, and a relative freedom from side effects. Each material has certain favorable characteristics and most often perform adequately. Since a totally satisfactory suture material has yet to be found, the choice remains with the individual surgeon.

Anesthesia

3:109 Ordinarily, general anesthesia is preferred in most extraocular procedures and when performing any intraocular operation. The type of general anesthesia used depends, of course, on the procedure and the individual preference of the surgeon.

3:110 It is generally agreed that a soft eye is essential for uncomplicated intraocular surgery. When the intraocular pressure is desirably low, the anterior chamber may be opened without a sudden marked change in the ocular dynamics. If the eye of the dog is firm and at or near its average normal pressure of between 15 and 25 mm Hg, the opening of the anterior chamber produces a forward shift of the iris-lens diaphragm. In glaucoma or cataract surgery the hyaloid face may rupture with resulting vitreous complications.

3:111 There are three ways of lowering intraocular pressure: medical, mechanical, and surgical. The medical method employs systemic drugs such as urea, mannitol, glycerine, carbonic anhydrase inhibitors and tranquilizers. The osmotic agents (mannitol and glycerine) have the added advantage of dehydrating the vitreous, thus reducing vitreous volume and further reducing the tendency for the iris and lens diaphragm to come

†Ethicon (Code R-51), Somerville, N.J.

‡Davis and Geck. (American Cyanamid, Pearl River, N.Y. 10965).

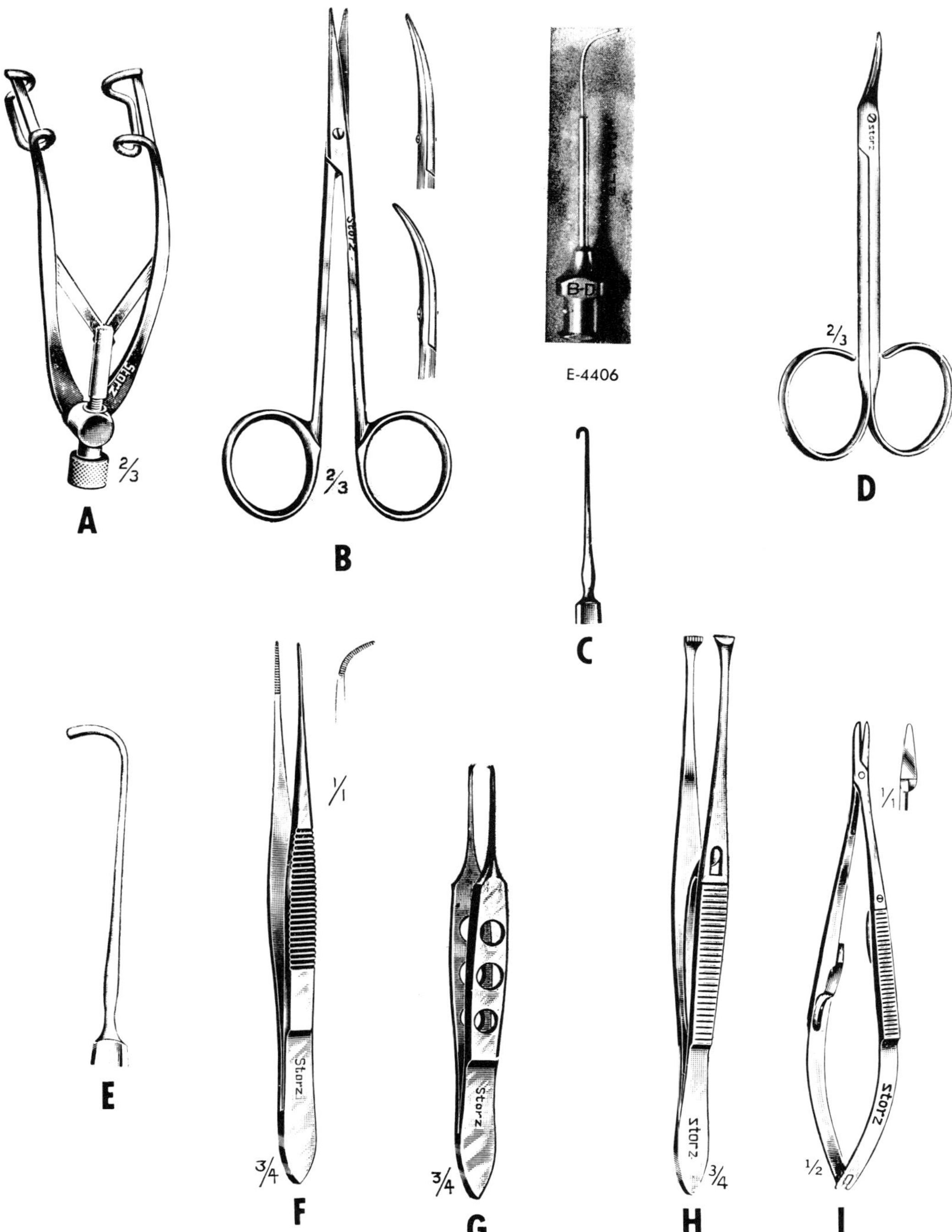

Fig. 3–15. Basic set of instruments. *A*. Castroviejo speculum. *B*. Strabismus scissors. *C*. Lacrimal cannula, curved. *C'*. Blunt iris hook. *D*. McGuire corneal scissors. *E*. Strabismus hook, medium. *F*. Dressing forceps. *G*. Tissue forceps (1 and 2 teeth). *H*. Fixation forceps with catch. *I*. Castroviejo needle holder.

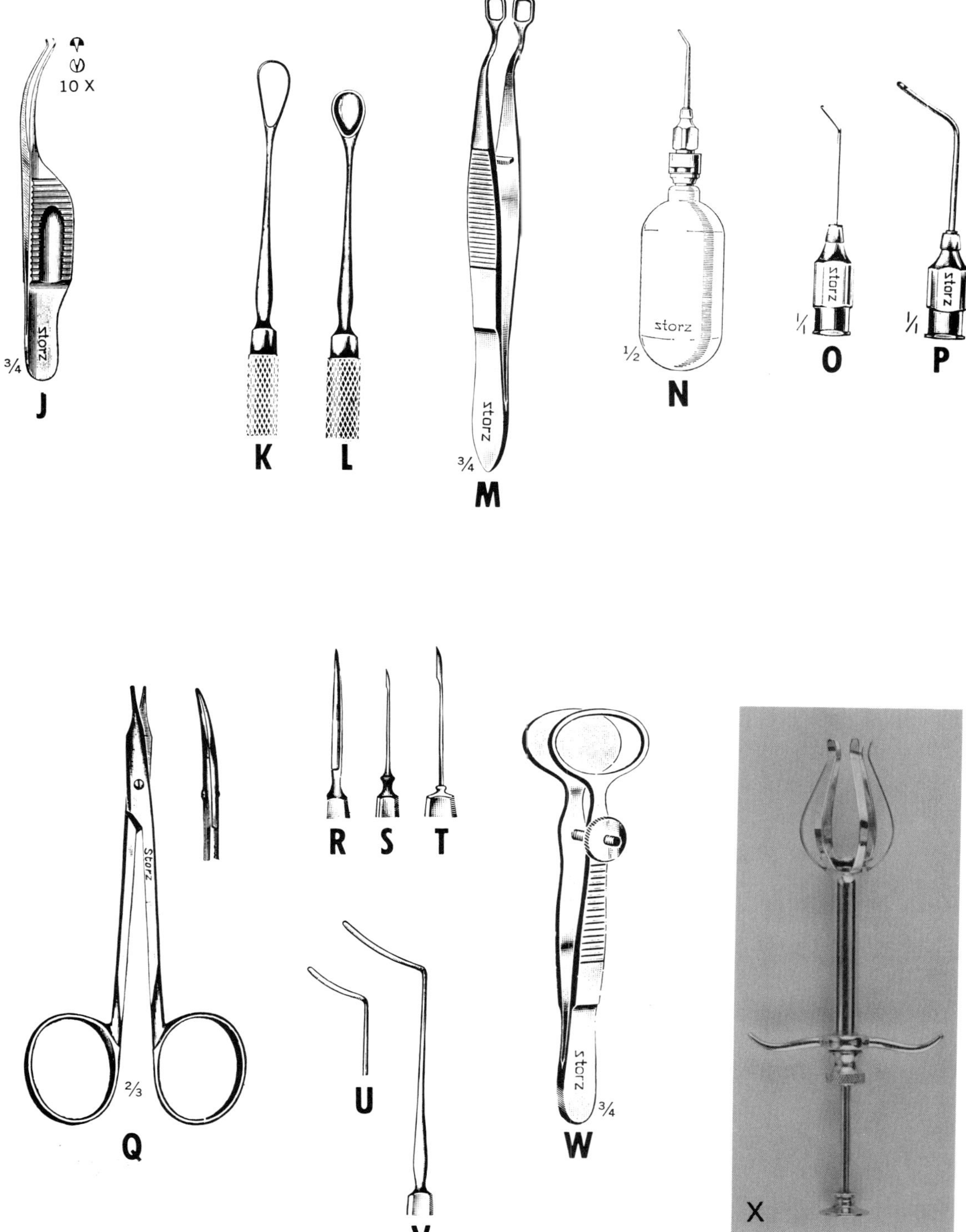

Fig. 3–15 *Continued.* *J*. Colibri type forceps. *K*. Lens loop. *L*. Lens spoon. *M*. McGannon lens forceps. *N*. Silicone irrigating bulb. *O*. Air injection cannula (27 ga). *P*. Irrigating canrula. *Q*. Tenotomy scissors. *R*. Castroviejo discission knife. *S*. Ziegler knife needle (3 mm). *T*. Ziegler knife needle (5 mm). *U*. Cyclodialysis spatula (10 mm). *V*. Cyclodialysis spatula (15 mm). *W*. Desmarres chalazion forceps. *X*. Sphere introducer.

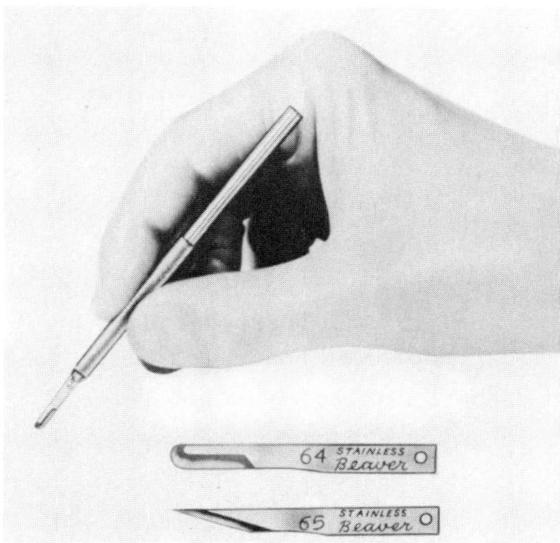

Fig. 3–16. Beaver mini-blades and handle.

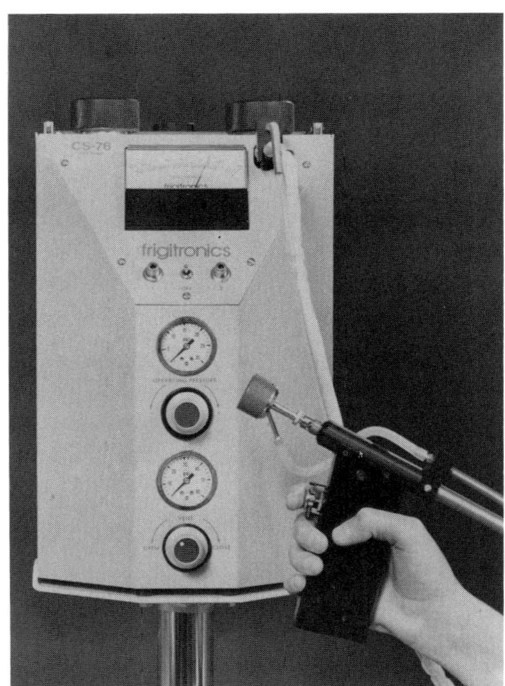

Fig. 3–17. Frigitronics CS-76 liquid nitrogen unit with attached nozzle for a defined spray. Cold probes can also be attached. (Frigitronics of Connecticut, Inc., 770 River Road, Shelton, CT 06484)

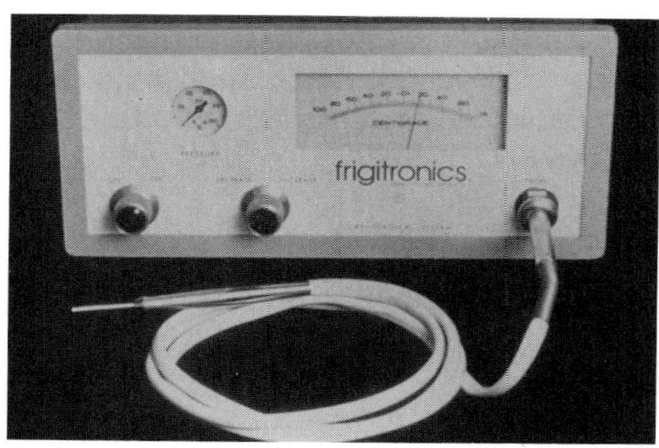

Fig. 3–18. Frigitronics N_2O Cryosurgical System with attached 3.5 mm glaucoma probe. (Frigitronics of Connecticut, Inc., 770 River Road, Shelton, CT 06484)

forward when the eye is opened. Mannitol (20% solution) at 3 to 5 ml/pound IV, just prior to opening the eye, or glycerine at 1 ml/pound orally, 30 minutes to 1 hour prior to anesthesia are most commonly used osmotic agents. (I prefer mannitol.) The mechanical method consists of exerting pressure on the globe for 5 minutes or more preoperatively. This procedure, however, often fails to reduce the ocular tension and is not without danger in some instances. A preliminary surgical procedure, *i.e.* posterior sclerotomy, has been used successfully in man but its use cannot be considered routine.

3:112 The use of Methoxyflurane (Metofane)* anesthesia has been helpful in lowering

*Metofane. Pitman-Moore Co., Box 1656, Indianapolis, Ind. 46206.

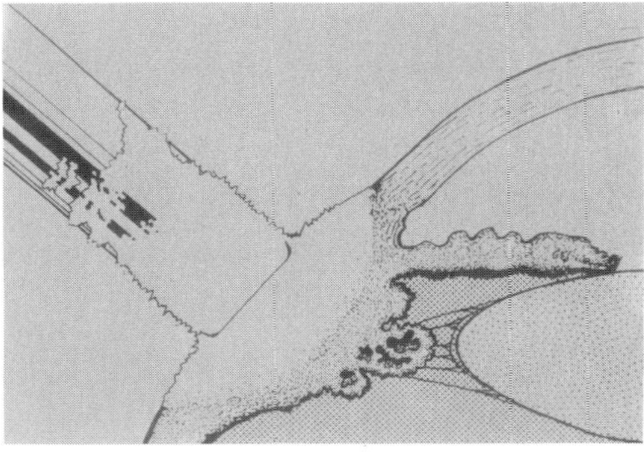

Fig. 3–19. The glaucoma probe applied to the conjunctiva about 6 mm back of the limbus freezes the ciliary body, including the ciliary epithelium.

the intraocular pressure and producing a relatively soft eye for intraocular surgery in the dog. Halothane (fluothane) anesthesia will achieve the same purpose, but I prefer Metofane because of a prolonged, smoother recovery and the relative freedom of cardiac side effects when epinephrine is used within the eye. As a further means of reducing intraocular tension, mannitol is used routinely (Par. 3:78).

3:113 Peripheral (palpebral) nerve blocks, though commonly used in man and in large animals, are seldom used in small animal practice because of the relative ease and safety of general anesthesia. The akinesia produced has been useful as an aid in diagnosis where blepharospasms make examination difficult, as an adjunct to general anesthesia, and as a temporary therapeutic measure (spastic entropion).[5]

REFERENCES

1. Beams, R. et al.: Effect of Topical Corticosteroids on Corneal Wound Strength, A.J.O., *66*:1131–1133, 1968.
2. Brightman, A.H.: Ocular Therapeutics in *Atlas of Veterinary Ophthalmology*, C. Peruccio, Editor, C.G. Edizioni Medico Scientifiche, Torino, Italy, Text in Italian, 43–57, 1985.
3. Brightman, A.H., Helper, L.C., Hoffman, W.E.: Effect of Aspirin on Aqueous Protein Values in the Dog, JAVMA, *178*:572–573, 1981.
4. Brightman, A.H., Vestre, W.A., Helper, L.C., Tomes, J.E.: Cryosurgery for the Treatment of Canine Glaucoma, JAAHA, *18*:319–322, 1982.
5. Bryan, G.M.: *Palpebral Nerve Blocks in Small Animals*, Proc. Am. Coll. Vet. Ophth., 1974.
6. Cole, D.F., Unger, W.G.: Prostaglandins as Mediators for the Responses of the Eye to Trauma, Exp. Eye Res., *17*:357–368, 1973.
7. Furgivele, F.P.: Penetration of Gentamicin into the Aqueous Humor of Human Eyes, Am. J. Ophth., *69*:481, 1970.
8. Havener, W.H.: *Ocular Pharmacology*, 3rd Ed. St. Louis, The C.V. Mosby Co., 1974.
9. Jones Barri, R.: Principles in the Management of Oculomycosis, Trans. Am. Acad. Ophthalmol. Otolaryngol., *79*:15–51, 1975.
10. Linn, M.L., Jones, L.T.: Rate of Lacrimal Excretion of Ophthalmic Vehicles, A.J.O., *65*:76–78, 1968.
11. Magrane, W.G.: Beta-Ray and X-ray Therapy in Diseases of the Eye, No. Am. Vet., *36*:295, 1955.
12. Magrane, W.G.: Cortisone in Ophthalmology, No. Am. Vet., *32*:763, 1951.
13. Magrane, W.G.: Investigational Use of Ophthaine as a Local Anesthetic in Ophthalmology, No. Am. Vet., *34*:568, 1953.
14. Magrane, W.G.: Ocular Physiology—Clinical Application, No. Am. Vet., *36*:389, 1955.
15. Magrane, W.G.: The Clinical Use of Chloromycetin in Canine Ocular Infections, No. Am. Vet., *34*:39, 1953.
16. Magrane, W.G.: The Use of Corticoids in Ophthalmology, Abstracts of First Veterinary Symposium on the Use of Meticorten and Meticortelone, Schering Corp., Bloomfield, New Jersey, 1956.
17. Magrane, W.G.: X-ray Therapy in Interstitial and Pigmentary Keratitis, No. Am. Vet., *29*:582, 1948.
18. Michaelson, S.: The Use of Beta Irradiation in Veterinary Ophthalmology, Vet Med., *49*:475, 1954.
19. Rubin, L.F. and Wolfes, R.L.: Mydriatics for Canine Ophthalmoscopy, J.A.V.M.A., *140*:137, 1962.
20. Schmidt, G., Vainisi, S., West, C., and Wolf, E.: Retrospective Survey of Cyclocryotherapy for the Control of Canine Glaucoma, Trans. ACVO, 55–61, 1983.
21. Severin, G.A.: *Veterinary Ophthalmology Notes*, 2nd Ed., Ft. Collins, Colorado State University Publication Service, 1976.
22. Wald, G.: The Photoreceptor Process in Vision, Am. J. Ophthal., *40*:36, 1955.

4

DISEASES AND SURGERY OF THE LIDS AND LACRIMAL APPARATUS

Anatomy and Physiology

4:1 The eyelids consist of movable folds of skin, loose connective tissue, muscular tissue, tarsus, and conjunctiva (Fig. 4–1). These dorsal and ventral folds form the *palpebral fissure*. The lids present protective eyelashes (cilia) at their margins, and contain numerous glands, blood vessels, lymphatics and nerves. They serve the purpose of excluding light from the eyes, sweep away foreign bodies reaching the cornea, spread lacrimal fluid and lubricant from their accessory glands over the cornea *(precorneal film)* and aid in the drainage of this fluid through the drainage channels by a pumping action. The upper eyelid is more movable than the lower.

4:2 The eyelids form a medial and lateral canthi. At the medial canthus is an island of skin known as the *caruncle*. Tactile hairs often originate from the area. Near this medial commissure (4 to 6 mm) are the two *puncta lacrimalia* (Fig. 4–2) through which the lacrimal fluid drains into the connecting *canaliculi*, then to the *lacrimal sac* and *nasolacrimal duct* (Fig. 4–3). This structure is known as the *excretory* portion of the lacrimal apparatus. The puncta are, in reality, slit-like openings set well back from the lid margins, in alignment with the most medial meibomian glands of the upper and lower lids, and turned in slightly toward the eye. The two openings are not always the same size and it is not uncommon for one or both to be absent (Par. 4:67). The lacrimal sac lies in the lacrimal fossa of the medial orbital wall. The sac is not as well developed in the dog as it is in man. From the sac area the fluid flows along the nasolacrimal duct within the nasolacrimal canal to the nasal punctum located 1 to 2 mm caudal to the opening of the external nares.

4:3 The secretory portion of the lacrimal apparatus that produces the watery portion of

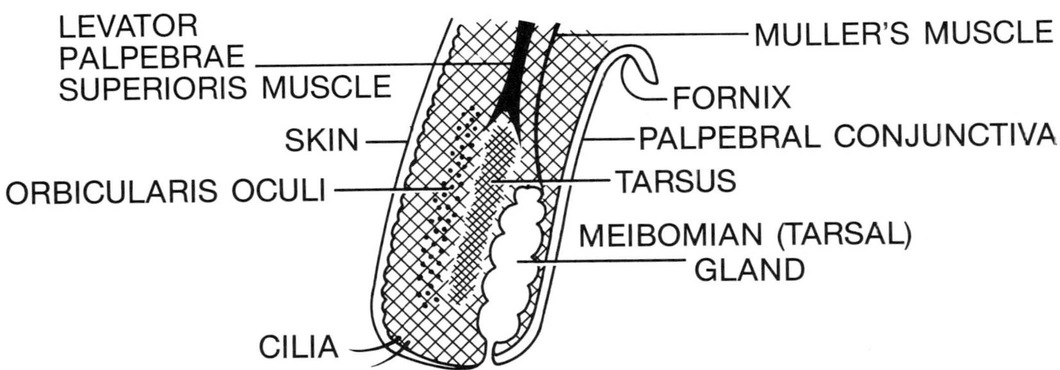

Fig. 4–1. Longitudinal section of the upper lid.

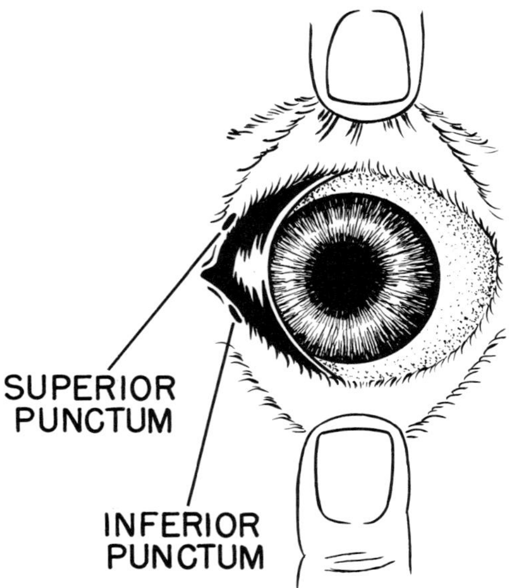

Fig. 4–2. The puncta lacrimalia.

the tear film and the 'tears' stimulated by eye irritation, includes the lacrimal gland and accessory glands. The lacrimal gland is located on the dorso-lateral aspect of the orbital cone behind the orbital septum (Par. 8:10) (Figs. 1–10 and 4–3). Excretory ducts empty into the conjunctival sac through openings in the upper fornix. The accessory glands of Krause and Wolfring, said to provide the base level of tear production in man, are evidently of little importance in the dog. The gland of the third eyelid is the other major source of tear production in the dog. Removal of either the lacrimal glands or the gland of the third eyelid reduces tear production, as measured by the Schirmer tear test, while removal of both glands eliminates the watery portion of the tear film.[16,18] The watery portion, in conjunction with the mucus produced by the goblet cells of the conjunctiva and the oil produced by the meibomian glands, comprises the precorneal film, so important to maintaining a normal cornea and conjunctiva (Par. 6:2). Tears are high in protein, have a low surface tension which enables them to wet the epithelial surfaces thoroughly, and are, in themselves, bactericidal.[21] The pH of lacrimal fluid ranges from 6.80 to 8.03 with an average of 7.56. There is a difference in the pH value among breeds, although the pH of tears in dogs with acute and chronic inflammations do not differ appreciably from the normal.[8]

4:4 The underlying structures of the eyelids include the well-developed *orbicularis muscle* (Fig. 1–9) which is found almost to the edge of each eyelid, and always nearest the anterior surface, thickening at the base of the eyelid.

4:5 Posterior to the orbicularis muscle is a layer of dense connective tissue called the *tarsus*. The tarsal plate serves to give the edge of the eyelid rigidity but is not as well developed in the dog as it is in man.

4:6 Dorsal to the tarsus is the levator palpebrae superioris muscle (Fig. 1–10). It is enervated by the oculomotor nerve, and acts to raise the upper lid. The enervation is closely associated with the enervation of the superior rectus muscle, so that when the eyeball is rotated upward, the lid is opened further. Deep to the levator is Muller's muscle (Fig. 4–1) which is enervated by sympathetics. Paralysis of this muscle in Horner's syndrome is responsible for the ptosis observed (Par. 12:24). In close apposition to the tarsus is a series of glands (tarsal or meibomian).

4:7 The *meibomian glands*[26] are plainly visible through the conjunctiva as pale parallel lines running vertically from the lid margins to the edge of the tarsal plate. Their outlets can be seen as tiny apertures along the lid margins. The oily secretion of the meibomian gland provides a monolayer of oil on the surface of the precorneal film and may provide surface tension along the lid margin to inhibit overflow of tears along the lid.

4:8 Finally, the inner surface of the eyelid is covered by mucous membrane, the *palpebral* conjunctiva.

Congenital Anomalies

4:9 A physiologic ankyloblepharon, with lid separation taking place 10 to 14 days following birth, is normal for the canine. A pathologic ankyloblepharon, with abnormal persistence

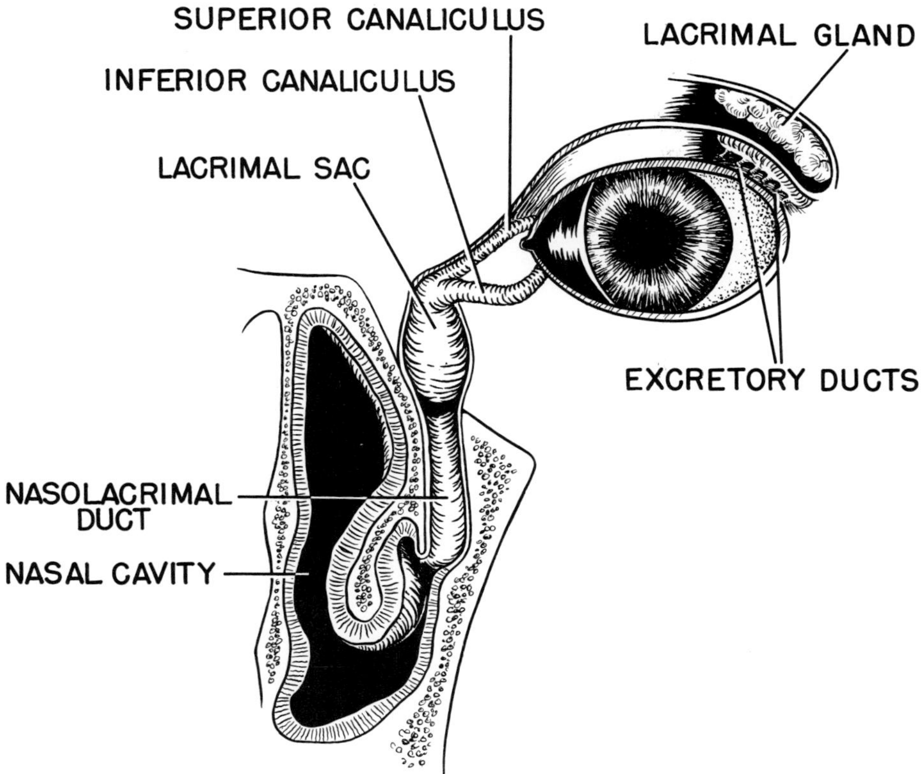

Fig. 4–3. The lacrimal production and drainage system.

of the upper and lower lid fusion, only occurs occasionally. *Coloboma* of the lid is a notching of the margin with an absence of the lashes and glands in the affected area. It is rarely encountered and can be treated, if necessary, by plastic methods. *Dermoid cyst,* a congenital tumor, occupies space at what would normally be the lateral canthus aspect of the lid commissure. This condition is more fully discussed in Paragraph 4:96.

4:10 *Narrow Palpebral Fissure* (blepharophimosis). This anomaly is not uncommon in terriers, *e.g.* Kerry blue terriers, and chows, and is often responsible for the development of a subsequent entropion. Enlargement of the palpebral fissure by *canthotomy* and *canthoplasty* will often suffice to correct the entropion without an additional entropion procedure.

4:11 Canthotomy is the temporary enlargement of the palpebral fissure by severing the lateral canthus and is used as a preliminary measure to other surgical procedures. A narrow palpebral fissure may be enlarged prior to or during intraocular or orbital operations.[2]

4:12 The technique is simple and consists of stretching the lateral canthus between the thumb and forefinger and cutting the canthus for the desired distance with heavy blunt-pointed scissors (Fig. 4–4). Hemorrhage attending the procedure can be minimized by first injecting a few minims of 1 to 5,000 epinephrine at the canthus or by crushing the canthus for 30 seconds or so with a hemostatic forceps. The latter is preferable especially if the dog is anesthetized with halothane since epinephrine may cause cardiac arrhythmias.

4:13 A canthotomy is commonly closed with 1 to 3 non-absorbable sutures. If dehiscence occurs due to the dog rubbing its face, the

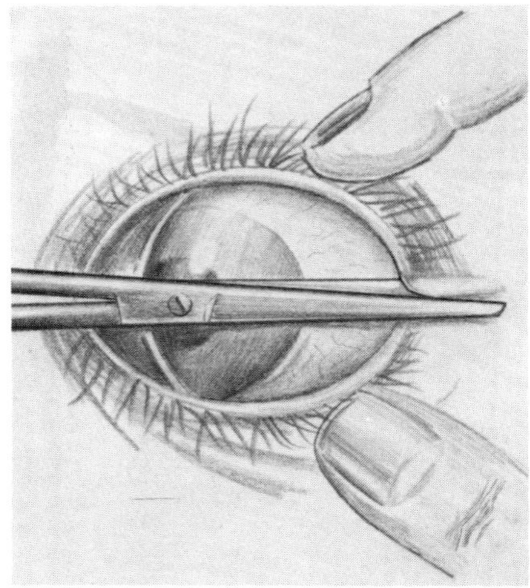

Fig. 4–4. Canthotomy.

canthotomy will close adequately without resuturing. Closing the conjunctiva first with 5 Ō or 6 Ō absorbable suture and the skin with 4 Ō non-absorbable or even absorbable suture is a preferred method of closure.

4:14 Canthoplasty results in a permanent lengthening of the palpebral fissure. If a permanent lengthening is desired, perform the canthotomy as shown in Figure 4–4, making the incision just a little longer than the desired lengthening; then suture the underlying conjunctiva to the upper and lower cut surfaces of the skin with 5 Ō or 6 Ō absorbable sutures, using an interrupted suture pattern.

4:15 *Large Palpebral Fissure.* Too large an opening may enclose a normal eye, *e.g.* in English bulldogs, spaniels, hounds, resulting in an ectropic condition. An owner seldom requests corrective measures. If, however, the anomaly poses a serious problem, the fissure is easily made smaller by removing the required portions of the upper and lower lid margins. The conjunctiva is then brought together with 6–0 chromic catgut. Apposition of the skin to form the new canthus completes the procedure (Figs. 4–7, 4–8).

Congenital or Acquired Conditions

Entropion (Plate 2A)

4:16 *Entropion* is simply defined as an inrolling of the lid (and with it the lashes). *Etiology.* It may be an acquired condition as a result of cicatricial contraction following injuries or be caused by blepharospasm associated with painful eye disease (spastic entropion). In the dog, it most often is seen as a congenital anomaly in the Chow, Shar-pei, English bulldog, St. Bernard, and the hunting breeds. Usually only the lower lid is involved, but occasionally, especially in the Shar-pei or chow, it becomes necessary to correct both upper and lower lids by one of several means.

4:17 *Symptoms.* Entropion results in superficial irritation of the bulbar conjunctiva and cornea producing a chronic discharge, vascularization and possible ulceration of the cornea. Neglect and/or rubbing by the animal can lead to erosion of the corneal stroma, prolapse of the iris and loss of an eye. Pain indicated by frequent blinking and blepharospasm, characterizes the subjective symptom.

4:18 *Treatment: Medical.* A mild acquired spastic entropion associated with a disease process may respond to treatment of the underlying disease. Mineral oil injections into the lid have been used in attempts to correct entropion. This procedure is not to be recommended because of the likelihood of producing foreign body granuloma at the site of the injection.[31]

4:19 *Surgery.* Many operative procedures with multiple variations have been advocated for the correction of entropion. The following embrace the principles of correction and are those with which the author is most familiar.

4:20 *Skin Excision.* Excision of an elliptical portion of the lid including a horizontal strip of the underlying orbicularis muscle (Fig. 1–9) still remains the most commonly performed and successful procedure. Predetermination of the correct amount of skin to be removed is accomplished by grasping a fold with straight hemostatic forceps, clamping tightly for 20 to 30 seconds, thereby producing a ridge of skin when the forceps is released (Fig. 4–5A). If the lid margin is still not in

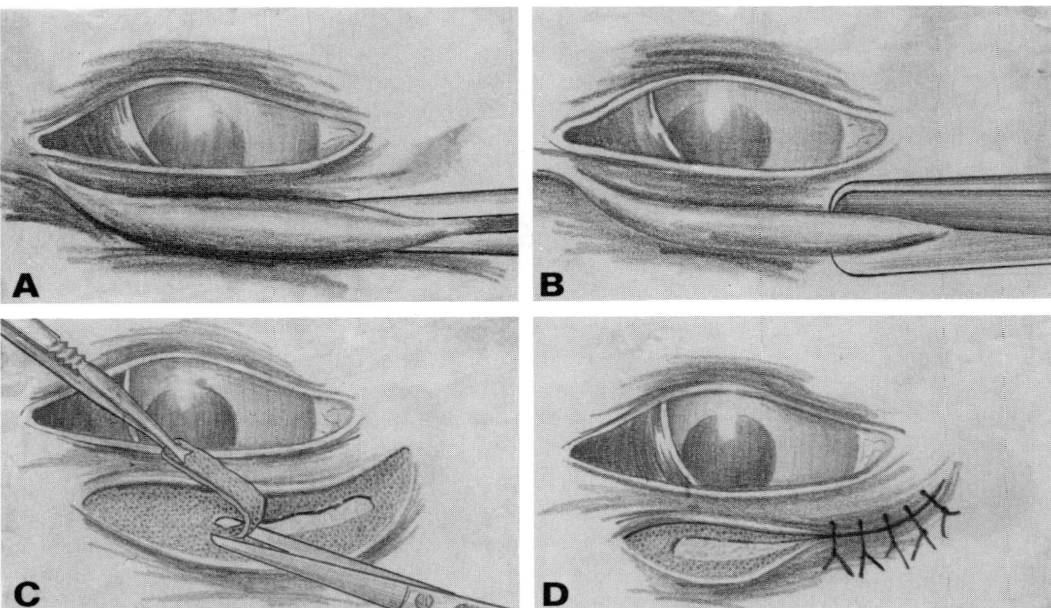

Fig. 4–5. Surgical correction of entropion. *A*. Ridge of skin is raised by clamping with hemostatic forceps. *B*. The ridge of skin is cut at its base with heavy scissors. *C*. Removing a strip of orbicularis muscle. *D*. Sutures being placed.

proper proximity to the globe, the fold can be smoothed out with the thumb and a bigger or lesser "bite" taken. When it appears that the amount of skin is adequate the ridge is cut at its base with heavy scissors (Fig. 4–5B). This produces a half moon or elliptical area. Then, commencing at one end of the wound the orbicularis is elevated with eye tissue forceps and a strip of muscle removed for the length of the incision (Fig. 4–5C). This step is attended by hemorrhage which is quickly controlled by the placing of interrupted sutures through the skin (Fig. 4–5D). I prefer 4 Ō silk in an interrupted pattern, with the first suture placed in the center of the wound to provide initial apposition of the skin edges, and then place additional sutures to provide adequate closure. Any non-absorbable suture could be used; however, silk is soft and will not cause corneal abrasion if a suture end gets misdirected. Removal of the strip of orbicularis muscle seems to be optional, as some surgeons who have deleted this step suggest similarly good results. Making the initial skin ridge and incision as close to the lid margin as possible allows the most eversion with the least skin removal and the best cosmetic result. A plastic collar (Fig. 4–6A) or plastic pail (Fig. 4–6B) affords the best protection against self-injury following any of the lid procedures. Sutures may be removed in 8 to 10 days.

4:21 *Canthoplasty* (Par. 4:14) alone or in combination with skin excision is usually the operation of choice in those instances where the entropion results from a narrow palpebral fissure.

4:22 The lateral canthoplasty technique (Fig. 4–10) described by Wyman[35] is indicated when there is entropion at the lateral canthus, usually involving both upper and lower lids, with an accompanying tendency toward ectropion more medially (Par. 4:29).

4:23 Congenital entropion is so severe in some puppies of some breeds, especially the Shar-pei, that correction is needed soon after the eyes open. "Lid tacking" is the procedure

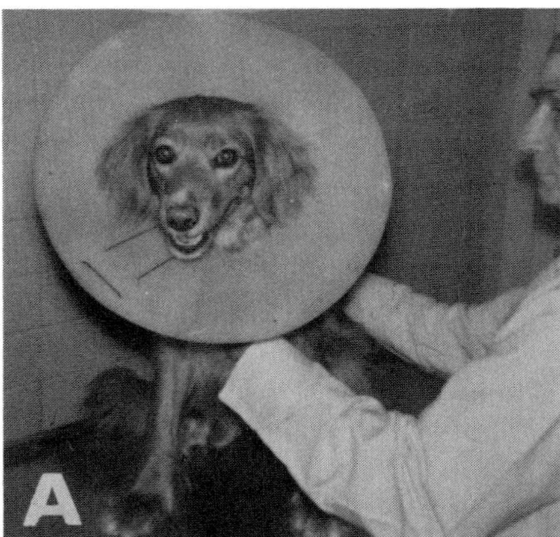

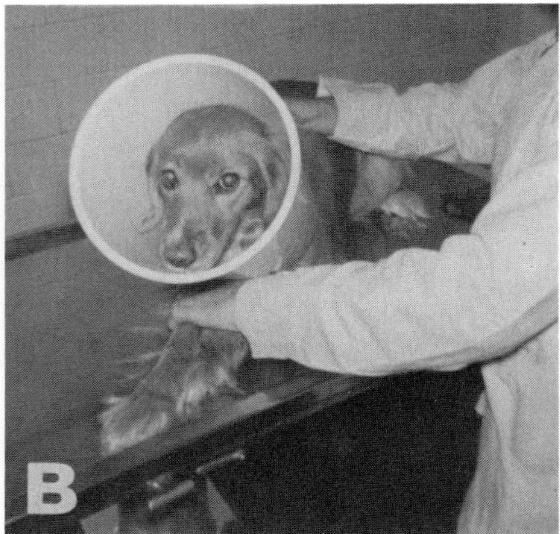

Fig. 4–6. *A.* Flexible plastic collar in place. *B.* Plastic pail in place.

of choice. Four Ō monofilament nylon suture with attached curved cutting edge needle is used to place 2 or 3 sutures along each upper and lower lid to roll the lids out to normal position. The needle is inserted through the skin, parallel to the lid margin along the edge of the tarsal plate, and then through the skin, parallel to the first insert, 1 to 2 cm away from the eye. Each suture is tied just tight enough to roll the lid out away from the cornea. Application of topical anesthetic in the eye, several times prior to surgery, will help relieve blepharospasm and aid in finding the lid margins. The procedure is done without sedation or general anesthesia, and does not seem to cause much pain, if an atraumatic cutting edge needle is used. The owner is advised to clean any discharge from the eyes or along the sutures, and to apply an antibiotic ointment without steroids, twice a day. The sutures are left in place for 3 to 4 weeks or until no longer needed. Some puppies will require surgical correction, but in some, the entropion no longer exists at 4 to 8 weeks of age. Since this appears to be a hereditary problem in the breed, owners should be strongly advised against breeding these dogs or repeating the breeding that produced the puppies.

Ectropion (Plate 2B)

4:24 This is simply an outrolling or eversion of the lid, just the opposite of entropion.

4:25 *Etiology.* The fault is most often congenital and hereditary in the cocker spaniel, St. Bernard, bloodhound and basset breeds. The acquired forms result from cicatricial contraction following accidents, overcorrection of entropion or prolonged blepharitis. A senile form results from relaxing of tissue and lack of tone. Eyelid paralysis, due to damage to the palpebral or auriculopalpebral nerve, or complete facial paralysis, results in ectropion most often, with an associated lagophthalmos. Exposure keratitis occurs in some of these dogs; however, dogs other than the exophthalmic breeds, can retract the eyeball, periodically, and cause the third eyelid to distribute the precorneal film and prevent corneal disease.

4:26 *Symptoms.* Exposure of conjunctival surface and eversion of the punctum thus causing epiphora (escape of tears) and a reddened, hypertrophied surface. An exposure keratitis may result in the marked cases, especially if the third eyelid has been removed.

4:27 *Treatment.* Only cases in which the ectropion is responsible for signs of eye disease, persistent conjunctivitis, keratoconjunctivitis or epiphora, need to be treated. Some owners request treatment for cosmetic purposes. One should advise owners that cosmetic surgery, such as entropion or ectropion repair, disqualifies dogs from the show ring. Repair

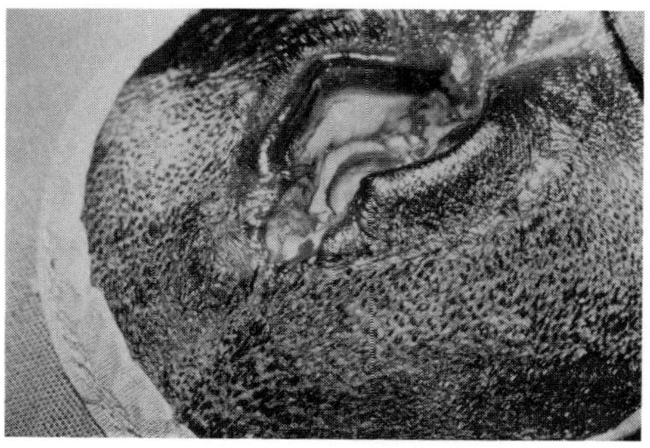

Fig. 4–7. A full thickness V-shaped piece of the lower lid is removed with scissors near the canthus. The incision may be free-hand or marked first by crushing with mosquito forceps.

procedures needed to control or prevent eye disease should, of course, be accomplished, but procedures strictly for cosmetic purposes should be discouraged, especially in dogs destined for the show ring.

4:28 Shortening of the lower lid is the most reliable technique for correction of the congenital ectropion. A full-thickness, V-shaped incision to remove the excess lower lid should be accomplished about 3 to 4 mm from the lateral canthus (Fig. 4–7). The conjunctiva is sutured with 6 Ō catgut (Fig. 4–8), and the skin with 4 Ō or 5 Ō silk. Cicatricial ectropion, caused by injury, can be corrected by excision of the lid scar, if it extends to the lid margin. If the scar is below the lid margin or the ectropion was caused by overcorrection of entropion, the V–Y technique (Wharton

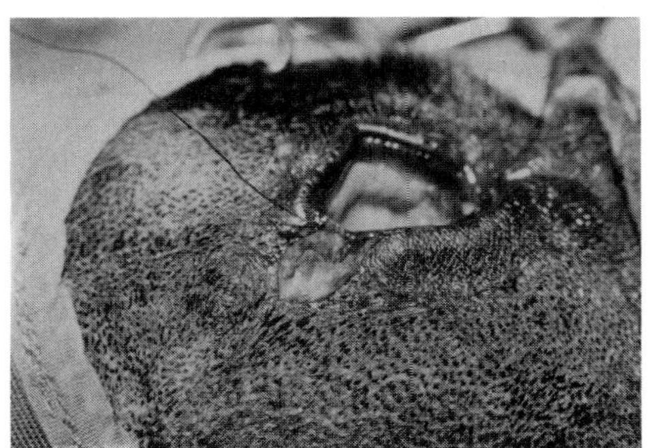

Fig. 4–8. The conjunctiva is first closed with continuous 6–0 catgut, followed by skin closure with 4–5–0 silk in an interrupted pattern.

Jones), with or without canthoplasty (Par. 4:14), is indicated. The V-shaped skin incision made from or near the lid margin should encompass the involved area of the ectropion and converge at the apex below it (Fig. 4–9). The triangle of skin is then undermined with tenotomy scissors in all directions (Fig. 4–9B). Any subcutaneous scar tissue must be excised. The base of the skin flap remains attached at the lid margin. Beginning at the apex or lowermost part of the V, transverse sutures of 5–0 Dermalon or silk are placed. Additional sutures on either side result in the Y closure, thus raising the lid border to its normal position (Fig. 4–9C).

Entropion-Ectropion (combined) (Plate 5A)

4:29 Lid anomalies also include a combination of entropion and ectropion within the structure of a single lid. Whereas the St. Bernard is the breed most commonly affected, surgical correction has been necessary in the English bulldog, Cocker spaniel, and several other of those breeds exhibiting a tendency towards both conditions. In most instances there is a lateral entropion associated with a central ectropion of either or both lids of both eyes. The term "roller coaster" lids is descriptive. The upper lid over the ectropic area resembles a "pagoda." A most serious keratoconjunctivitis leading to blindness can result from this lid anomaly.

4:30 It is thought that a poorly functional or absent lateral retractor anguli oculi muscle (Fig. 1–9) is responsible for the relaxation of the lid.[35] The lateral retractor muscle of the dog takes the place of the lateral canthal ligament of the human.[26] This muscle inserts in the orbicularis oculi muscle superiorly and inferiorly and originates on the anterior tip of the inferior orbital process of the temporal bone. To replace a poorly developed or absent lateral retractor muscle, bundles of orbicularis muscle can be utilized.[35] When anchored properly into the periosteum of the zygomatic arch, the lids are drawn into a more normal position.

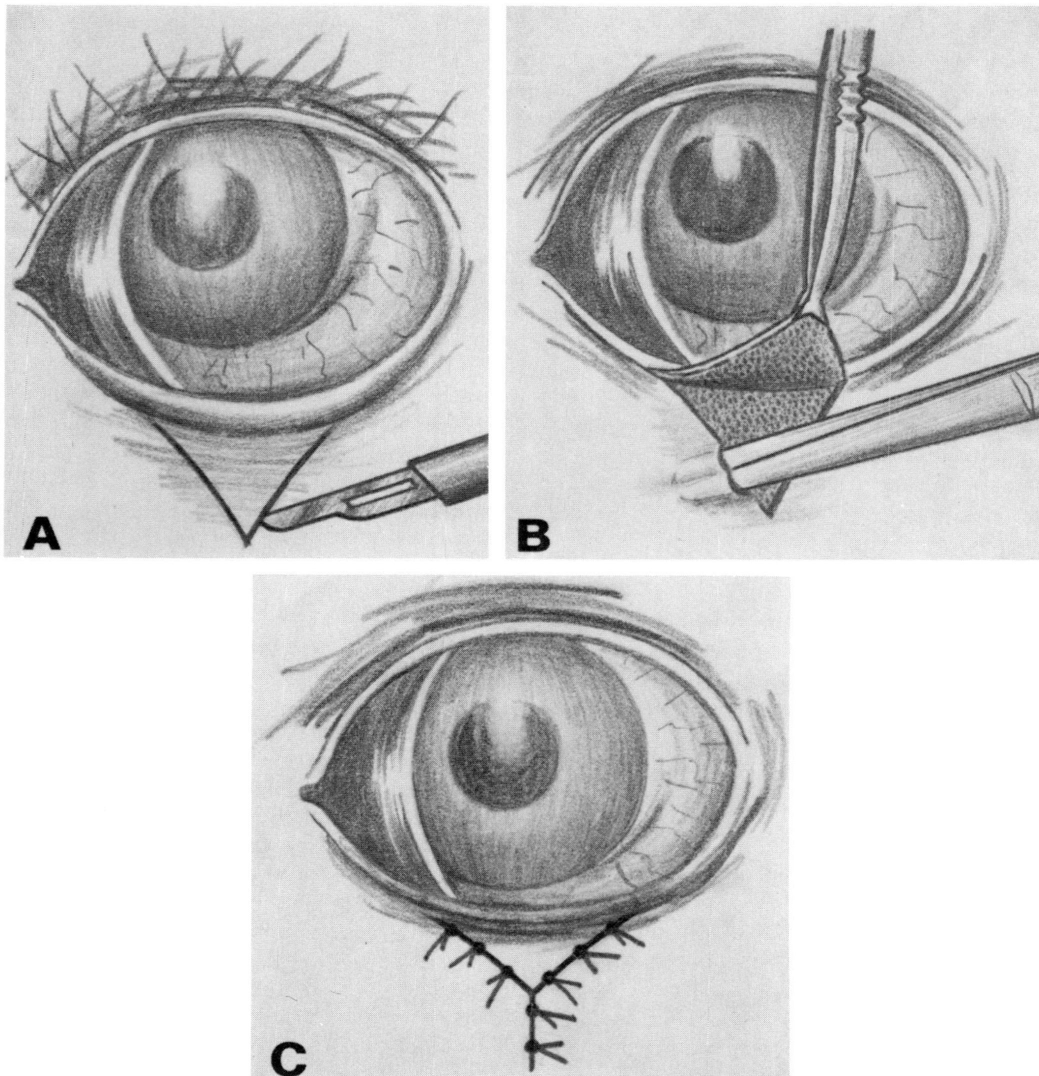

Fig. 4–9. Surgical correction of ectropion. *A*. V-shaped skin incision from lid margin. *B*. Undermining of skin. *C*. Resultant Y closure.

4:31 The operation: Wyman lateral cantho-plasty (modified)

1. A lateral fold of both upper and lower lid is prepared by grasping with a straight hemostatic forceps in the manner described for entropion (Par. 4:20). These folds are made to meet opposite the lateral canthus (Fig. 4–10A).

2. The folds are excised with heavy scissors, a "boomerang" incision resulting (Fig. 4–10B).

3. Commencing at apex (a) and (b), upper and lower strips (tongues) of orbicularis muscle are dissected with tenotomy scissors to terminate in a single bundle base (c) (Fig. 4–10C).

4. A skin incision is made from the base of the muscle bundle opposite the lateral canthus to an area over the temporal bone (Fig. 4–10D). Undermining on either side of the incision is helpful for the eventual placement of the muscle bundle.

5. The two tongues are brought together at the base with 4–0 double armed chromic gut. One needle traverses the base and is then turned and brought up through the length of the opposite tongue (Fig. 4–10E). The second needle is brought up through the length of the other tongue in the same manner (Fig. 4–10F).

6. One or both needles are then used to tack and suture the bundle to the periosteum over the zygomatic arch (Fig. 4–10G). To assure adequate tension, shortening of the muscle bundle may be necessary before the sutures are placed.

7. Skin closure completes the procedure (Fig. 4–10H). With the bundle buried and the overlying skin replaced, the lateral entropion and central ectropion are corrected. The palpebral fissure assumes a near normal appearance.

Distichiasis

4:32 In *distichiasis* a second, abnormal row of eyelashes is present. This row is usually incomplete, with one to a dozen or so lashes arising from the orifices of the meibomian glands. Usually only the upper lid is involved but both may well be (Fig. 4–11).

4:33 *Etiology.* Although considered primarily a congenital condition involving more commonly the Pekingese, Cocker Spaniel, Poodle and Bedlington terrier breeds, we have noted that these lashes may occur spontaneously at any age and in any breed. Distichia is often an incidental finding without any evidence of irritation or corneal involvement. These fine, soft cilia need not be removed.

4:34 *Symptoms.* When the lashes are bristle-like, considerable damage to the conjunctiva and cornea may result (Plate 2C). Epiphora is a most constant accompaniment. Distichiasis is not uncommon to the dog and is often missed because the examiner fails to use magnification in his examination of the orbital structures. Very fine cilia are most easily detected by inspecting the lid margin in profile.

4:35 *Treatment.* Unwanted lashes may be plucked from their orifice or cut flush with the lid margin but this provides only temporary relief. Permanent correction can be achieved by several means. (1) *Electro-epilation* (Fig. 4–12). This is applicable when only a few lashes are present. The Cameron-Miller unit is set on a reading of 1 on the coagulation side. With a special fine epilation needle (Fig. 3–3) the orifice alongside the lash is entered and the needle inserted to the base of the cilia. The current is turned on as soon as it becomes difficult to insert the needle farther toward the base. Often the cilia will then cling to and be extracted in the withdrawal of the needle. Otherwise, when it is felt that the root has been destroyed, the lash is easily removed with epilation or tissue forceps. The globe is protected by inserting a tape-padded tongue depressor between lid and cornea. Similarly, epilation by electrolysis utilizes a small milliamp direct current with a fine wire electrode which is inserted into the lash follicle (Fig. 4–13). Either method is tedious and exacting, demanding accurate placement of the electrode. This can

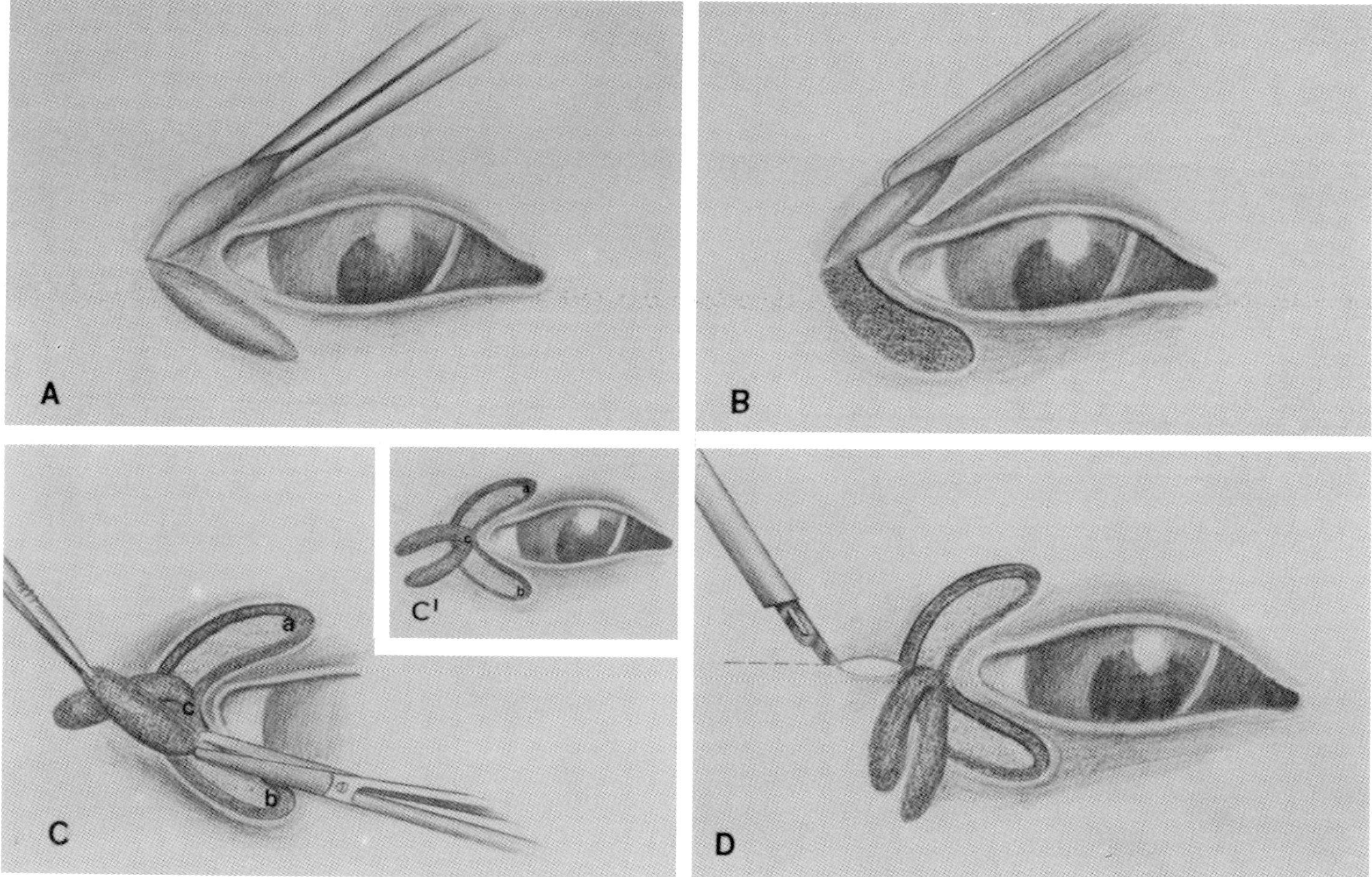

Fig. 4–10. Wyman lateral canthoplasty (modified) for correction of combined entropion-ectropion. *A.* Folds of upper and lower lids are made to meet opposite the lateral canthus. *B.* Excision of folds. *C.* Commencing at (a) and (b) tongues of orbicularis muscle are dissected to terminate in a single bundle base. Step completed (inset) (C'). *D.* Skin incision is made from the base of the muscle bundle to an area over the temporal bone.

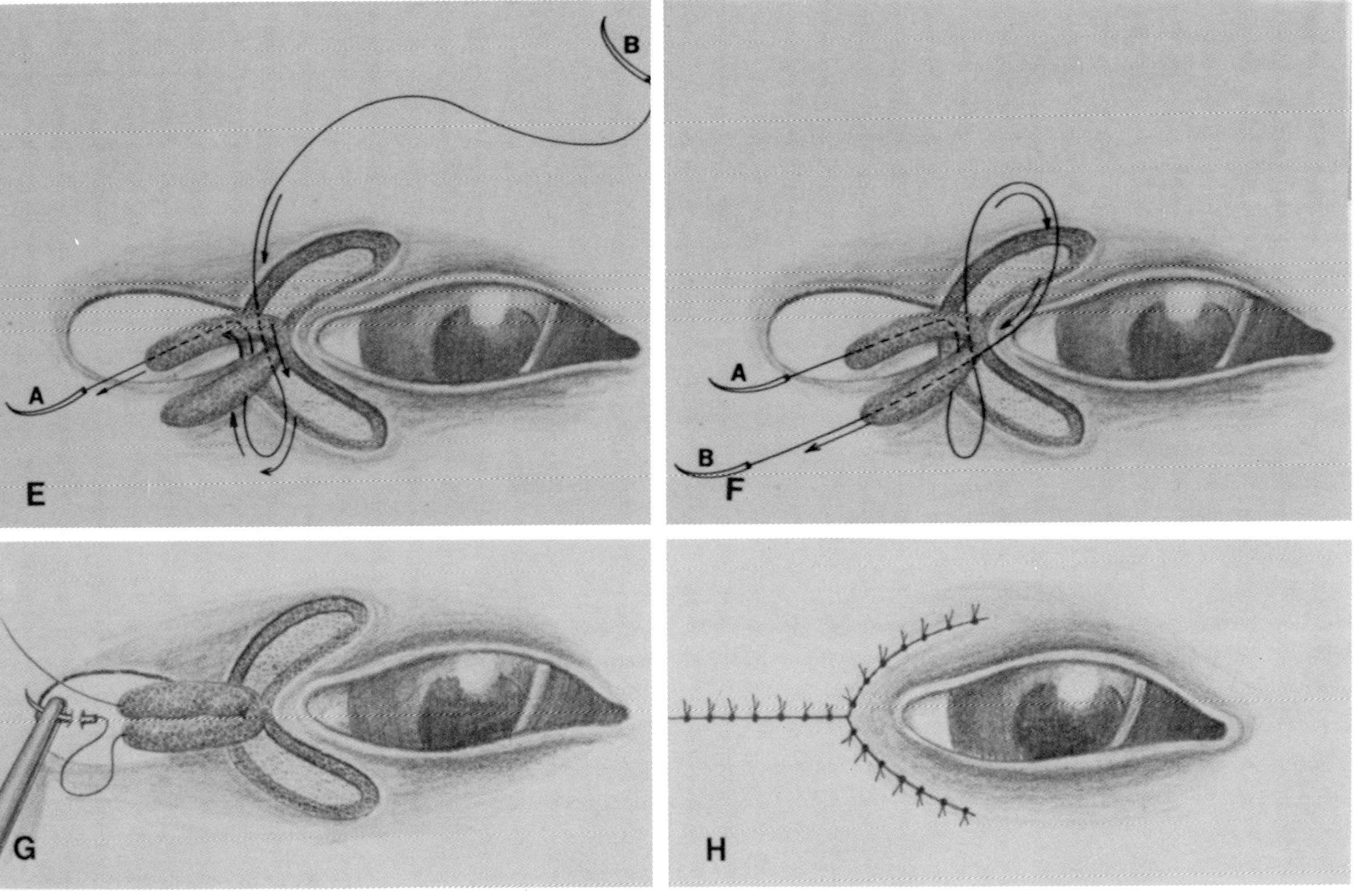

Fig. 4–10 *Continued.* *E*. Tongues are brought together at the base. One needle (A) traverses the base, is turned and brought up through the opposite tongue. *F*. The second needle (B) is brought up the length of the other tongue. *G*. The bundle is "tacked" to the periosteum over the zygomatic arch of the temporal bone. *H*. Skin closure.

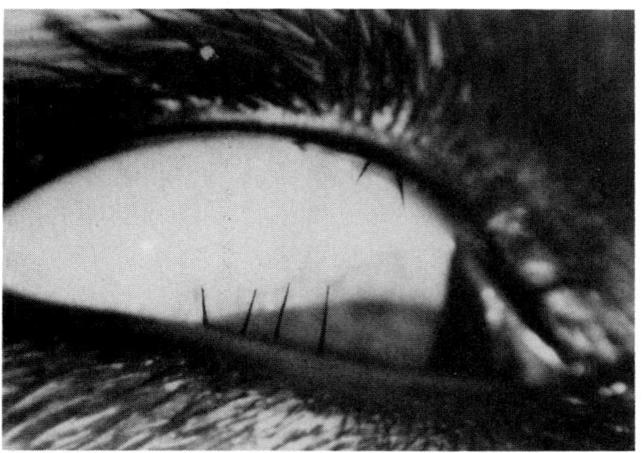

Fig. 4–11. Distichiasis involving both upper and lower lids.

only be accomplished with good magnification, preferably the use of the operating microscope. Growth of new eyelashes from other meibomian glands at a later time is not uncommon.

4:36 (2) *Lid Splitting.* The anatomy of the eyelid allows for it to be split into two lamina by an incision anterior to the tarsal plate. When the major portion of a lid contains aberrant lashes, resection of the cilia-bearing tarsoconjunctiva is preferred. Gelatt[10] describes a procedure that, with modification, has worked well. It is easily performed in breeds with relatively thick eyelids, such as the Cocker Spaniel or the St. Bernard; however, it is difficult in small breeds with thin eyelids, and may result in trichiases, caused by the loss of eyelid rigidity. I, therefore, have limited this procedure to thick eyelids. On thick eyelids, it is also possible to make a vertical incision on the conjunctival side of the meibomian gland, parallel to the first incision and to the same depth, and then remove the lash-bearing glands by cutting out the block of tissue with tenotomy scissors, leaving the conjunctival surface in place. No sutures are needed.

Technique: When the entire eyelid con-

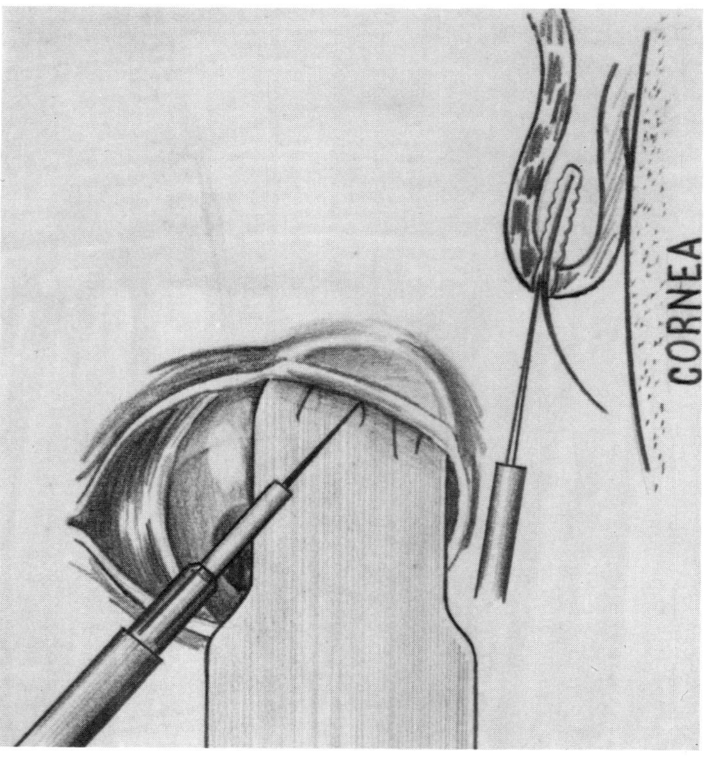

Fig. 4–12. Electro-epilation. Needle inserted to base of cilia. Eye protected by tongue depressor.

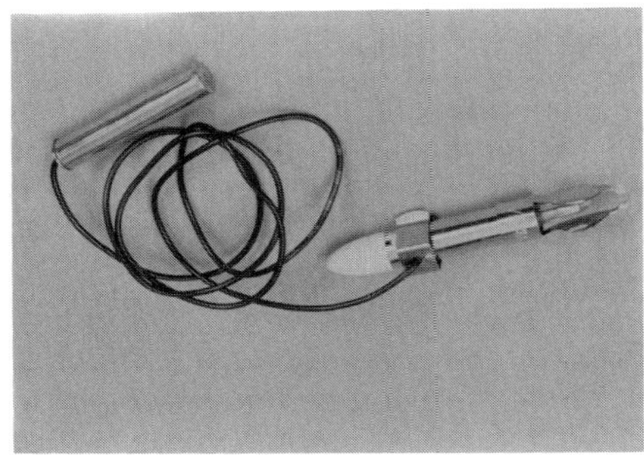

Fig. 4–13. Perma-Tweez instrument for epilation of distichia.

tains extra cilia the complete lid is split. Care must be exercised to locate and avoid the puncta and canaliculi so as not to interfere with lacrimal drainage. The eyelid is held by chalazion or entropion forceps (Fig. 3–15). This tends to minimize hemorrhage attending the incision. In addition, the immobilization and tautness achieved are helpful in acquiring accuracy. The lid is then split (anterior to the cilia) into two layers by incising to a depth of 3 to 5 mm between the skin-orbicularis oculi muscle and the tarsoconjunctiva (Fig. 4–14, *left*). A #64 Beaver blade (Fig. 3–16) is used for the splitting. When the proper incision length and depth have been reached the clamp is released. Eye tissue forceps (teeth) and tenotomy scissors are then used to cut the posterior "wedge" of cilia-bearing tarsoconjunctiva from the intact anterior aspect of the lid (Fig. 4–14, *right*). Topical epinephrine and compresses are used to control hemorrhage. No sutures or tarsoconjunctival flaps[13] are used. The posterior aspect of the lid heals very rapidly by granulation and without disfigurement.

4:37 A newer procedure that has provided good results in a limited number of cases is the electrosurgical procedure described by Riis.[27] After giving general anesthesia, the Cameron Miller or similar unit is used to make an incision through the conjunctival surface, at the base of the meibomian gland of the lid to destroy the lash-producing follicles (Fig. 4–15A–C). Good magnification to allow accurate placement of the incision is important. The Cameron Miller unit should be set at 2.5 to 3.5, and the conjunctival surface should be dry. A smooth even stroke with a fine electroscalpel blade should be accomplished to get an even depth and width of incision. The depth of the incision should be ½ the lid thickness. Following the lid incision, the distichia should lift out of the meibomian glands quite easily (Fig. 4–15D). It is important to make the incision at the base of the glands to destroy the hair follicle. If made on the hair shaft (Fig. 4–15E), a new hair or hairs may grow through the incision, producing a form of ectopic cilia. Aftercare consists of antibiotic and steroid ointment topically for 5 days. DMSO ointment or solution may be applied once after surgery to minimize swelling. Considerable lid distortion with notching in one area occurred in one small dog with thin eyelids, probably because we cut too deeply or did not have the conjunctival surface dry. This implies the care that must be used if this technique is employed.

4:38 I have not used cryosurgery for treating distichiasis; however, Wheeler and Severin[34] report satisfactory results. Their procedure is as follows. Pretreatment: acepromazine maleate, .05 mg/kg, SQ; atropine, .05 mg/kg, SQ; flunixin meglumine, 1.1 mg/kg, IV, 20 minutes prior to treatment. Local anesthesia is used if only a few lashes are to be treated; otherwise, general anesthesia. The lid is everted with a chalazion forceps, so that the meibomian glands are visible within the loop of the forceps. A Kryomed nitrous oxide unit, set at 625 mm Hg probe-line pressure is used. The 2 mm attached glaucoma probe is applied to the conjunctival surface over the meibomian gland for 45 seconds for the first freeze; the area allowed to thaw; and a 20-second application is used for a second freeze. If a row of distichia are to be treated, two to three areas are frozen in sequence, and then refrozen in a similar order. Aftercare consists of topical antibiotic steroid ointment, 3 times a day for 5 days.

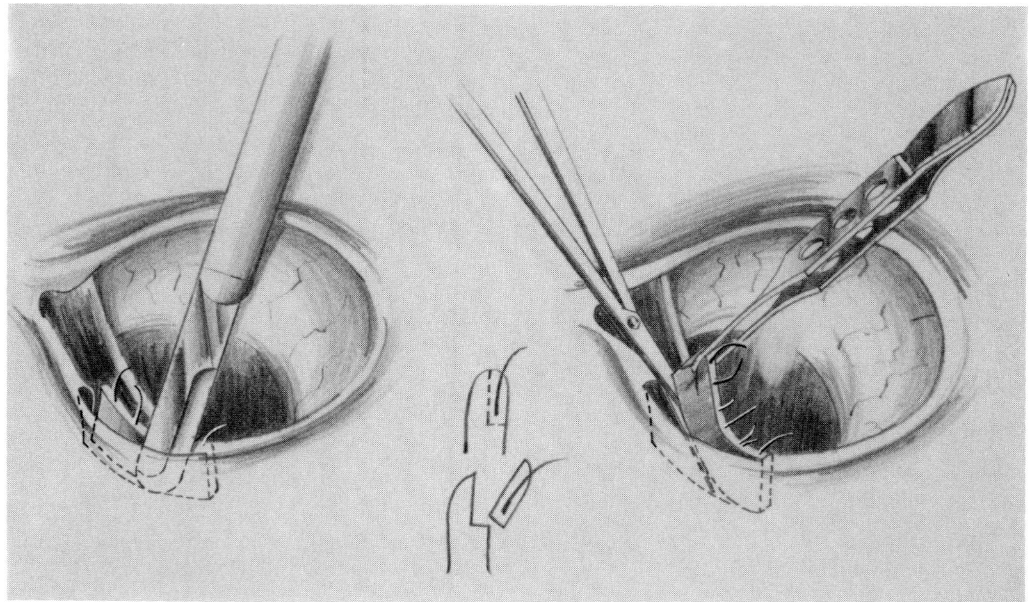

Fig. 4–14. Lid splitting. *Left.* Incision between skin and tarsoconjunctiva. *Right.* Wedge of cilia-bearing tarsoconjunctiva being removed.

Considerable swelling of the lid and some eyelid depigmentation are common sequelae. The non-painful swelling subsides over several weeks, and the repigmentation occurs by 3 months. They report good owner acceptance. The tissue temperature reached during freezing is important. The goal is $-20°$ C to $-25°$ C. Temperatures warmer than $-15°$ C are thought to be ineffective, while colder than $-30°$ C may cause tissue damage and scarring.

Trichiasis

4:39 In *trichiasis* (Fig. 4–16), the regular eyelashes assume an abnormal deviation so that they set up a conjunctival or corneal irritation.

4:40 *Etiology.* Sometimes congenital, but often the deviation is acquired and is due to a moderate entropion or blepharospasm. Trichiasis can also be caused by lid splitting in thin eyelids.

4:41 *Symptoms.* There is epiphora and possible corneal damage (*e.g.* superficial vascularization and scarring) with an accompanying mucoid discharge.

4:42 *Treatment.* Electro-epilation and/or surgical eversion of the lid margin and other plastic procedures can be used depending upon the cause. If from the nasal fold, the nasal fold may be removed (Par. 6:89).

Ectopic Cilia (Figs. 4–17, 4–18)

4:43 Ectopic cilia of the lids are lashes or clusters of lashes that grow through the conjunctiva. Those usually encountered in the dog are on the upper palpebral surface and are thought to originate from lash follicles or a misdirected hair follicle. The history, signs and physical findings have been almost identical in each case presented.[17] These include a unilateral blepharospasm, epiphora or mucoid discharge (Fig. 4–18A), slight to moderate inflammation of the superior bulbar conjunctiva, and vascularization of the adjacent cornea (Fig. 4–18B). When the upper lid is everted one or more short, stiff cilia will be seen protruding through the palpebral conjunctiva at the center position, 4 to 6 mm

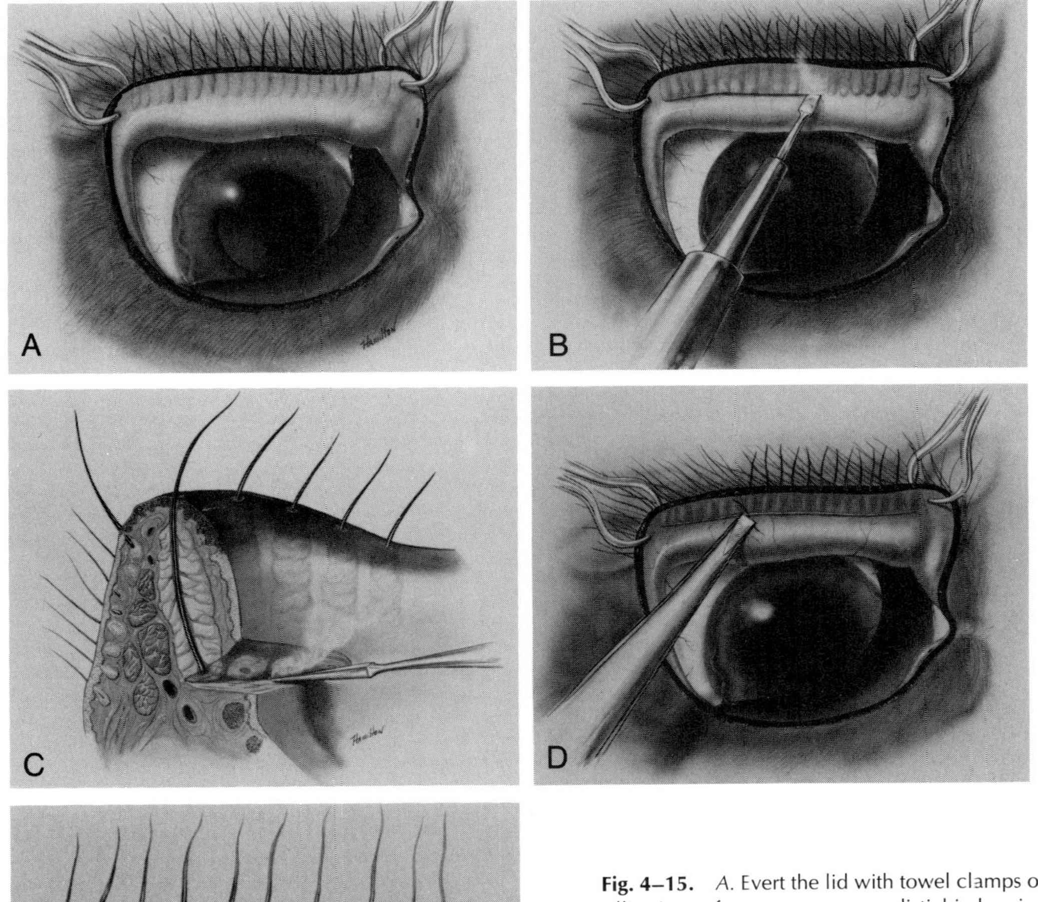

Fig. 4–15. *A.* Evert the lid with towel clamps or Allis tissue forceps to expose distichia-bearing meibomian glands, carefully avoiding the lacrimal punctum. *B.* Incise along the base of the distichia-bearing meibomian glands with a fine electroscalpel blade. *C.* A cut-away view showing the depth of incision. *D.* Distichia should lift out easily if the incision is correct. *E.* Improper incision may result in aberrant growth of distichia. (Courtesy of Dr. Ron Riis, Cornell University.)

posterior to the lid margin. Although most often unilateral, both eyes may be afflicted with follicles producing four to eight cilia.[1] Good magnification and short acting anesthesia are often required to properly examine this structure.

4:44 *Treatment.* Ectopic cilia are best removed by electro-epilation (Par. 4:35). After epilation, the hole should be probed with a fine forceps for other submerged cilia.

Diseases and Surgery of the Third Eyelid (Membrane Nictitans) (Palpebral Tertia) (Fig. 4–19)

4:45 *Anatomy and Physiology.* The third eyelid is also called the membrana nictitans,

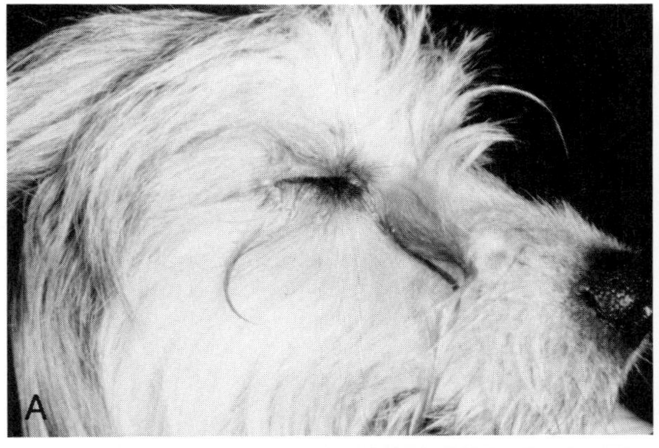

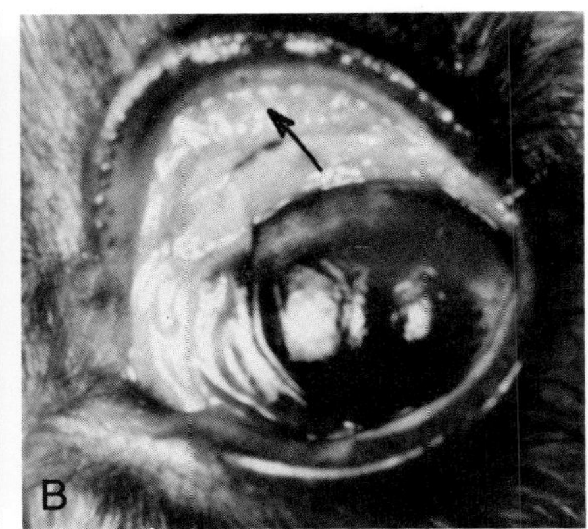

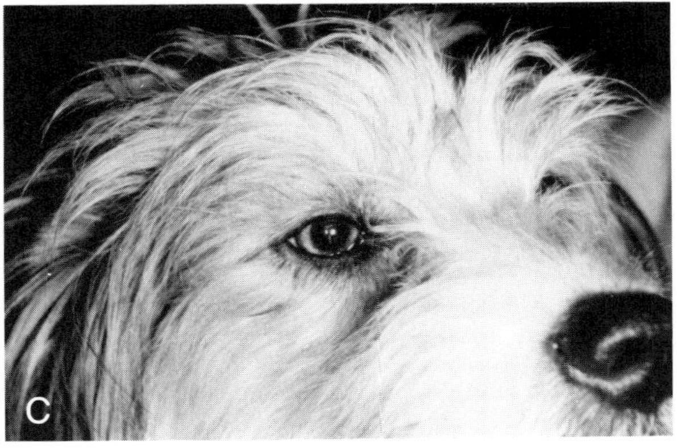

Fig. 4–18. *A*. Blepharospasm and epiphora associated with ectopic cilia. *B*. Cilia protruding through the conjunctiva at the middle of the upper lid. Upper cornea abraded by the cilia (arrow) with accompanying superficial vascularization. *C*. Immediate relief of symptoms following removal of cilia.

inversion of the third eyelid itself are not excuses for its extirpation. The third eyelid and its gland does serve a useful purpose and its absence can predispose to chronic conjunctivitis, keratoconjunctivitis sicca, lid defects and keratopathies (Plate 3B). This procedure, then, should only be performed as a last resort, or, *e.g.* in the case of a malignancy.

4:47 *Inversion or Eversion of the Third Eyelid.* Although dogs are not commonly born with deformity of the third eyelid, certain breeds, including St. Bernards, Great Danes, Weimaraners and English Bulldogs seem to be predisposed to inversion or eversion of the third eyelid while young. Deformity appears to be caused by bending of the cartilage during growth. Eversion seems to be more common than inversion (Plate 2D). Deformity is often bilateral. Similar deformity caused by injury is seen occasionally in hunting dogs. It is unilateral.

4:48 *Signs.* The presenting sign is often increased visibility of the third eyelid and a watery to mucoid ocular discharge. Close examination reveals deformity of the T-shaped cartilage (Fig. 4–20A). The free edge of the third eyelid is hidden in the lower fornix in the case of eversion. In long-standing cases, there may be marked follicular conjunctivitis.

4:49 *Treatment.* Surgical correction consists of removal of the curved portion of the cartilage. After giving general anesthesia, the free edge of the third eyelid is grasped with a fixation forceps and gently elevated. A small bleb of saline solution is injected in the area of the deformity to separate the outer surface of the third eyelid from the cartilage (Fig. 4–20B). An incision is then made through the conjunctiva on the inner surface of the third eyelid and carefully through the cartilage proximal to the deformity (Fig. 4–20C). The cartilage is then grasped with a small forceps

A

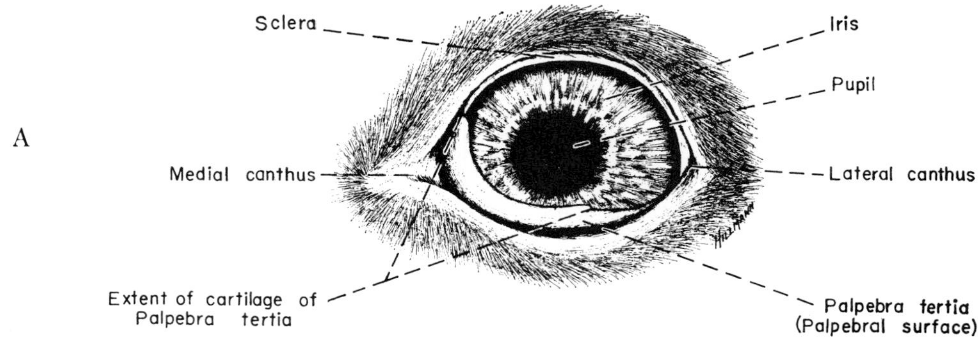

B

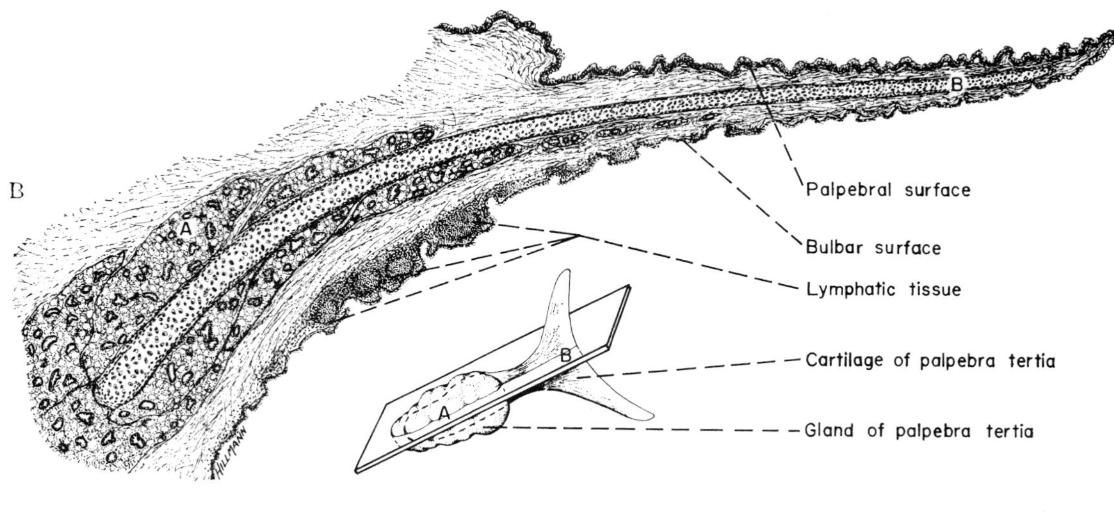

C

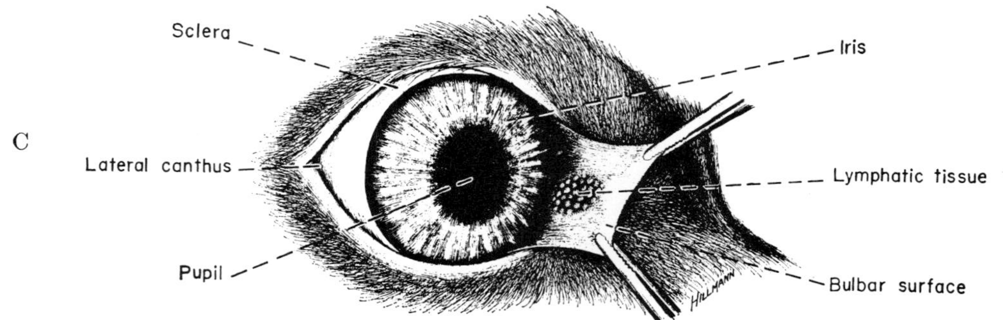

Fig. 4–19. *A.* The membrane nictitans. *B.* The membrane nictitans in histological section. *C.* The membrane nictitans reflected to reveal lymphatic tissue. (Miller, Christensen and Evans, *Anatomy of the Dog,* courtesy of W.B. Saunders Co.)

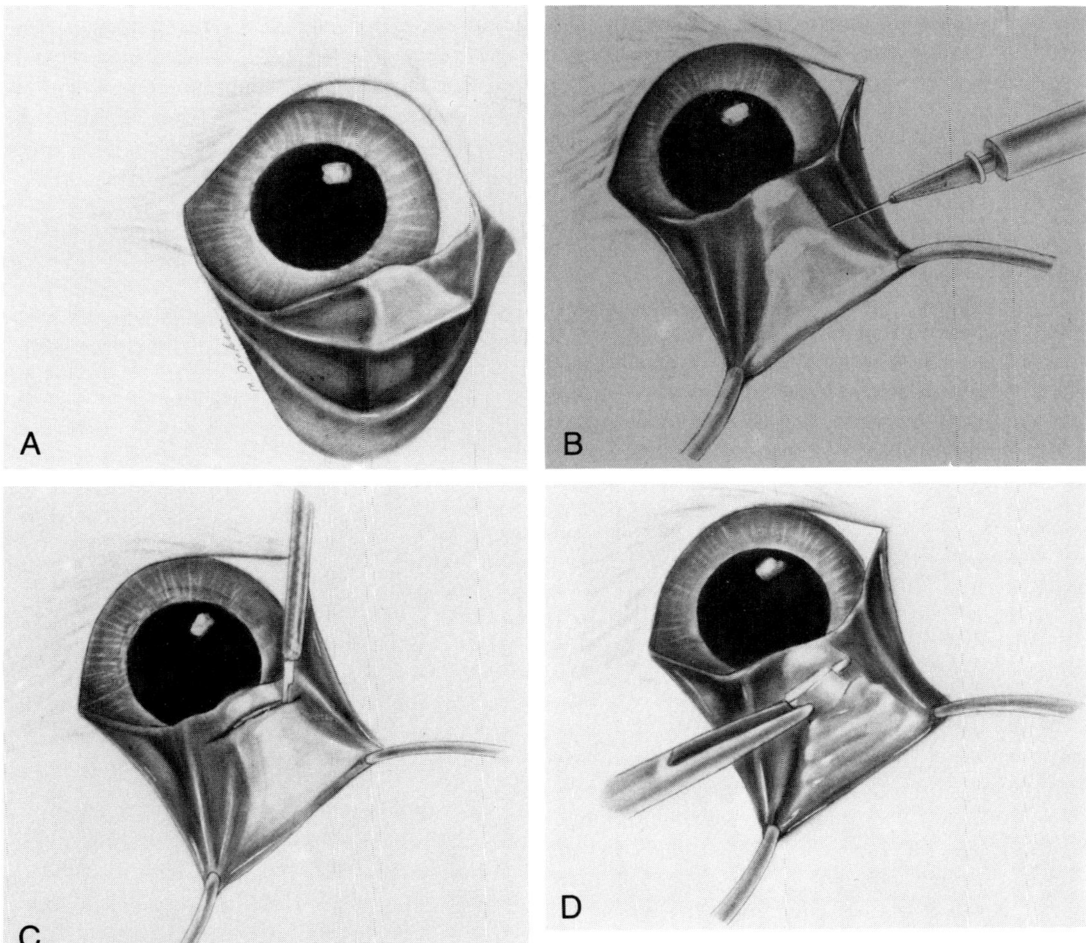

Fig. 4–20. *A.* Eversion of the nictitating membrane. *B.* Injection of saline solution between the cartilage and the anterior conjunctival surface after straightening the nictitating membrane. *C.* Incision of the posterior conjunctival surface and cartilage just proximal to the deformity. *D.* Grasping the deformed segment of cartilage to be dissected free and removed with tenotomy scissors.

and dissected carefully from the conjunctiva with tenotomy scissors (Fig. 4–20D). After the deformed cartilage is exposed, it is excised with scissors or scalpel. It is seldom necessary to dissect past the junction of the cross-piece and stem of the T of the cartilage, even if there is some distortion of the cross-piece. If the gland of the third eyelid has been exposed by the surgery, the incision is closed with 6 Ō catgut. Aftercare consists of a topical antibiotic steroid ophthalmic ointment twice a day for 5 to 7 days.

4:50 *Prolapse of the Gland.* Protrusion of the gland over the free edge of the third eyelid called hypertrophy, hyperplasia or adenoma, and commonly termed "cherry eye" by dog breeders is actually a prolapse of the base of the gland up and out past the free edge of the third eyelid. A congenital, perhaps hereditary, weakness of the connective tissue band between the cartilage and glandular portion of the third eyelid (Plate 2G) and the globe has been suggested.[30] If only one eye is involved, the other should be evaluated concerning potential for prolapse. The tear production should also be evaluated with the Schirmer tear test.

4:51 *Treatment.* The ideal treatment is to return the gland to normal position. Blogg[4] and Gross[12] suggest reducing the prolapse and maintaining the reduction by suturing. In my experience, the procedure is successful unless the stem of the cartilage is seriously deformed. After general anesthesia, the third eyelid is grasped with fixation forceps to expose the inner surface. Tenotomy scissors are used to make an incision through the inner conjunctival surface, starting at the tip of the prolapsed gland and extending down to the fornix, between the third eyelid and the globe. A small-toothed forceps, such as a Bishop-Harmon forceps, is used to reach through the incision in the fornix and grasp some fibrous tissue attached to the globe. 5 ō catgut, Dexon or other absorbable suture is placed through this tissue and through the tip of the prolapsed gland exposed by the upper end of the incision. A second suture is similarly placed before tying the first suture, and then each is tied. A steroid antibiotic ointment is dispensed to be used for 7 to 10 days. Removal of the gland should not be the first choice if the Schirmer tear test value is less than 20 mm/min, or if in a breed predisposed to keratoconjunctivitis sicca, such as the English Bulldog. But it is necessary if the suturing technique is not possible or fails. Removal is facilitated by crushing the junction of the gland and the third eyelid with a hemostatic mosquito forceps prior to excising the gland with small scissors (Fig. 4–21). Hemorrhage, if any, following excision can be controlled by light pressure on the eyelids for a few minutes. General anesthesia is required for this surgery in most dogs; however, excision may be accomplished with only topical anesthesia, such as Ophthaine in docile dogs if the topical anesthetic is instilled 3 or 4 times over a 5- to 10-minute period. Aftercare following gland removal, consists of a steroid in antibiotic ophthalmic ointment applied twice a day for 5 to 7 days.

4:52 *Prominence of the Third Eyelid.* The prominence of the third eyelid varies from breed to breed and is mentioned in some breed standards. The owner's impression of prominence also is influenced by pigmentation. A non-pigmented third eyelid often causes a complaint of increased prominence or persistent conjunctivitis. Explanation to the owner is all that is needed.

4:53 Congenital causes of elevations of the third eyelid include microphthalmos and rarely Horner's Syndrome.[5] In the latter, the elevation of the third eyelid is accompanied by the other signs, ptosis, and miosis.

4:54 Elevation of the third eyelid can also be acquired. As mentioned earlier in this chapter, any disease that causes retraction of the globe will cause increased prominence of the third eyelid. Acquired Horner's syndrome, corneal injury or any other disease causing a painful eye should be considered. One should always examine behind the third eyelid for a foreign body (Plate 2H).

4:55 In rare instances, a bilateral progressive enophthalmos, with accompanying elevation of the third eyelid, develops without the other signs of Horner's syndrome. It may be accompanied by atrophy of the masseter and temporal muscles. The elevation of the third eyelid can be severe enough to cause impairment of vision (Fig. 4–22 and Plate 2E). Elevation is most pronounced when the dog is relaxed. The cause of the elevation is the enophthalmos, but the exact cause of the enophthalmos is obscure. It most often occurs in middle-aged to old dogs.

4:56 *Treatment.* Elevation of the third eyelid itself seldom requires treatment. Treatment of underlying eye disease, if present, will alleviate this sign. If the elevation is primary as in Figure 4–22A, and excision seems desirable to improve vision or for cosmetic purposes, it is best to remove only the edge, not the entire third eyelid. The amount to remove should be planned carefully before anesthesia (Fig. 4–22B) and that amount excised carefully with tenotomy scissors (Fig.

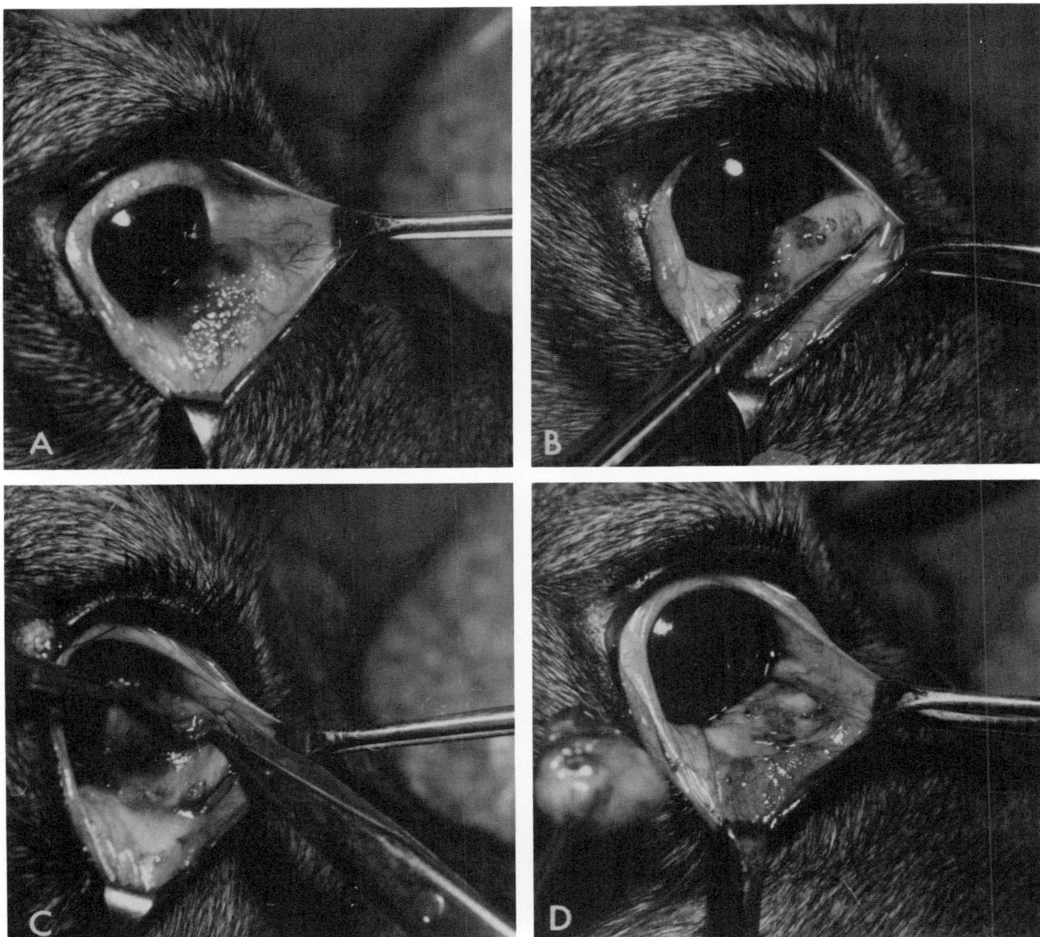

Fig. 4–21. Removal of nictitans gland. *A.* Nictitans gland exposed. *B.* Base of gland compressed by mosquito forceps. *C.* Removal of gland (eye tissue forceps and tenotomy scissors). *D.* Gland removed.

4–22C), after anesthesia. The resulting wound is closed with 6 Ō chromic catgut, continuous suture to prevent prolapse of the remaining cartilage and gland. The results (Fig. 4–22D) are good and the function of the third eyelid and its glands is not sacrificed. Aftercare consists of application of a steroid antibiotic ointment BID for 5 days.

Inflammation

4:57 Plasma cell infiltration or Plasmoma as first described by Teichert[32] (Plate 3A) is a specific inflammatory and degenerative disease of the third eyelid of German Shepherds. The first sign is bilateral inflammation and depigmentation of the edge of the third eyelid. A mucoid discharge is evident. As the inflammation progresses, there is thickening of the third eyelid and development of a nodular irregular surface and finally a scalloped or irregular edge. Some dogs have concurrent chronic superficial keratitis (pannus) and some develop it later. Corneal disease does not, however, develop in all cases. The cause is not established, but is probably an immunologic defect similar to the cause of chronic superficial keratitis in the German Shepherd. Biopsy or deep conjunctival scraping reveals plasma cells in addition to other

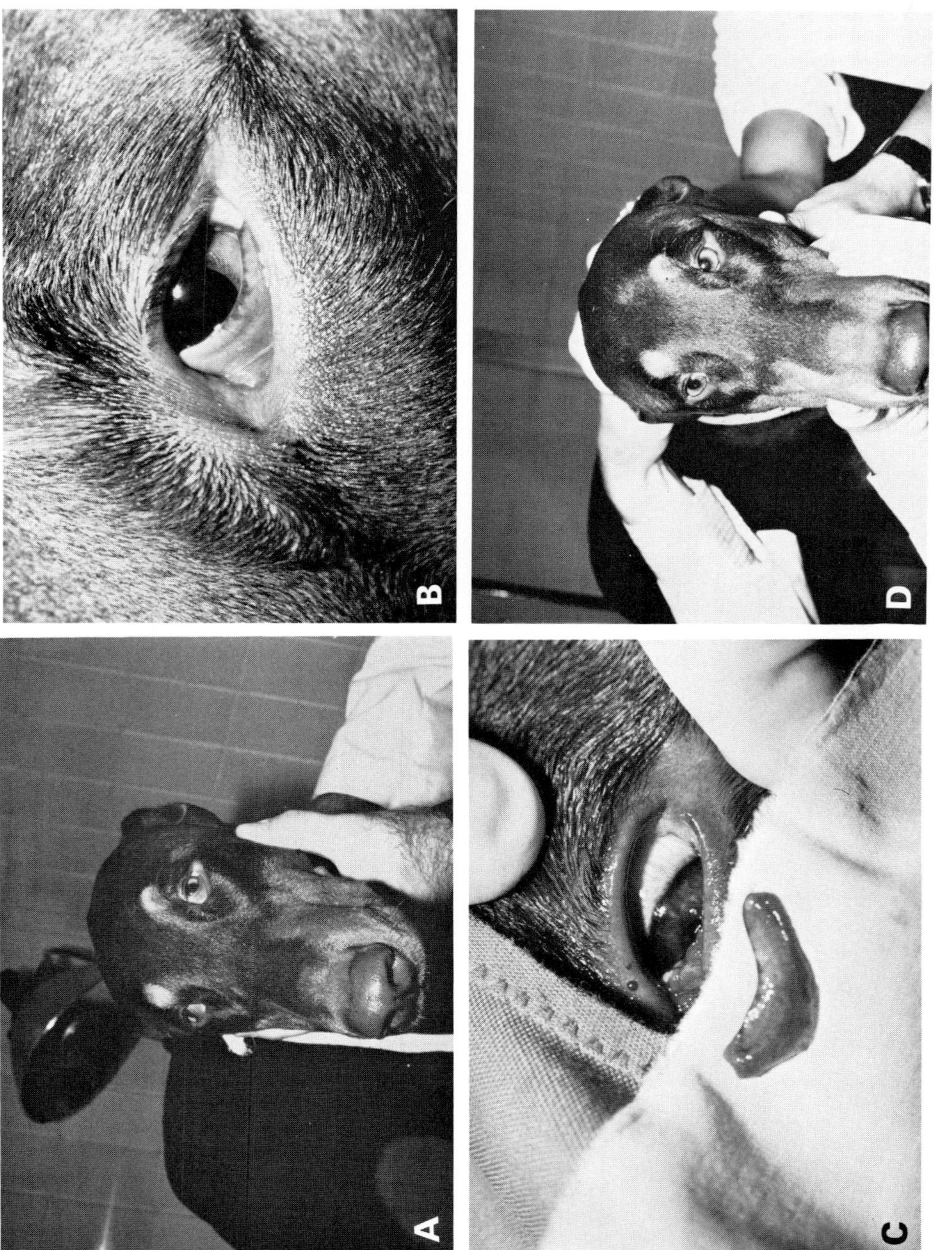

Fig. 4–22. *A.* Doberman with bilateral elevation of nictitating membrane. *B.* Close-up of left eye prior to general anesthesia. *C.* Excised edge of the nictitating membrane and eye after excision and suturing of nictitans. *D.* After recovery from general anesthesia.

inflammatory cells. One should consider chronic infections or allergy to medication in the differential diagnosis, especially if the above signs develop in dogs on topical treatment for chronic superficial keratitis. Culture and antibiotic sensitivity should be accomplished and a change in the antibiotic should be considered if an antibiotic steroid drop is being applied.

4:58 *Treatment.* Treatment of plasma cell infiltration like treatment of chronic superficial keratitis consists of suppressing the inflammatory response with continued steroid application. The owner must be impressed that treatment is for control and must be continued indefinitely. A subconjunctival injection of 10 mg of triamcinalone acetonide (Kenalog) to each eye for initial control followed by steroid-antibiotic drops twice a day will usually provide control. The alternative is to apply steroid-antibiotic drops 6 to 8 times a day for 10 to 14 days, followed by twice a day application.

Neoplasms

4:59 Neoplasms of the membrane nictitans or of its gland are rarely seen. Those reported include adenoma, lipoma, endothelioma, carcinoma and sarcoma. A mastocytoma involving these structures was successfully excised without losing the integrity of the third eyelid.[14]

Third Eyelid Flap (TEF) Technique

4:60 Various conjunctival flap procedures are employed in man to protect or strengthen a damaged cornea. These same techniques can be employed in the dog (Par. 5:55), but unless the third eyelid has been removed, a TEF can be used more easily and is as effective. The more common uses include:

1. An impending iris prolapse (deep ulceration) (Par. 6:125)
2. Following an iris prolapse (after the iris has been snipped off flush with the cornea) (Par. 6:133)
3. To bring a blood supply to a nonhealing ulcerated area. The inner surface of the membrane is first scarified.
4. In indolent ulcers or bullous keratitis (Par. 6:65).
5. To add support to corneal wounds that have been sutured (Par. 6:143), or following corneal surgery, *e.g.*, superficial keratectomy.

4:61 This is an especially useful operation in short-nosed breeds were snug bandaging (which might serve the same purpose) is difficult to achieve. Mechanical support for the eye is obtained through the pressure immobilization provided by this technique.

Technique

4:62 Instrument requirements: three double armed sutures (*e.g.*, 3 Ō or 4 Ō monofilament nylon or other nonabsorbable sutures), needle forceps, eye fixation forceps, knife blade (if scarifing indicated).

4:63 Three mattress sutures are placed through the superior edge of the nictitans at its medial, central and lateral aspects (Fig. 4–23A). The needle must penetrate both surfaces of the membrane to incorporate the cartilage. The needles are then brought through the upper conjunctival fornix area to the outside skin (Fig. 4–23B). The membrane is then pulled up snug over the eyeball and the sutures tied down over buttons for better retention and to prevent pressure necrosis (Fig. 4–23C and D). The globe is now fully enveloped and immobilized by the third eyelid and the sutures are not in contact with the corneal surface. A newer technique developed by Blogg[4] (Fig. 4–24), has several advantages: (1) it is less traumatic and better tolerated by the dog, (2) it is quicker, and (3) it allows the flap to be let down to examine the eye and pulled back up again if indicated. We use the Blogg technique commonly now in the dog, cat, and horse. Figure 4–24 outlines the technique.

4:64 If scarifying is indicated (Fig. 4–25), this is done just prior to the pulling up of the membrane. Ordinarily the immobilization

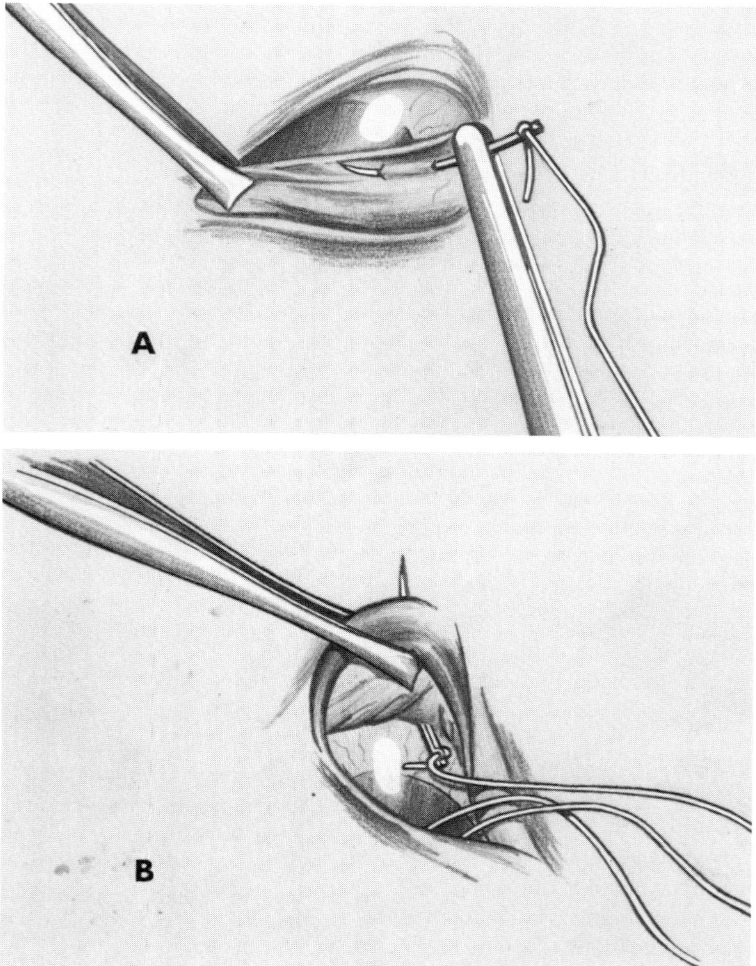

Fig. 4–23. Third eyelid flap (TEF). *A.* Placement of sutures in the nictitans. *B.* Needle through the fornix to the outside skin.

and protection afforded the cornea by the flap make scarification unnecessary except in the most refractory ulcerative keratopathies.

4:65 The sutures are left in place for 10 to 14 days. During this time, the eye can be cleansed and medication used through the partial lid opening (Fig. 4–23D). The use of a protective collar (Fig. 4–6) may or may not be necessary, depending upon the nature of the patient. If the sutures are placed properly, three are used, and the anterior aspect of the globe is fully enveloped by the third eyelid, it is seldom that the "flap" will release prematurely—even when the patient is under home care. Failures are usually the result of insufficient sutures, tying the sutures too tight, and/or attaching the membrane to the bulbar conjunctiva above as opposed to the method described here. Regardless of the purpose (Par. 4:60) for the procedure, the clinician will almost invariably be pleased with the results.

4:66 If the membrane has been scarified, it may remain adhered to the ulcerated cornea following suture removal. Thus will usually pull loose of its own within a few hours to a

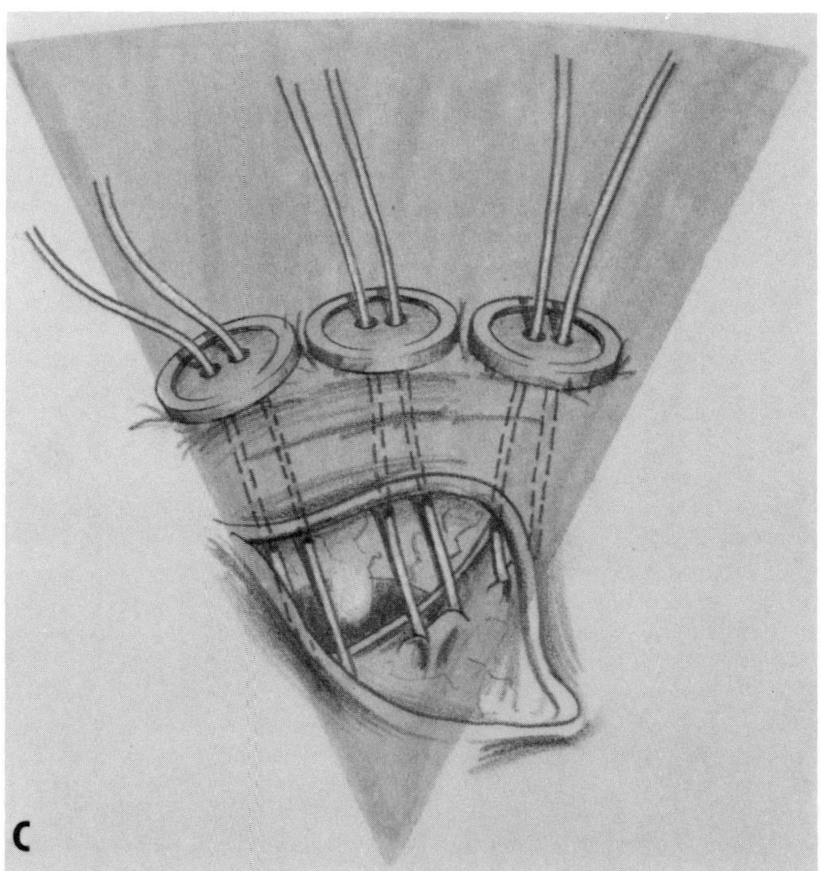

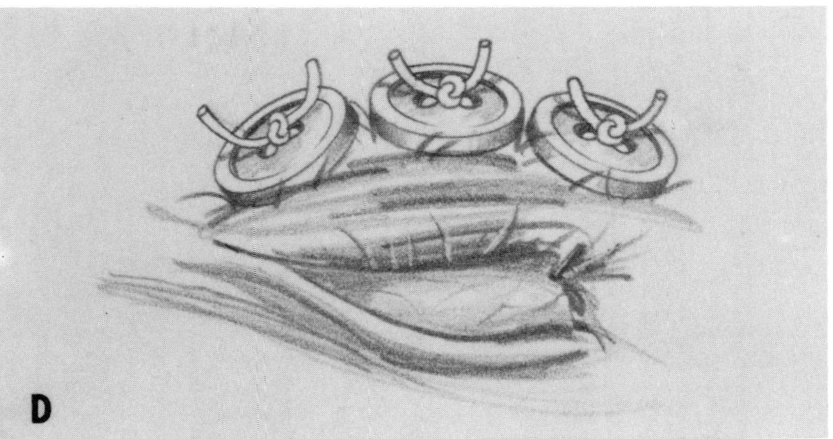

Fig. 4–23 *Continued.* *C.* Sutures prior to pulling up and tying over buttons. *D.* Completed operation.

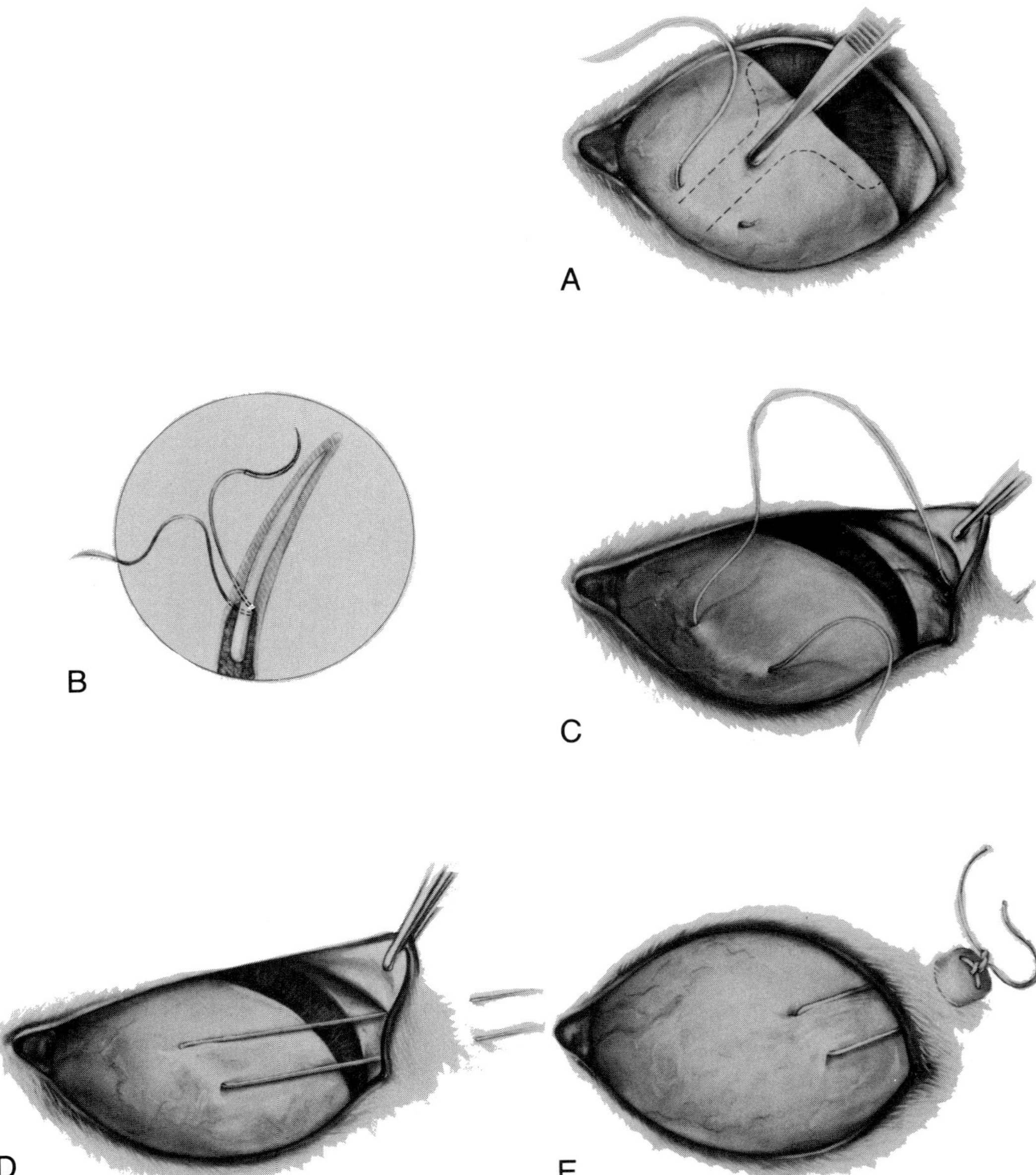

Fig. 4–24. *A*. The 3rd eyelid is elevated with a forceps and the needle is directed so that the suture passes behind the cartilage about midway between the free edge and base of the 3rd eyelid. *B*. The suture encompasses the stem of the T but does not penetrate the conjunctiva on the inner surface of the 3rd eyelid. *C*. The needles of the double-armed suture are passed through the upper fórnix and out through the skin dorsal to the lateral canthus. *D*. By traction on the suture the 3rd eyelid is elevated until the free edge is in the upper fornix. *E*. The suture is passed through a button and tied. The ends are cut long enough to allow the 3rd eyelid to be lowered after untying the knot if re-examining the cornea is desired.

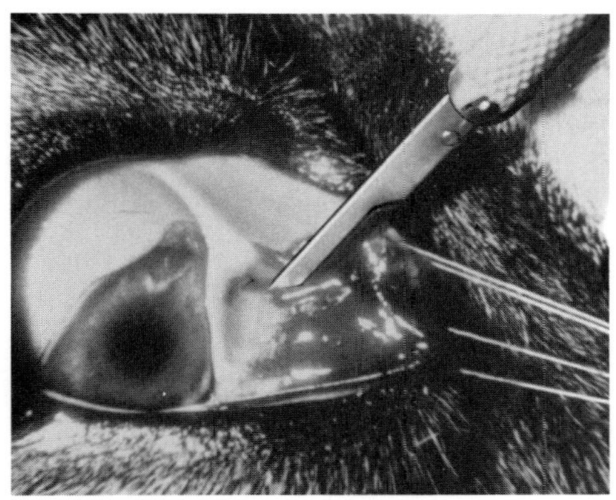

Fig. 4–25. Scarifying inner glandular surface of the membrane nictitans. Note pre-placed sutures.

day, but can be separated with a smooth spatula if one desires. Or, the superior border of the third eyelid may stay adhered to the fornix area. This too will soon release on its own. If not, following topical anesthesia, a spatula or muscle hook is used to free the adhesion.

Atresia

4:67 *Atresia* or congenital absence of the openings to the lacrimal canal is not uncommon, especially to the Bedlington, Sealyham, and miniature Schnauzer breeds. Either or both the upper and lower punctum may be absent or covered by a thin membrane (Plate 5D). It is, however, more common to find the inferior opening occluded in this manner.

4:68 *Symptoms.* Epiphora (spillage of tears) producing a rust colored tear streak at the nasal fold is to be expected. Many dogs, however, may go through life with occluded or absent punctae showing little evidence of this "wet eye" anomaly. In many dogs, epiphora is evident only when some ocular irritation causes increased tear production.

4:69 *Treatment.* It is often possible to reestablish patency of an inferior opening when the punctum is covered by a membrane. By irrigating through the superior opening a ballooning will be noted at the intended origin of the inferior opening (Fig. 4–26A). This ballooned area is "nicked" or a small piece is cut away, allowing the solution to escape (Fig. 4–26B). Careful observation usually reveals a normal appearing punctum under the area of excision. Aftercare consists of twice daily application of antibiotic-steroid drops (Fig. 4–27) for 5 days. Daily irrigation is not needed.

4:70 Complete surgical restoration of the nasolacrimal drainage apparatus by means of a dacryocystorhinostomy and plastic drainage tubes is a most specialized procedure, often important to man's well-being, but seldom indicated in the dog. Although one report[7] details a successful conjunctivorhinostomy procedure, our results both in a clinical trial and a research project were unsatisfactory.

Epiphora

4:71 Roberts[28] concluded that chronic epiphora in dogs is related not to overproduction of tears, but rather to anatomic defects or functional disturbances that interfere with drainage through the nasal lacrimal canals. This may ordinarily be the case, but irritation of one sort or another will certainly provoke excess tear formation. Once the source of the irritation is eliminated, the excess tearing stops.

4:72 *Etiology.* Causes include: atresia, plugged ducts, allergens, distichiasis, trichiasis, ectopic cilia, entropion, ectropion, eversion and/or hypertrophy of the membrane nictitans, and contact with hair from the nasal skin folds and periorbital skin. Epiphora in poodles, as well as other toy breeds, occurs in the absence of any of the above causes. Kerpsack[19] found hypertrophy and inflammatory elements in the nictitans gland on histopathologic examination, although this seems to me unlikely as the cause of epiphora. Peiffer and Gelatt[25] suggested that the cause of epiphora is improper drainage, associated with a slight entropion of the medial aspect of the lower lid, and outlined a surgical procedure for correction.

4:73 *Treatment.* Oxytetracycline, given orally, was found to be effective in preventing

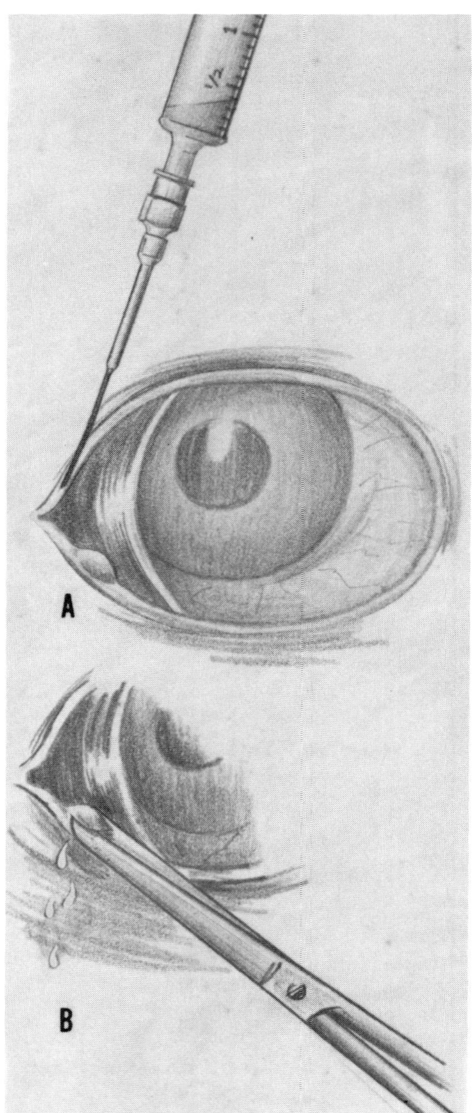

Fig. 4–26. *A*. Atresia. Ballooning of membrane which covers the opening. *B*. Cutting membrane to correct the atresia.

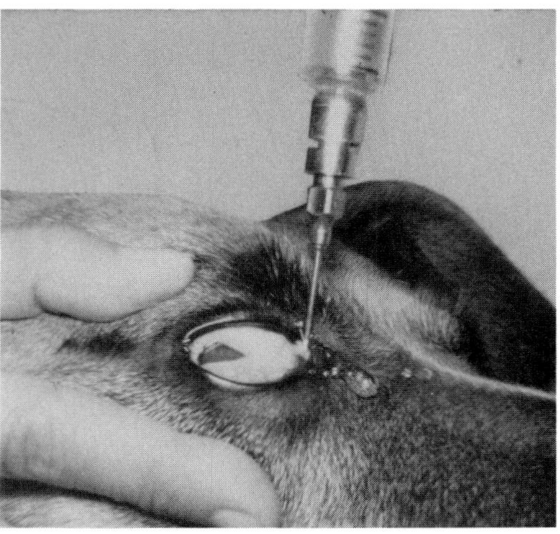

Fig. 4–27. Irrigation of the lacrimal drainage system.

the hair staining common in epiphora.[15] Schirmer tear tests conducted prior to and during a 60-day period in which five dogs were given tetracycline HCl at 6 to 8 mg per kg orally daily revealed no change in tear production associated with the drug administration.[33] Tetracycline probably reduces hair staining associated with epiphora either by affecting the composition of the tears or interaction of the tears, skin, and perhaps surface bacteria that produce the reddish-brown discoloration of the hair.

4:74 In using tetracycline or oxytetracycline, I use 25 mg per day in toy breeds (up to 15#), and 50 mg per day for larger dogs. The powdered animal formulas can also be used at ½ tsp. daily for toy breeds and 1 tsp. daily for larger breeds. It is given for about a month and then discontinued for 2 to 4 weeks, and used symptomatically. If no improvement is seen in the initial 4 weeks, discontinue. It seems to work in 75 to 80% of the cases.

4:75 Excision of the gland of the third eyelid was the commonly employed treatment in the past. With the discovery of the function of the gland of the third eyelid as the source of part of the tears,[16,18] and the realization that a few dogs developed keratitis sicca following gland removal, this procedure is now reserved for selected severe cases. After eliminating all other causes, removal of the gland of the third eyelid, as described in Par. 4:51, is considered in dogs with Schirmer values over 20 mm/min. Even these dogs could develop keratoconjunctivitis sicca, in the unlikely instance that the lacrimal gland production diminishes. In my experience, very few have developed KCS. I have little experience with the procedure described by Peiffer,[25] but it deserves serious consideration.

Other Lid Diseases

4:76 Other common affections of the eyelids not associated with inheritance or breed predisposition include edema, blepharitis, periorbital dermatitis, chalazion, hordeolum, lid abscess, wounds, foreign bodies, and tumors.

Edema

4:77 *Etiology.* Simple edema of the lids is usually of allergic origin (insect bites, pollen); however, trauma, infection, periorbital dermatitis or demodex mange may be excitatory factors. Muller[24] lists Microsporum canis, Microsporum gypsum, Trichophyton mentagrophytes, Sarcoptes and Staphylococcus aureus as additional causes of infectious dermatoses affecting the eyelids.

4:78 *Treatment.* Treatment directed at the cause will usually afford quick relief. Antibiotic-steroid combinations are effective in those cases of allergic or infectious origin. Amitraz (Mitaban),* .2 ml to 1 ml/oz of mineral oil, applied every third day is for demodex mange of the lids.

Blepharitis (Plate 2F) (Plate 5E,F)

4:79 *Symptoms.* The symptoms are inflammatory edema with reddening and thickening of the palpebral conjunctiva and lid margins, sticky discharge, blepharospasm.

4:80 *Etiology.* Etiology consists of contact with irritating weeds, mange dermatitis, association with hordeolum, chalazion, accompanying or following distemper, or in combination with conjunctivitis or keratoconjunctivitis.

4:81 *Sequelae.* Sequelae include hypertrophy of the lid margins, trichiasis, entropion and ectropion.

4:82 *Treatment.* The disease is often obstinate. A determination of the causes and their removal are important. It is well to have the lid hair cut closely. The secretions should be cleaned thoroughly from the conjunctival sac before instillation of an antibiotic-steroid ointment to the outer and inner lid margins. Surgical drainage and curettage (Par. 4:86) or manual expression of the purulent material is often indicated in those instances in which the sebaceous or meibomian glands are involved. Expression of material from the meibomian glands is accomplished by placing a tongue depressor behind the lid and pressure milking the contents towards the margin. Expressed material should be examined for demodex mites, and collected for bacteriologic culture and antibiotic sensitivity. The use of hot packs twice daily, in addition to systemic as well as topical antibiotics, as indicated by sensitivity testing, is often necessary for infections involving the meibomian or other lid or skin glands. The antibiotics should be continued for at least 3 weeks.

*Upjohn Co., Kalamazoo, MI

Chalazion

4:83 If a duct of a meibomian gland becomes obstructed, the oily secretion produces a swelling of the gland and inflammation of the surrounding tissue. The inflammatory enlargement is termed a chalazion.

4:84 *Symptoms.* A painless, pea-like swelling in the upper or lower eyelid (Fig. 4–28, Plate 3H). It develops slowly and the contents are usually a cheesy material. When the lid

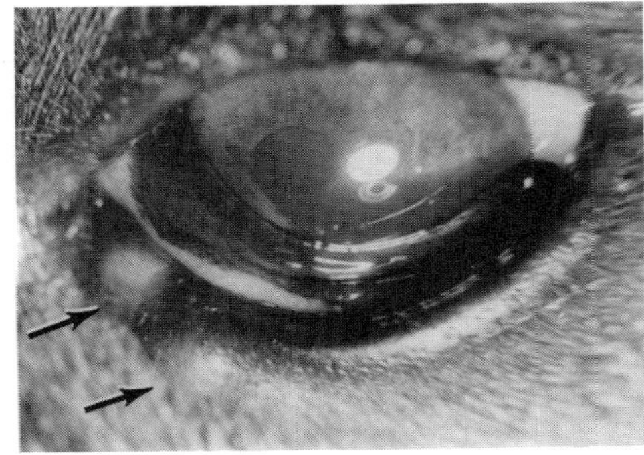

Fig. 4–28. Chalazion of lower lid. Note the two pea-like swellings.

is everted, the conjunctiva over the chalazion is seen to be reddened and elevated. A conjunctival irritation may result or if the chalazion becomes chronic, it may involve the lid margin in the form of a granuloma.

4:85 *Treatment.* Treatment consists of incision and curettage. A chalazion clamp is applied and the eyelid is everted. An incision is made through the conjunctiva over the swelling (Fig. 4–29A) and the walls of the chalazion thoroughly curetted (Fig. 4–29B). The clamp is released and an antibiotic ointment applied for several days postoperatively. In the chronic form (granuloma), electrocoagulation may be necessary.

Hordeolum

4:86 An external hordeolum or 'stye' is an infection of the skin glands of the lid. An internal hordeolum is an infection of the meibomian gland. Staphylococcus aureus and Beta hemolytic streptococci are the most common bacteria involved.

4:87 *Symptoms.* Hordeolum is usually painful and apt to provoke a blepharospasm and lacrimation. The condition is frequently associated with a blepharitis and an abscess ordinarily develops.

4:88 *Treatment.* Incision and rubbing of an antibiotic ointment thoroughly into the lid margins will usually suffice. If there are recurrences, systemic antibiotics and hot packs, 3 to 4 times a day, are of value.

Lid Abscess (Fig. 4–30)

4:89 Abscess of the lid can result from penetrating wounds, embedded foreign bodies, chalazion, hordeolum, or chronic meibomitis. Immediate relief and correction are usually attained by surgical drainage, flushing of the abscess sac and the instillation of an antibiotic ointment. Most abscesses involve the upper lid and the fornix offers the best incision site (Fig. 4–30B). Enlarging of the incision to provide adequate drainage is accomplished by

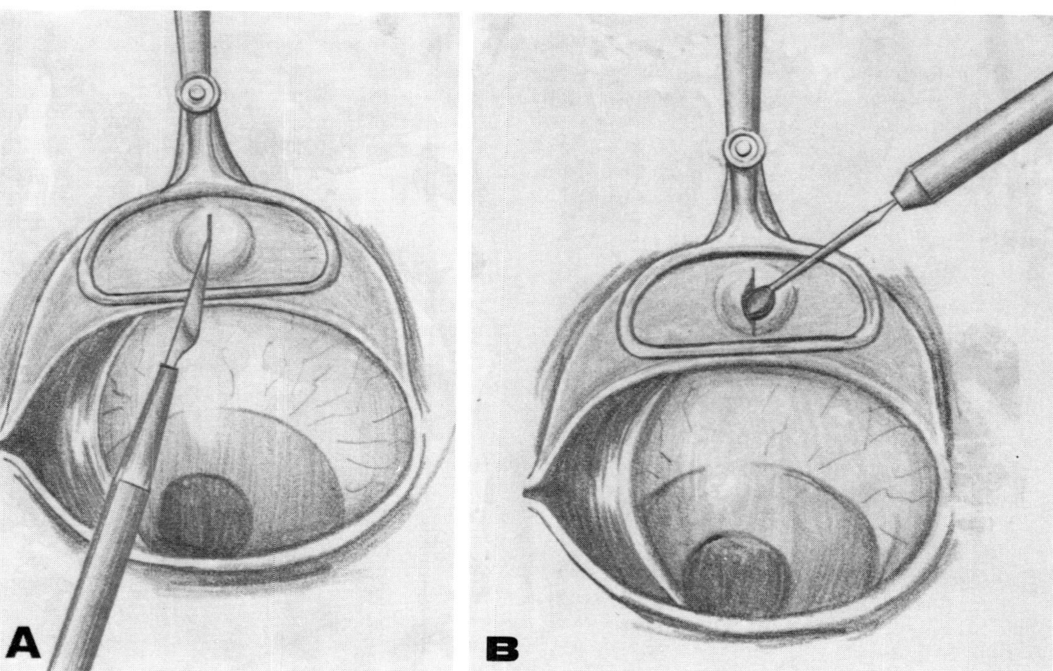

Fig. 4–29. Surgical correction of chalazion. *A.* Lid everted and incision. *B.* Curettage.

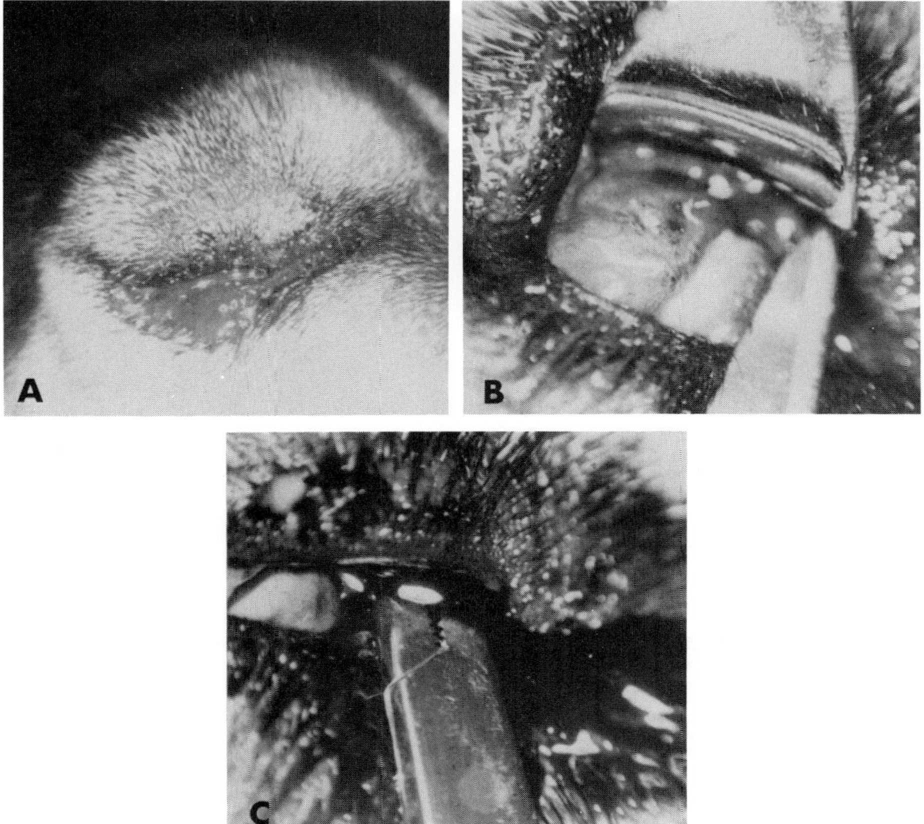

Fig. 4–30. *A.* Abscess of lid. *B.* Incision into the fornix area with upper lid retracted. *C.* Drainage established by inserting and spreading blades of a mosquito forceps.

inserting and spreading the blades of the mosquito forceps (Fig. 4–30C).

Wounds

4:90 Lacerations of the eyelids are not uncommon and result from bites, cat scratches, automobile injuries and entanglement with hooks and wire. These injuries produce a variety of tears, the surgical correction of which often proves a challenge. The possibility of injury to the globe must not be overlooked.

4:91 Wounds should be repaired as soon as possible after they have been sustained. The general principles of repair include:

1. Thorough cleansing of the wound and removal of all foreign material.
2. Minimal debridement. Nonviable appearing tissue often may be saved.
3. Eyelid must be sutured in layers. It is important to close the conjunctiva (5–0 chromic catgut) and to repair the orbicularis muscle when needed.
4. The use of fine needles and suture material (5–0 dermalon), immobilization by bandaging and prevention of self-mutilation by use of a plastic collar (Fig. 4–6A) or pail (Fig. 4–6B) are essential to success.

4:92 In the repair of eyelid wounds in which there has been considerable loss of tissue, plastic surgery employing a sliding flap technique is occasionally necessary.

Tumors

4:93 Meibomian gland adenomas (Fig. 4–31) are the most common lid tumors. Papillomas, adenocarcinomas and melanomas are also moderately common.[3,12] Interestingly, the melanomas or adenocarcinomas seldom metastasize, even if incompletely removed. Other less commonly encountered tumors include squamous cell and basal cell carcinoma, mastocytoma and histiocytoma (Plate 3C). Whereas the other tumors occur most commonly in older dogs, histiocytomas are more likely in younger dogs, develop rapidly, are often multiple and seem to be most common in the Collie. Most often, they regress spontaneously in 3 to 8 weeks.

4:94 *Treatment.* Small papillomas are superficial. After several applications of topical anesthesia, they may be snipped off, and a silver nitrate stick applied. Tumors of the conjunctival surface or skin surface of the lid can be removed quite nicely with a biopsy loop on an electrosurgical unit. Tumors involving the full thickness of the eyelid (Plate 4F) can also be removed with the biopsy loop. An electrosurgical unit needle can be used to destroy the base, but regrowth occurs in some cases. Full thickness excision is my choice for tumors involving the full thickness of the lid. Up to ⅓ of the eyelid can be removed without obvious deformity of the palpebral fissure.

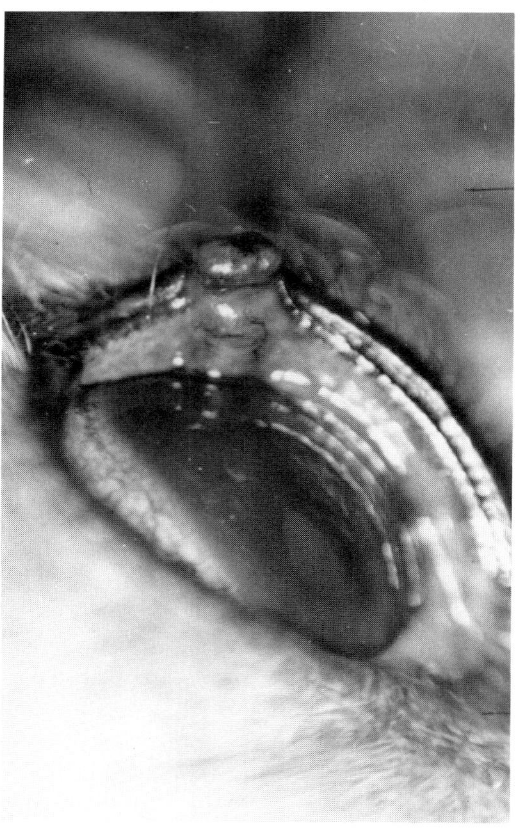

Fig. 4–31. Meibomian gland adenoma.

4:95 *Procedure.*[5] A Chalazion clamp is placed over the lid (Fig. 4–32A). A wedge of lid containing the tumor is excised (Fig. 4–32B). The Chalazion clamp is loosened enough to allow the remaining tarsal plate to be apposed and then retightened. The conjunctiva is sutured from the apex of the V to the lid margin with 6 Ō catgut (Fig. 4–32C). The edges of the lid margin are apposed with 4 Ō silk (Fig. 4–32D) and the skin is closed (Fig. 4–32E). It is important to make certain the dog does not damage the area for 7 to 10 days. A collar, with or without a bandage, should be used for protection. The sutures are removed in 10 to 12 days.

4:96 We and others have recently been using cryosurgery (Par. 3:90) to treat meibomian gland tumors. Treatment can most often be accomplished with topical and local anesthesia, thus avoiding general anesthesia in these older dogs. Sedation may be needed in some cases.

4:97 Our procedure is to apply a chalazion clamp (Fig. 3–15W) around the lid tumor after application of topical anesthesia and injection of local anesthetic. After excising a biopsy sample, the tumor, including an adjacent few millimeters around it, is frozen, either by spraying with liquid nitrogen (Fig. 3–17) or by application of a cold probe (Fig. 3–18). The tissue is allowed to thaw and a second freeze is accomplished.

4:98 Aftercare consists of a steroid-antibiotic ointment applied to the conjunctival sac

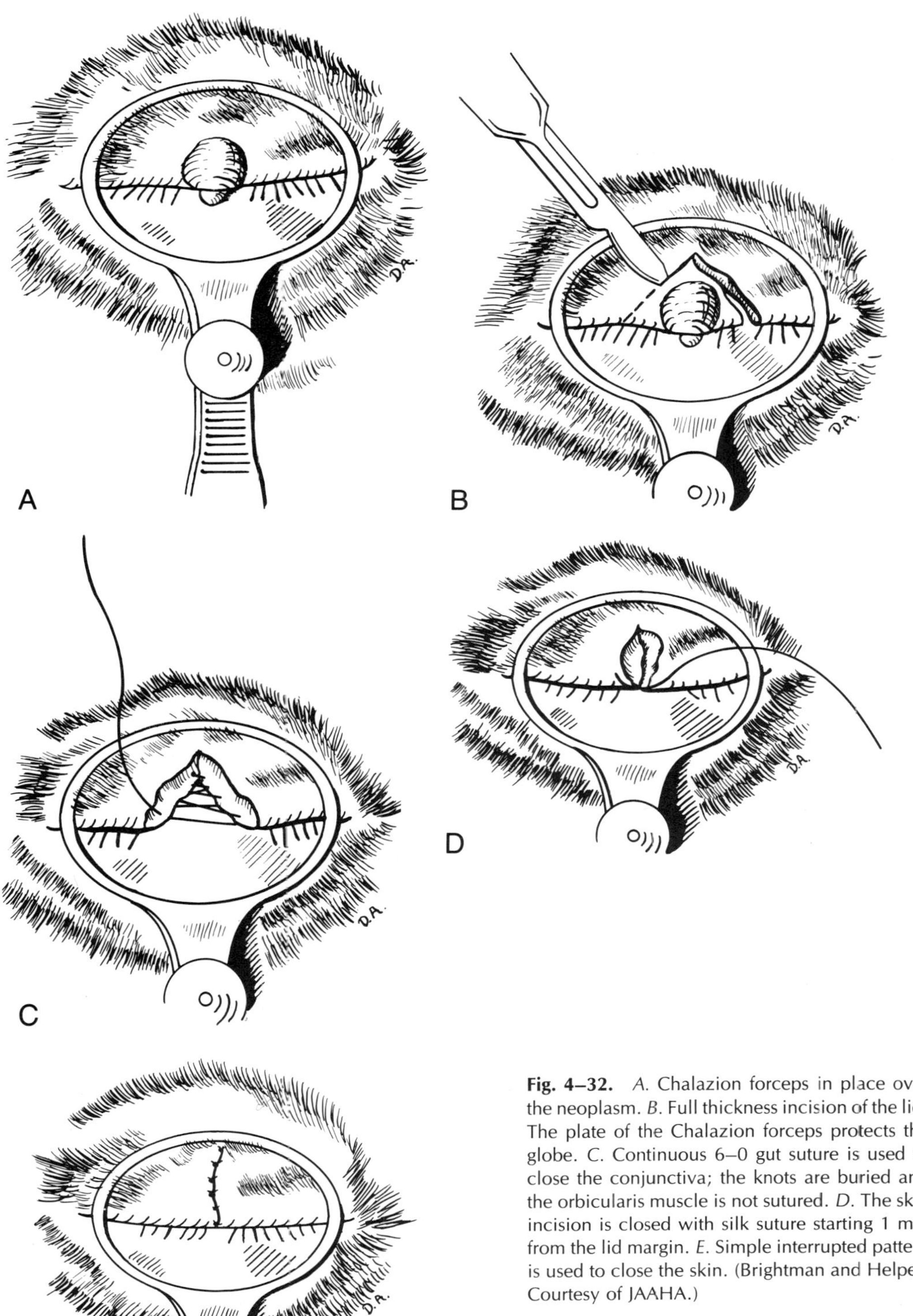

Fig. 4–32. *A.* Chalazion forceps in place over the neoplasm. *B.* Full thickness incision of the lid. The plate of the Chalazion forceps protects the globe. *C.* Continuous 6–0 gut suture is used to close the conjunctiva; the knots are buried and the orbicularis muscle is not sutured. *D.* The skin incision is closed with silk suture starting 1 mm from the lid margin. *E.* Simple interrupted pattern is used to close the skin. (Brightman and Helper, Courtesy of JAAHA.)

BID for 7 to 10 days. Considerable lid swelling is to be expected within 24 hours, and the area will become depigmented in 2 to 3 weeks. Return of pigment can be expected in 2 to 3 months.

4:99 Severin uses a similar procedure, except he incises the tumor through the conjunctival surface and scrapes out as much of the tumor mass as possible, and then inserts a small cryoprobe into the cavity created. He then freezes the surrounding tissue with a single or double freeze.

4:100 Although there is more swelling than with conventional excision, discomfort seems to be minimal and the danger of general anesthesia and the stress of hospitalization are avoided.

4:101 Dermoid cyst (congenital) (Fig. 4–33) removal is easily performed by simple excision. The scalpel incisions are made through the skin and down to the underlying bulbar conjunctiva. These upper and lower incisions are made to meet at what should be the lateral canthus (Fig. 4–34A). The skin and dermoid are then undermined and dissected free of the conjunctiva. The resulting wound is allowed to heal "open" (Fig. 4–34B), or can be closed by suturing the conjunctiva and skin to form the appropriate sized palpebral fissure.

Tarsorrhaphy

4:102 Closure of the eyelids may be achieved on a temporary or permanent basis, depending on the indications. A temporary tarsorrhaphy (Fig. 9–15) is routinely employed at the close of all intraocular procedures and involves placing a mattress type suture through the skin only of the upper and lower lids. This suture is ordinarily removed on the sixth or seventh postoperative day.

4:103 Permanent tarsorrhaphy, a union of the lids by means of intramarginal adhesions, is performed when the lids are to be closed for some time but ultimately to be separated again. This is an especially useful operation following prolapse of the globe when a lagophthalmos (incomplete lid closure) and neuroparalytic keratitis are present and the cornea needs to be kept centrally covered for a lengthy period. Even following a successful replacement of the globe (Par. 8:73), eyeball and lid innervation may be such that an exposure keratitis is in the offing (Plate 9G). The protection afforded the cornea by the lids for a two or three month period is usually sufficient.

4:104 *Technique.* The procedure for performing the closure is to place the two lids in a clamp or chalazion forceps with the lid edges nearly touching (Fig. 4–35). A 5 to 7

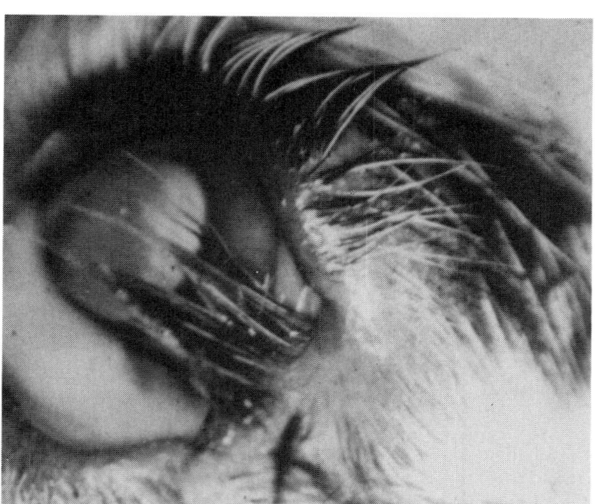

Fig. 4–33. Dermoid of the lower lid and lateral canthus.

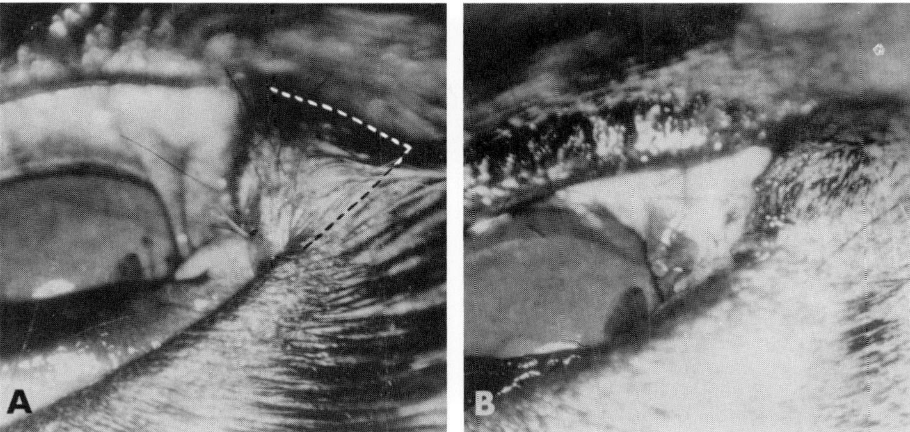

Fig. 4–34. *A.* Dermoid of the lateral canthus area. *B.* Lateral canthus reformed.

mm length of marginal lid skin is removed above and below. Needles (5–0 to 6–0 monofilament nylon suture) are passed deep, but not through the conjunctiva. The clamp holds the lids firmly and protects the underlying cornea. Also, the use of the clamp permits accurate wound apposition and controls bleeding. The clamp is then removed and the sutures tied, thus bringing the raw lid edges into firm apposition.

4:105 The sutures are removed on the eighth to tenth postoperative day, and the intramarginal adhesions are permitted to remain as long as necessary. If medication is indicated, openings at the medial and lateral aspect allow for its instillation and escape of secretions. With the passage of time the attachment stretches somewhat, but this is unimportant. Severing the adhesions is done after achieving good topical anesthesia. One

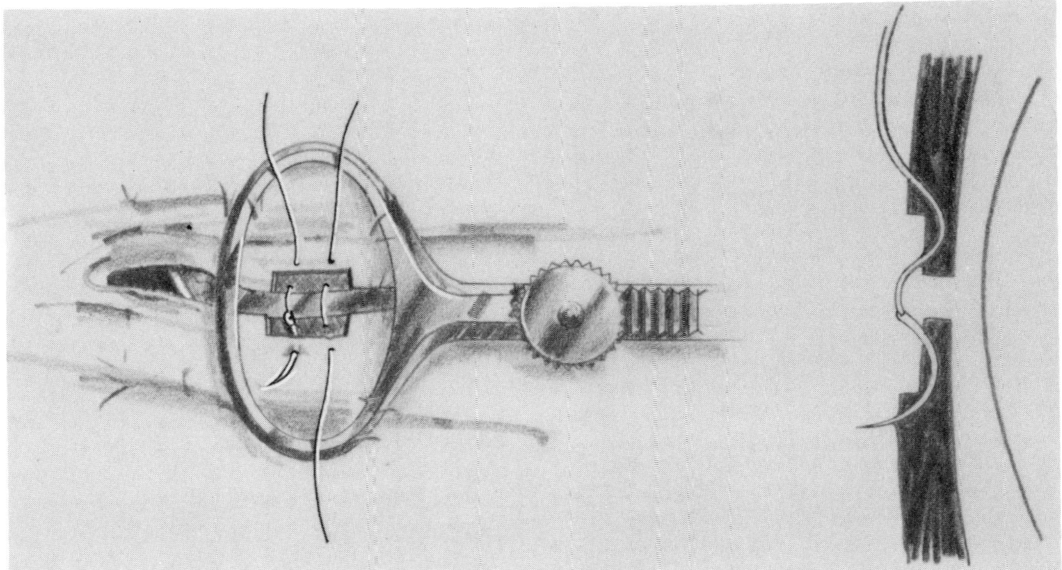

Fig. 4–35. Tarsorrhaphy. A strip of marginal lid skin is excised. Sutures are placed so, when tied, the raw lid edges become apposed.

blade of a blunt tenotomy scissors is placed under the adhesion on the corneal side and the snip is made. The severed lid edges heal rapidly and with a good cosmetic result [Tarsorrhaphy (Plate 3G)].

Infections of the Lacrimal Apparatus

4:106 Occlusion of the lacrimal canal (Par. 4:67) and epiphora (Par. 4:72) have been discussed.

Dacryoadenitis

4:107 Inflammation, abscess formation or new growths in the lacrimal gland (Par. 8:10) are uncommon in the dog. Xerophthalmosis, denoting a condition of the lacrimal gland when it ceases to secrete tears, is frequently encountered on a temporary or permanent basis. Causes include distemper, senility, and injuries to the gland with subsequent deenervation, degeneration with loss of function (Par. 6:72). An immune-mediated inflammation probably occurs in certain breeds, such as the West Highland White and, perhaps, Cocker Spaniel and English Bulldog.

Dacryocystitis

4:108 Inflammation of the lacrimal sac is usually due to an obstruction in the nasolacrimal duct followed by infection of the sac. The condition cannot be considered common in the dog probably because the sac is underdeveloped as compared to that of man. ***However, it is often the cause of a seemingly obscure unilateral conjunctivitis which fails to respond to any treatment*** (Par. 5:48). The sac serves as a reservoir of infection, continually inoculating the conjunctiva via the inferior lacrimal opening (puncta). Also, because there is no adequate drainage from the sac to the nasolacrimal duct, there remains but this one escape route for the infected discharge.

4:109 *Diagnosis.* A positive diagnosis can usually be established by irrigation of the nasolacrimal duct (Par. 2:19) (Fig. 4–26). Topical anesthesia is generally adequate but the intractable patient may require sedation or general anesthesia. Irrigation through the upper punctum causes thick material to come out of the lower punctum (Plate 3F). If the irrigating solution does not reach the nose, an obstruction exists in the duct.

4:110 Dacryocystorhinography[9,36] may be a valuable adjunctive measure for defining disorders of the lacrimal system. This radiographic procedure may confirm a dacryocystitis by identifying the level of obstruction and reveal the size and position of the lacrimal sac. Dacryostograms may also be useful for the determination of congenital anomalies, the possible neoplastic involvement of the lacrimal drainage system, damage done by facial fractures, and to reveal an obstruction which cause chronic epiphora.

4:111 *Treatment.* Thorough irrigation (Fig. 4–26) of the drainage apparatus and establishment of patency, if possible, are important. Instillation of a repositol or suspension type antibiotic through the lacrimal needle often suffices to clear up the sac infection. Ideally an antibiotic sensitivity test should first be conducted. "Pen-strep," gentacin and Panolog have been used at different times to effect recovery. The instillation should be made on a daily or, better still, twice daily basis for about 4 days. It can be done following topical anesthesia.

4:112 If medical treatment proves ineffective, one of several surgical procedures can be considered. Surgical extirpation of the sac has proven successful. A probe placed in the upper opening and extending to the sac area offers a good landmark for the incision site (Fig. 4–36). It is difficult to define the actual sac but infected tissue will be found just inside the orbital rim. Its removal by dissection and scraping will ordinarily offer permanent relief. As would be expected, following removal of the sac the patient no longer has an avenue for the escape of tears, but epiphora, if present, is less objectionable than the purulent discharge from dacryocystitis.

4:113 Severin[29] recommends nasolacrimal

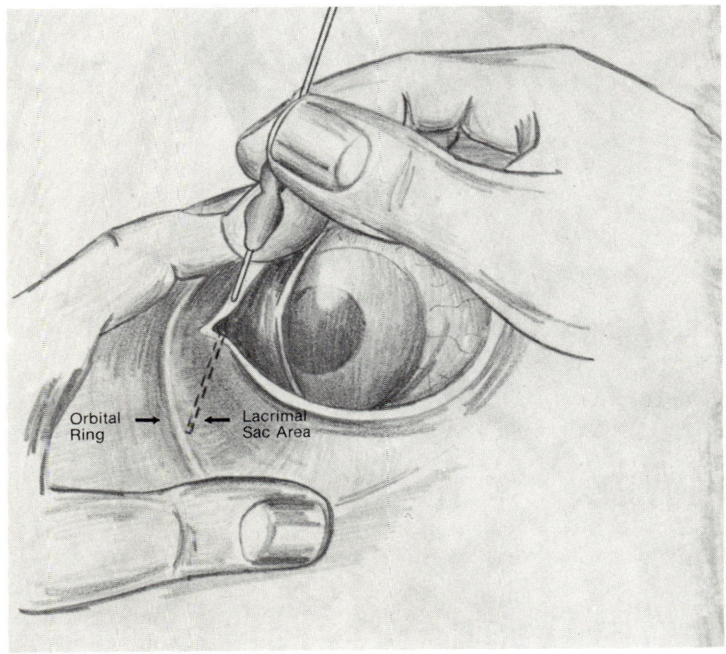

Fig. 4–36. Cut away view of probe extending to lacrimal sac area.

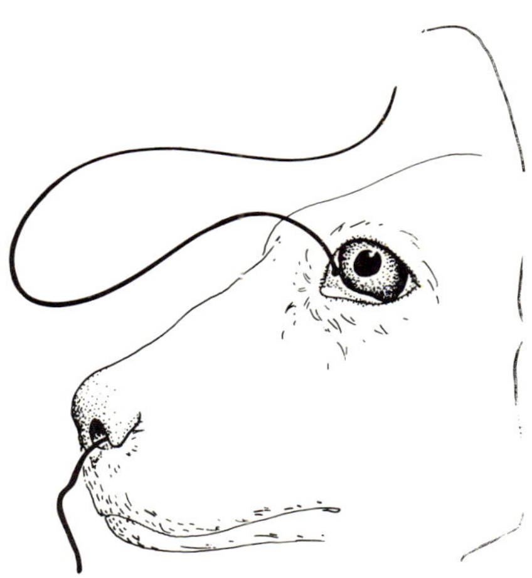

Fig. 4–37. Lateral view of the head showing monofilament nylon suture passed through the upper punctum and the lacrimal duct and emerging from the nose.

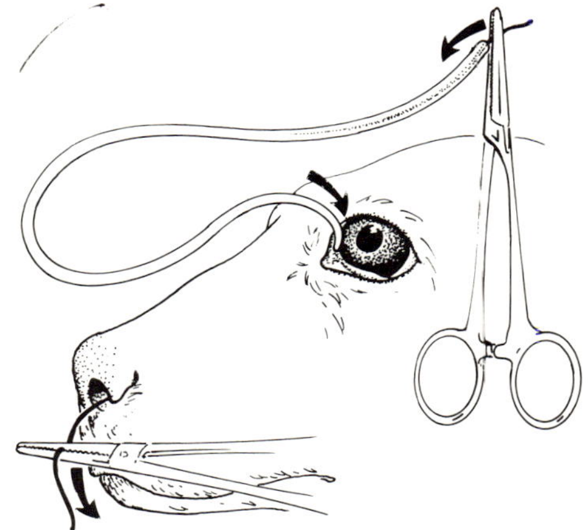

Fig. 4–38. Lateral view of the head with plastic tubing slipped over the monofilament catheter. A mosquito forceps is positioned on the catheter so that the tubing can be pulled into the upper punctum by applying traction with the forceps near the nose.

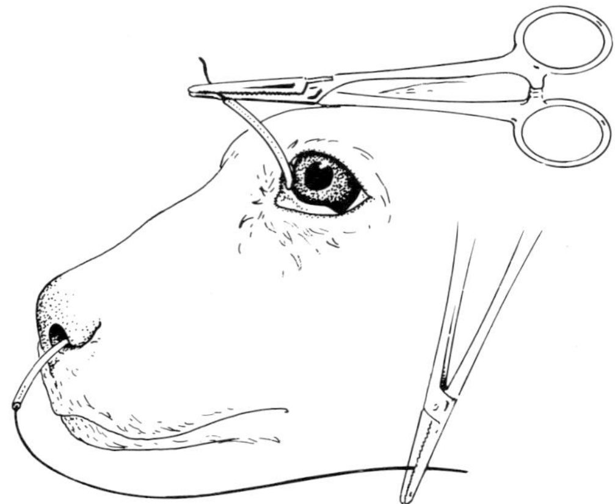

Fig. 4–39. Lateral view of the head with tubing pulled through the duct.

duct catheterization in treating acquired obstructions and chronic dacryocystitis. A 0 or 00 monofilament nylon suture is flamed to make a blunt point. This end is passed into the upper punctum, down the duct and out through the opening at the external nares (Fig. 4–37). Retention tubing is placed by slipping plastic tubing* over the suture and sliding it to the punctum. Next, mosquito hemostatic forceps are placed on the suture next to the tubing and where it comes out the nose (Fig. 4–38). Traction is then applied to the forceps near the nose. This pulls the tubing through the duct (Fig. 4–39). After the tubing is in place, the suture is slipped out. Knots are tied in the end of the tubing and it is sutured to the face (Fig. 4–40). The tubing is left for 2 to 3 weeks. During this time the lower punctum is flushed daily until the discharge stops. The eye is medicated with an antibiotic-corticosteroid solution.

*PE 50 or 90. Intramedic Polyethylene (Clay Adams, Inc., New York, N.Y.).

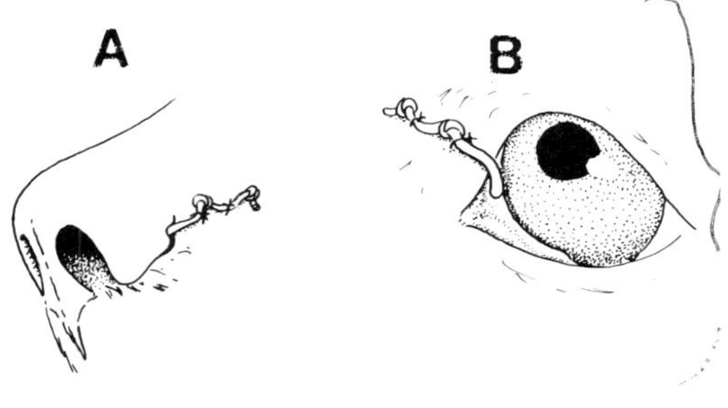

Fig. 4–40. The nose (A) and eye (B) with tubing sutured in place with nonabsorbable suture.

REFERENCES

1. Bedford, P.G.: Eyelashes and Adventitious Cilia as Causes of Corneal Irritation, J.S.A.P., *12*:11–17, 1971.
2. Berens, C. and King, H.J.: *An Atlas of Ophthalmic Surgery*, Philadelphia, J.B. Lippincott Co., p. 42, 1961.
3. Blodi, F.C. and Ramsey, F.K.: Ocular Tumors in Domestic Animals, A.J.O., *64*:627, 1967.
4. Blogg, R.: *The Eye in Veterinary Practice, Extraocular Diseases*, Philadelphia, W.B. Saunders Co., 1980.
5. Brightman, A.H., Helper, L.C.: Full Thickness Resection of the Eyelid, JAAHA, *14*:483–485, July/Aug, 1978.
6. Campbell, Karen: Personal Communication, Sept., 1987.
7. Covitz, D., Hunziker, J., Koch, S.A.: Conjunctivorhinostomy: A Surgical Method for the Control of Epiphora in the Dog and Cat, JAVMA, *171*:251, 1977.
8. Dörr, G.: Personal Communication. From a thesis, College of Veterinary Medicine, U. of Munich, W. Germany (1973).
9. Gelatt, K.N. et al.: Dacryocystorhinography in the Dog and Cat, J.S.A.P., *13*:381–397, 1972.
10. Gelatt, K.N.: Resection of Cilia-Bearing Tarsoconjunctiva for Correction of Canine Distichia, J.A.V.M.A., *155*:892, 1969.
11. Gelatt, K.N.: *Textbook of Ophthalmology*, Philadelphia, Lea & Febiger, Chapter 10, 1981.
12. Gross, S.L.: Effectiveness of a Modification of the Blogg Technique for Replacing the Gland of the Canine Third Eyelid, Trans. ACVO, 38–40, 1983.
13. Halliwell, W.H.: Surgical Management of Canine Distichia, J.A.V.M.A., *150*:874, 1967.
14. Hallstrom, M.: Mastocytoma in the Third Eyelid of a Dog, J.S.A.P., *11*:469–472, 1970.
15. Harrison, V.A.: Clinical Observations on Epiphora, Vet. Rec., *76*:437, 1964.
16. Helper, L.C.: The Effect of Lacrimal Gland Removal on the Conjunctiva and Cornea of the Dog, J.A.V.M.A., *157*:72–74, 1970.
17. Helper, L.C. and Magrane, W.G.: Ectopic Cilia of the Canine Eyelid, J. Sm. An. Pract., *11*:185, 1970.
18. Helper, L.C., Magrane, W.G., *et al.*: Surgical Induction of Keratoconjunctivitis Sicca in the Dog, J.A.V.M.A., *165*:172–174, 1974.
19. Kerpsack, R.W. and Kerpsack, W.R.: The Orbital Gland and Tear-staining in the Dog, VM/SAC, *61*:121, 1966.
20. Krehbiel, J.D. and Langham, R.F.: Eyelid Neoplasms of Dogs, Am. J. Vet. Res., *36*:115–119, 1975.
21. Magrane, W.G.: Ocular Physiology, No. Am. Vet., *36*:388, 1955.
22. Martin, C.L.: Everted Membrane Nictitans in German Shorthaired Pointers, J.A.V.M.A., *157*:1229–1232, 1970.
23. Muller, G.H., Amitraz Treatment of Demodicosis, JAAHA, *19*:435–441, 1988.
24. Muller, G. and Kirk, R.: *Small Animal Dermatology*, 2nd Ed., Philadelphia, W.B. Saunders Co., 1976.
25. Peiffer, R.C., Gelatt, K.N., Gwin, R.M.: Inferior

Medial Entropion as a Cause of Epiphora and Its Correction in the Dog, J. Can. Pract., 5:27, 1978.

26. Prince, J.H., Diesem, C.D., Eglitis, I. and Ruskell, G.L.: *Anatomy and Histology of the Eye and Orbit in Domestic Animals*, Springfield, Charles C Thomas, 1960.
27. Riis, R.C.: Basal Meibomian Gland Cautery, A Surgical Technique for Distichiasis, Proceedings of ISVO/ASVO meeting, Las Vegas, NV, 88–93, 1982.
28. Roberts, S.R.: Abnormal Tear Secretion in the Dog, Mod. Vet. Practice *43*:37, 1962.
29. Severin, G.A.: Nasolacrimal Duct Catheterization in the Dog, J.A.A.H.A., *8*:13–16, 1972.
30. Severin, G.A.: Veterinary Ophthalmology Notes, 2nd Ed., Ft. Collins, Colorado State University Publications Service, 107, 1976.
31. Symposium on Granulomatous Diseases—Part I: J.A.V.M.A., *127*:334, 1955.
32. Teichert, G.: Plasmazellulare Infiltration des dritten Augenlides beim Hund, Berl. Münch. tier. Wschr., *79*:449, 1966.
33. Thun, R., Abraham, R.S., Helper, L.C.: Effect of Tetracycline on Tear Production in the Dog, J.A.A.H.A., *11*:802–804, 1975.
34. Wheeler, C.A., Severin, G.A.: Cryosurgical Epilation for the Treatment of Distichiasis in the Dog and Cat, JAAHA, *20*:877–884, Nov/Dec, 1984.
35. Wyman, M.: Lateral Canthoplasty, J.A.A.H.A., 7:196, 1971.
36. Yakely, W.L. and Alexander, J.E.: Dacryocystorhinography in the Dog, J.A.V.M.A., *159*:1417–1421, 1971.

5

DISEASES AND SURGERY OF THE CONJUNCTIVA

Anatomy and Physiology

5:1 The conjunctiva is a mucous membrane composed of an epithelial layer and a substantia propria. The bulbar portion covers the eyeball except for the cornea, and is reflected at the fornix to form the palpebral conjunctiva which covers the third eyelid and lines the upper and lower eyelids. Except for the tarsal plate of the lids, and near the limbus on the globe, the subconjunctival tissue is areolar and the conjunctiva is freely moveable which allows for mobility of the eyeball. The firm adherence of the conjunctiva, Tenon's capsule and the sclera at the limbus makes surgical separation of these structures difficult in this area.

5:2 The multilayered columnar epithelium of the palpebral portion of the conjunctiva contains mucus producing goblet cells more numerous toward the fornices of the conjunctival cul-de-sac than near the lid margins or limbus.

5:3 The substantia propria consists of two layers: (1) the adenoid layer and (2) the fibrous layer. The fibrous layer is closely adherent to the subconjunctival tissue and could be classed with it. The adenoid layer is a fibrous network infiltrated with aggregates of lymphocytes and a few mast cells and histocytes. One author[21] suggests that the conjunctiva could be viewed as a lymph node split and lined with epithelium. Proliferation of lymphocytes in the adenoid layer is a normal defense response of the conjunctiva. The adenoid layer is not present in the newborn. In the human, it begins to develop at 2 to 3 months of age. The absence of the layer is one reason the conjunctiva of the newborn is not as resistant to infection.

5:4 The nerve supply to the conjunctiva (and cornea) from the first and second divisions of the trigeminal nerve is also important in the conjunctival-corneal defense system. These sensory nerves by reflex action initiate tear secretion and the blink reflex when irritated by any noxious substance or tactile stimulation.

5:5 The thin and nearly transparent nature of the conjunctiva allows easy observation of the blood vessels of the conjunctiva and visualization of the subconjunctival episcleral vessels. Hyperemia of the conjunctival vessels is an essential feature of a red eye commonly and often erroneously termed "conjunctivitis." Differentiating conjunctival and episcleral (ciliary) hyperemia is essential in assessing the cause and seriousness of a red eye. Six signs that are helpful in such assessment are as follows:

(1) *Distribution of vessels.* Conjunctival vessels are more intense at the fornix and fade out toward the limbus. Ciliary injection is most intense at the limbus.

(2) *Branching of vessels.* Conjunctival vessels branch profusely; ciliary vessels radiate out from the limbus with little branching.

(3) *Movability.* Conjunctival vessels move when the conjunctiva is moved; ciliary vessels remain stationary with the conjunctiva moving over them.

(4) *Color.* Conjunctival vessels are bright red; ciliary are deep red or violet.
(5) *Direction of blood flow.* Conjunctival vessels—fornix to limbus; ciliary—limbus to fornix. Place a finger on a vessel and slide it toward the fornix to empty the vessels. Conjunctival vessels will not refill immediately behind the finger, ciliary vessels will.
(6) *Possible extension into the cornea.* Conjunctival vessels are superficial and cross the limbus onto the cornea. Episcleral ciliary vessels appear to stop short of the limbus. Ciliary vessels extending into the cornea appear as short straight vessels that appear to originate at the limbus.

5:6 Hyperemia of ciliary vessels is a common sign in serious eye diseases such as glaucoma, uveitis, or intraocular neoplasia. Hyperemia of conjunctival vessels, in addition to ciliary hyperemia, is not uncommon. It is, therefore, important to determine whether there is ciliary hyperemia, *in addition to* conjunctival hyperemia, not just which is most obvious. Ciliary hyperemia is an indication for a thorough eye examination and careful monitoring of response to treatment. *Deep vascular hyperemia often implies deep trouble in the eye.*

5:7 Conjunctival hyperemia can be active or passive. Causes of active hyperemia include:
(1) *Direct irritation.* Wind, dust, bright light, extreme heat or cold. A deficient tear film may aggravate the irritation.
(2) *Reflex irritation.* Paroxysmal conjunctival hyperemia and recurrent transient conjunctival or ciliary hyperemia caused by irritation of the trigeminal nerve due to sinus infection, tooth infection, etc. has been reported in man.
(3) *Primary vasodilation.* Vasodilator drugs, inhalation of oxygen or paresis of sympathetic nerves, causing loss of adrenergic vasoconstrictor effect in the conjunctiva, such as caused by severing of the sympathetic trunk or the presence of a mediostinal or cervical tumor.
(4) *Skin diseases.* Lid tumors, Staphylococcal blepharitis, seborrhea of lid margins.
(5) *Local infection.* Infection of conjunctiva or cornea.
(6) *Systemic infection.* Conjunctival injection is common with many febrile infectious diseases.
(7) *Allergic conditions*

5:8 Passive hyperemia of the conjunctiva is the result of engorgement of the circulation from mechanical venous obstruction or increased viscosity of the circulating blood. Causes include:
(1) *Mechanical venous obstruction.* Glaucoma-pressure blocks anterior ciliary veins, causing them to be engorged. Uveal neoplasm may cause passive congestion of overlying area of sclera and conjunctiva.
(2) *Systemic diseases.* Generalized passive congestion due to heart failure; increased viscosity of blood due to polycythemia or increased plasma viscosity, such as in multiple myeloma or macroglobulinemia; marked increase in sedimentation rate associated with any cause.

5:9 In active hyperemia, the conjunctival vessels look bright red, and the dog most often exhibits signs of discomfort; whereas, in passive hyperemia, the vessels have a darker strangulated appearance, but discomfort is usually less obvious.

5:10 *Chemosis.* Edema of the conjunctiva occurs easily because of the loose subepithelial arrangement of the conjunctiva. Local or systemic allergic reactions or inflammation due to infection or trauma can cause sudden dramatic chemosis.

5:11 *Conjunctival Hemorrhage.* Hemorrhage, like chemosis, can be quite dramatic because of the loose arrangement of the conjunctiva. Minute hemorrhages can be easily seen, because blood vessels in the conjunctiva are so prominent. Trauma and acute inflammation are common causes, while thrombocytopenic purpura and other hemorrhagic blood dyscrasias should be considered in obscure cases. Petechial hemorrhages in the conjunctiva can also be caused by any of several of the infectious diseases.

CONGENITAL DISEASES

5:12 *Dermoid Cyst.* This congenital tumor may involve the conjunctiva alone (Plate 5G), the conjunctiva, subconjunctival and adjacent subcutaneous tissue of the lid (Fig. 4:33A) or the conjunctiva and cornea (Plate 6A). The mass is usually dark brown to black and contains variable number of hair follicles with hairs growing from them. The caruncle at the medial canthus that may contain a few hair follicles in some breeds, especially, St. Bernards, should not be mistaken for a conjunctival dermoid.

5:13 *Treatment.* Excision of a conjunctival dermoid is indicated if the tumor is causing ocular discharge or discomfort, or if it is considered unsightly by the owner.

INFLAMMATION

5:14 Conjunctivitis can range from a single, self-limiting inflammation to a protracted inflammation that challenges the diagnostic and therapeutic ability of the practitioner. Careful examination with at least 2.5× magnification, plus the use of conjunctival scraping and culture techniques, will aid immeasurably in establishing rational therapy. The use of the Schirmer tear test is essential in evaluating tear production, since diminished tear production is a common primary cause or contributing factor in many cases of protracted conjunctivitis.

Conjunctivitis—General Considerations

5:15 Because of its exposed position the conjunctiva comes in contact with more microorganisms than any other mucous membrane.[19] Thus, conjunctivitis is the commonest of all eye diseases encountered. It is well, however, to rule out an accompanying keratitis, glaucoma and iritis as the conjunctival changes are marked and may be misleading in these diseases.

5:16 In general most of the cases of conjunctivitis are caused by bacterial or virus infection, contact allergens, irritation from foreign bodies or chemical substances and trauma. Decreased tear production is a common cause of protracted conjunctivitis and should always be considered. An etiologic diagnosis is not always easy. Often distinctive clinical signs which are diagnostic in the early stages of a disease have disappeared by the time the dog is presented for treatment. In these instances the clinical examination must be supplemented with laboratory studies if the etiology of the condition is to be determined.

5:17 The use of conjunctival scrapings and smears as an aid in diagnosis and treatment has been well documented by Cello[5] and others. Smears are samples of the exudate found in the conjunctival sac, while scrapings are really limited biopsies in which cells of the conjunctiva are removed and examined. In preparing a scraping, a small platinum spatula is held at right angles to the conjunctiva and drawn over the surface lightly enough to avoid bleeding, but firmly enough to contact the epithelium. It is convenient to combine smears and scrapings on different sections of the same slide.

5:18 Two slides are prepared so that both a Gram stain and a Giemsa stain can be made. Cello[5] emphasizes the importance of having a standardized method of making the Giemsa preparation since the stain is very sensitive and it is possible to get wide color variations on scrapings from the same eye if the time, concentration, or pH of the stain is changed. Since color differences are used as criteria for degenerative changes, technical errors can lead to false interpretations. A method which has proved satisfactory is as follows:

1. Fix the smear in acetone-free methyl alcohol for 15 minutes.
2. Flood the smear with stain which has been prepared by adding 1 drop of the

Giemsa stock solution to each ml of glass distilled water (pH 7.0–7.1). Stain for 1 hour.
3. Decolorize in 95% alcohol for 5 seconds.
4. Air dry and examine.

5:19 The slides are examined for the presence, number and type of bacteria, changes in the epithelial cells, and number and type of leukocytes. Bacteria are rarely seen in scrapings taken from normal conjunctiva and infrequently in smears made from secretions found in the sac. This is in contrast to surveys in which studies of cultures revealed a small percentage of sterile eyes.[5,6,10] Cello[5] believes that these apparent discrepancies might be explained on the basis of small numbers of bacteria existing in the healthy conjunctival sac.

5:20 In conjunctivitis, smears and scrapings show an increased number of bacteria, epithelial changes, and an infiltration of leukocytes with or without tissue cells. Scrapings most frequently show only one type of organism and are more accurate than are cultures and smears as a means of determining the bacterium most likely to be primarily involved in the infection.

5:21 Conjunctival scrapings also enable the clinician to evaluate results of treatment. The presence of keratinized cells, goblet cells, bacteria, and leukocytes in an eye which has been under treatment indicates a need for a change in therapy. This is particularly true in infections which show frequent remissions and exacerbations.

5:22 Bistner[1] describes a method of culturing bacteria from the inferior conjunctival cul-de-sac and lower lid. The technique uses moist, sterile swabs and blood agar and mannitol plates as isolating media. He is of the opinion that the wet swab method offers a better bacteria recovery than the dry method. The lower lid is everted (palpebral surface), a wet swab taken and streaked on the two plates. No topical anesthetic should be used because they are often bactericidal. A lid margin swab is also taken and the same plates inoculated in two areas. Commercially prepared swabs* prepared with a transport medium in a modified ampule within the sterile container are convenient to use.[8] Crush the ampule of transport media prior to removing the swab to moisten the tip. Plating should be done immediately. Bacteria collected are often few in number and may die if left in the transport media to be plated later.

5:23 Studies vary as to type and percentage of bacteria isolated from the conjunctival sacs of clinically normal dogs.[6,17,18] Most agree that bacteria are often present on the conjunctiva or lids of over 50% of dogs, and that staphylococcus albus is commonly present. The utilization of different techniques, breed selection, and time of year undoubtedly influenced these findings.

5:24 Organisms frequently isolated included *S. albus*, *S. aureus*, *alpha-hemolytic streptococci*, *diphtheroids*, *Neisseria* spp., *Pseudomonas* spp., nonhemolytic streptococci and beta-hemolytic streptococci. The bacteria isolated are the ones usually incriminated in disease so clinical judgment has to be made as to their significance. Other factors involving the host would be expected to produce clinical signs of disease. These include the virulence and numbers of organisms, the animal's resistance, and associated local or systemic conditions. Antibiotic sensitivity tests can be conducted in further diagnosis and selection for treatment.

5:25 In clinical evaluation of an inflamed eye, one should keep in mind the old adage, *Conjunctivitis itches, keratitis hurts*, and be especially careful in examining for corneal irritation or injury and for intraocular disease when blepharospasm, photophobia or other evidence of eye pain is present.

5:26 There are several changes in the conjunctiva that occur in the development of conjunctivitis:

(1) *Active hyperemia*—as mentioned earlier (Par. 5:7) is an early change in response to nearly any external stimuli.

---

*Culturette. (Scientific Products, Evanston, Ill.)

(2) *Papillary hypertrophy* of the conjunctiva in which there is thickening of the conjunctiva and increased vascularity, gives the conjunctiva a less transparent red velvety appearance.
(3) *Increased mucus production*—occurs due to stimulation of the goblet cells present in the conjunctival epithelium and from proliferation of goblet cells.
(4) *Proliferation of lymph follicles.* A small cluster of lymph follicles in the conjunctiva on the inner surface of the third eyelid is normal. Development of lymph follicles on the outer surface of the third eyelid on the bulbar conjunctiva or in the upper or lower fornix, in addition to proliferation at the normal sites, is not uncommon in conjunctivitis, since lymphocyte proliferation is one defense mechanism. Lymphocyte proliferation is especially common in chronic or persistent allergic conjunctivitis. Infiltration by neutrophils is common in bacterial infections, but can also occur in severe conjunctivitis of most any cause.

5:27 Conjunctivitis has been classified in many ways. The following discussion of conjunctivitis is organized by type of discharge present. A general discussion is followed by a discussion of specific types of conjunctivitis causing the discharge.

5:28 *Catarrhal Discharge.* Conjunctivitis with this type of discharge, increased tear production and/or mucus production accompanying active hyperemia. Follicular conjunctivitis is a specific clinical type of conjunctivitis causing this type of discharge.

5:29 *Etiology.* One should first consider the causes listed under active hyperemia. All listed except perhaps local bacterial infections, which generally cause a purulent discharge, should be considered. In persistent cases, especially if discharge is minimal, conjunctival scrapings should be used to detect whether inflammation is present or if just hyperemia is present. An increase in mucus production is often the first sign of diminishing tear production, so a Schirmer tear test should be accomplished in all persistent cases. It is also important to observe closely for entropion distichiasis, ectopic cilia or other mechanical factors that cause irritation.

5:30 *Treatment.* In many cases, acute cataractal type of conjunctivitis recovery would occur without treatment, but since potentially pathogenic bacteria are present in the conjunctival sac of many dogs,[18] it is best to treat the animal with antibiotic drops or ointment for 4 to 5 days. If allergy is considered to be the primary cause, steroid-antibiotic drops or ointment is indicated.

5:31 *Follicular Conjunctivitis.* A persistent grayish mucoid discharge from an eye that appears normal on casual observation is a classic sign of follicular conjunctivitis. Close examination, however, reveals hypertrophy of lymphoid follicles on the inner surface of the third eyelid, and perhaps some follicle formation in the outer surface of the third eyelid and in the upper or lower fornix. (Plate 4C).

5:32 *Etiology.* Nearly any prolonged irritation of the eye is capable of stimulating lymphoid follicle proliferation. Common causes include pollens and other allergens, dust or other irritants and previous infection, since these lymphoid follicles are centers of antibody production ready to react when stimulated. The antigen antibody interaction that results is, at least in part, responsible for the inflammation. In many instances, the major cause of the initial stimulation of the follicle development is gone, or can be eliminated with proper management, but the eye is still reactive and capable of response to minor stimulation. This minor stimulation results in protracted low-grade inflammation and mucus production.

5:33 *Treatment.* Debriding the follicles with a curette, or the end of the handle of a Bard-Parker scalpel or other blunt instrument is helpful in removing these centers of antigen-antibody reaction (Fig. 5–1). Debridement should be followed by 7 to 10 days of topical steroid antibiotic ophthalmic ointment therapy. The steroid-antibiotic therapy

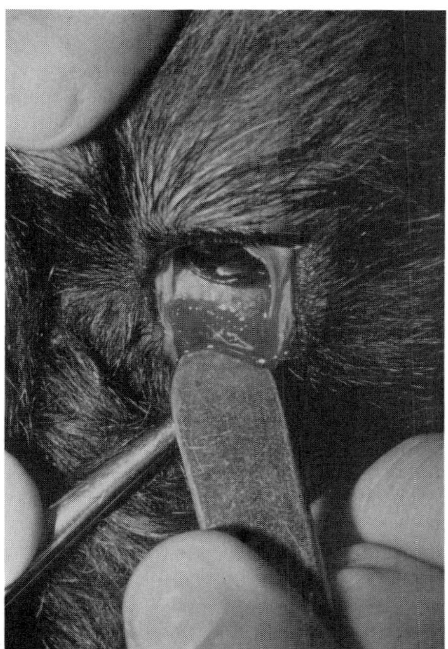

Fig. 5–1. Debriding follicles on the inner surface of the third eyelid with the end of a Bard-Parker scalpel handle can be accomplished after two instillations of topical anesthesia.

alone is adequate in mild cases, but rapid recurrence after therapy is discontinued is common in severe cases when topical therapy alone is used. Continued topical therapy may be needed in cases continually exposed to an allergen. Recurrence may be seasonal.

5:34 *Mucopurulent or Purulent Discharge.* Purulent discharge implies exudation of serum, fibrin and inflammatory cells from the conjunctiva and conjunctival blood vessels, in addition to the mucus production and tear secretion (if present). There is also increased desquamation of epithelial cells from the conjunctiva, and these materials combined, make up the discharge.

5:35 *Etiology.* Although other causes of severe inflammation could result in a mucopurulent or purulent discharge, bacterial infection is by far the most common cause. Since the defense mechanisms of the conjunctival sac are normally quite effective in preventing infections, one should examine carefully for factors that lower such defense. These factors include systemic diseases, eyelid deformities, obstructed nasolacrimal duct—especially if accompanied by infection in the duct (dacryocystitis)—conjunctival foreign bodies and diminished tear production.

5:36 *Treatment.* If careful evaluation reveals no inciting or aggravating cause, antibiotic ophthalmic ointment applied 2 to 4 times a day or antibiotic drops applied at least 4 times a day should be applied for 7 days. Neomycin, bacitracin-polymixin, or chloromycetin-polymycin combinations are good, because they have a broad therapeutic spectrum. I prefer to reserve the use of chloromycetin for cases where specifically indicated because of the slight risk to the owner. If the nasolacrimal duct is occluded and a concurrent dacryocystitis is present, treatment will not be successful unless the dacryocystitis and occluded duct are also treated (Par. 4:108). If the tear production is diminished, treatment for keratoconjunctivitis sicca (Par. 6:71) should be instituted.

5:37 In unresponsive cases, culture for bacteria and fungi and antibiotic sensitivity should be accomplished. In addition, conjunctival scrapings should be prepared and examined (Par. 5:17–5:24).

5:38 *Chronic Purulent Conjunctivitis or Keratoconjunctivitis.* There appears to be a syndrome in dogs, primarily Cocker Spaniels and English Bulldogs, in which chronic conjunctivitis or keratoconjunctivitis occurs in conjunction with generalized seborrhea and chronic ceruminous otitis. The syndrome starts in middle-aged dogs as a purulent or mucopurulent conjunctivitis. Superficial corneal ulcers may be a concurrent problem and vascularization and melanin infiltration of the cornea develops as the ulcers heal, or more insidiously without a history of ulceration. Whereas the tear production as measured by the Schirmer tear test is normal early in the disease, it gradually diminishes over several months or even longer, and keratoconjunctivitis sicca becomes a part of the problem. Staphylococcus aureus, Beta hemolytic streptococcus and occasionally other bacteria are isolated on culture of the conjunctiva.

5:39 One author[21] suggests that there is a seborrheic blepharitis and staphylococcal blepharoconjunctivitis and epithelial erosions of the cornea in man associated with seborrhea. Another author[3] suggests that in these cases of seborrhea the meibomian gland secretion can be irritating to the cornea and conjunctiva and that this abnormal meibomian gland secretion is the underlying cause of the syndrome he terms the *Triple S syndrome:* 1. Seborrheic staphylococcal blepharoconjunctivitis, 2. *Sicca* (Keratoconjunctivitis sicca) and 3. Superficial (punctate) keratitis.

5:40 *Treatment.* The goal of treatment should be to control the conjunctival and corneal disease while determining the cause, and establishing treatment for the seborrhea and ceruminous otitis. Since in many cases, the underlying cause of the skin disease cannot be eliminated or the disease even completely controlled, it is often necessary to establish long-term treatment for control rather than elimination of the eye disease. Examination should include culture and antibiotic sensitivity, and, of course, evaluation of tear production. Initial treatment should consist of neomycin- bacitracin- polymycin ophthalmic ointment 3 times a day, following thorough cleansing of the conjunctiva and lids with eyewash. If sensitivity testing reveals no resistant bacteria, topical steroids and/or a subconjunctival injection of 5 mg Kenalog or Depo-Medrol should be given if corneal vascularity and melanosis is present. Continued topical medication with antibiotic-steroid drops once or twice a day, in addition to cleansing the lids and conjunctiva of the now minimal discharge, is often needed indefinitely, unless the underlying disease process, causing the skin, ear, and eye disease, is alleviated. If tear production is subnormal, treatment for keratoconjunctivitis sicca, including parotid duct transposition, should be considered, with realization that restoring tear production will not alone alleviate all of the corneal and conjunctival disease. A general work up of the skin disease, including thyroid function tests should be conducted, and the skin disease treated. Systemic treatment to alleviate the seborrhea, if indicated, may help the eye disease as well.

Ophthalmia Neonatorum

5:41 An acute purulent conjunctivitis occurs in the newborn puppy before lid separation takes place. The lid area appears swollen and an exudate is soon noted exuding from a small lid opening (Fig. 5–2). Both eyes are usually involved. If the condition is not recognized early or is left untreated, severe corneal infection and perforation may result with a subsequent iris prolapse and loss of an eye.

5:42 *Treatment.* It is imperative that, on noting the first symptoms, a lid separation is performed. This is easily accomplished with a muscle hook or other blunt instrument inserted at the medial canthus (Fig. 5–2). Slight traction will cause separation at the lid junction. Using scissors or other sharp instruments should be avoided, because the lids may be damaged. By thus exposing the conjunctival surfaces and globe, topical antibiotic therapy can be instituted. The prognosis then is generally favorable. Ophthalmia neonatorum sometimes accompanies a generalized

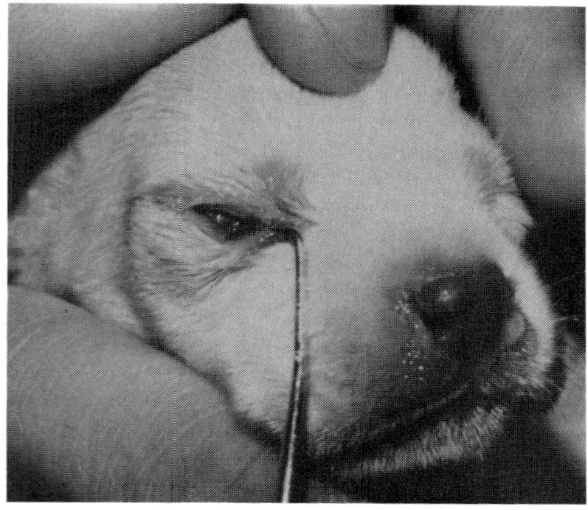

Fig. 5–2. Ophthalmia neonatorum. Note the discharge around the right eye just after opening with a muscle hook, and the swelling of the still closed left eye.

septicemia in puppies, so examine the rest of the puppy as well.

Other Conditions of the Conjunctiva

Inflammatory Hyperplasia (Plate 5H)

5:43 An apparent allergen-producing inflammatory process resembling pterygium of man results in a conjunctival encroachment and overgrowth onto the cornea. There appears to be a predisposition to its occurrence in the collie breed, especially those kept in an outdoor environment with above average exposure to sunlight.

5:44 *Treatment.* In the early stages use of the steroids by subconjunctival injection (Par. 3:65) and topical instillation will cause regression and clearing. If there is considerable corneal involvement (Fig. 5–3 and Plate 4D), a superficial keratectomy is indicated (Par. 6:166). It may be necessary to continue steroids indefinitely to prevent recurrence. Severe cases may require systemic steroids to maintain regression.

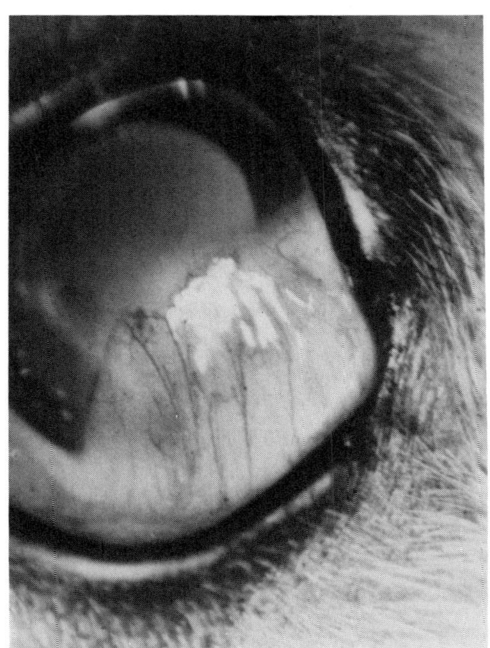

Fig. 5–3. Pterygium-like lesion invading the superficial cornea.

Injuries

5:45 *Foreign bodies.* Weed seeds, awns and other loosely attached or imbedded conjunctival foreign bodies are not uncommon, especially behind the third eyelid of hunting dogs. A conjunctival discharge, usually unilateral and accompanied by ocular discomfort are the usual signs. Removal can usually be accomplished with thumb forceps following instillation of topical anesthesia. An antibiotic ointment should be instilled for 4 to 7 days.

5:46 *Wounds.* The conjunctiva heals quite rapidly if uncomplicated by infection. Torn conjunctiva adheres within 1 hour to the episcleral tissue and healing begins by sliding of cells from the conjunctiva adjacent to the injury. In 24 hours, epithelial proliferation begins, and a smooth layer of conjunctiva covers the defect in a few days. It may be advisable to suture large tears in the conjunctiva, but use of an antibiotic ointment or drops to prevent infection is all that is required in most cases. Conjunctival wounds should be examined closely for retained penetrating foreign bodies.

5:47 *Symblepharon* (Fig. 5–4) (Plate 3E). The rapid healing properties of the conjunctiva can lead to adhesion of the bulbar to the

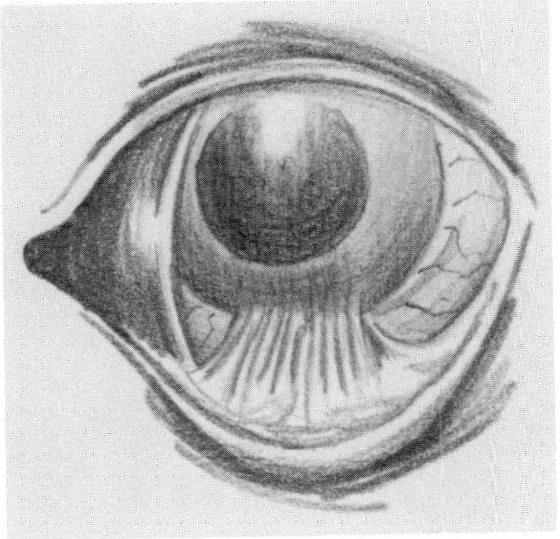

Fig. 5–4. Symblepharon (adhesion of bulbar to palpebral conjunctiva).

palpebral conjunctiva or palpebral conjunctiva to the cornea, if raw surfaces remain in contact following injury or severe infection. Small adhesions can be severed and reformation discouraged by movement and application of antibiotic ointment. A buccal mucosa graft can be used for repair in the cases of extensive symblepharon.

5:48 The first step in the repair of an eye in this condition (symblepharon) is to loosen and dissect away the scarred and vascularized tissue from the underlying sclera until the globe rotates freely. The defect is then lined with a thin graft of buccal mucous membrane. The graft is sutured to the adjacent conjunctiva with interrupted 5–0 catgut, all stitches being *anchored* to the sclera to prevent contraction of the graft.

5:49 The graft is easily obtained from inside the lip or from the gum (Fig. 5–5). The graft should be scraped and thinned down enough so that it consists only of epithelium and a minimum of supporting tissue.[4] Preparation and use of a graft in this manner may also be indicated in instances in which there is extensive loss of conjunctiva, *e.g.* wounds or following new growth removal.

Erosion of the Medial Canthus (Plate 5C)

5:50 A peculiar condition involving the conjunctiva (catarrhal discharge) and the lids and skin (erosion) has an obscure etiology. It is thought to be caused by a hypersensitivity reaction to tears but may have a bacterial component. A rather constant epiphora leads to ulceration or excoriation of the medial canthus, sometimes with destruction of the lower punctum.

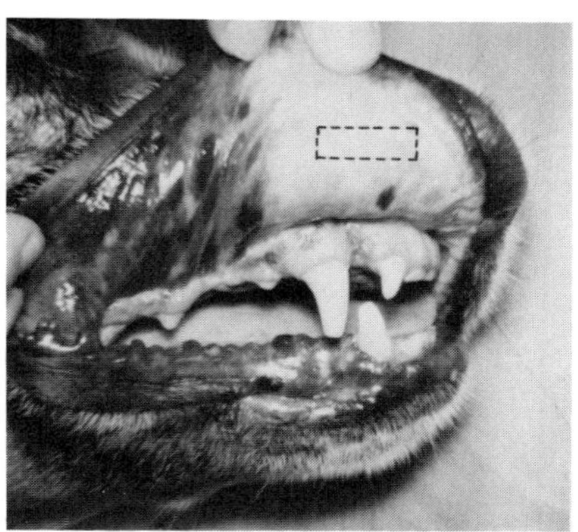

Fig. 5–5. Area from which a mucous membrane graft may be obtained.

5:51 *Treatment.* Correction of the epiphora is essential for long-term success. The causes of epiphora should be evaluated (Par. 4:71). If there is no apparent cause for excess tear production, and the lacrimal duct and lower punctum are patent, the procedure[15] for correction of medial canthus entropion should be considered. If the lower puncta has been eroded, one should conduct a Schirmer tear test to be certain that the value is over 20 mm/min; then, the gland of the third eyelid should be excised (Par. 4:51) to lower tear production.

Cysts

5:52 Inclusion cysts of the conjunctiva are rather uncommon. They may occur after inflammation or injury or may be of obscure etiology.

Parasites

5:53 Thalesia californiensis, a white thread-like nematode, is occasionally found in the conjunctival sac of dogs in the west coast states (Fig. 5–6). Lacrimation or a mucopurulent ocular discharge, blepharospasm and even a keratitis or a corneal ulcer may be found. The parasites can easily be seen, especially with 2.5× magnification. Infections have been reported in sheep, deer, horse, cat, dog, coyote, bear, and humans. The house fly of the genus Muscus or Fannia probably serves as the intermediate host.[4]

Treatment. Mechanical removal by flushing or with forceps after application of topical anesthesia can be accomplished in most cases. Aftercare consists of symptomatic treatment of the conjunctivitis and keratitis if present.

Neoplasia

5:54 Neoplasms of the conjunctiva of the dog are much less common than neoplasms

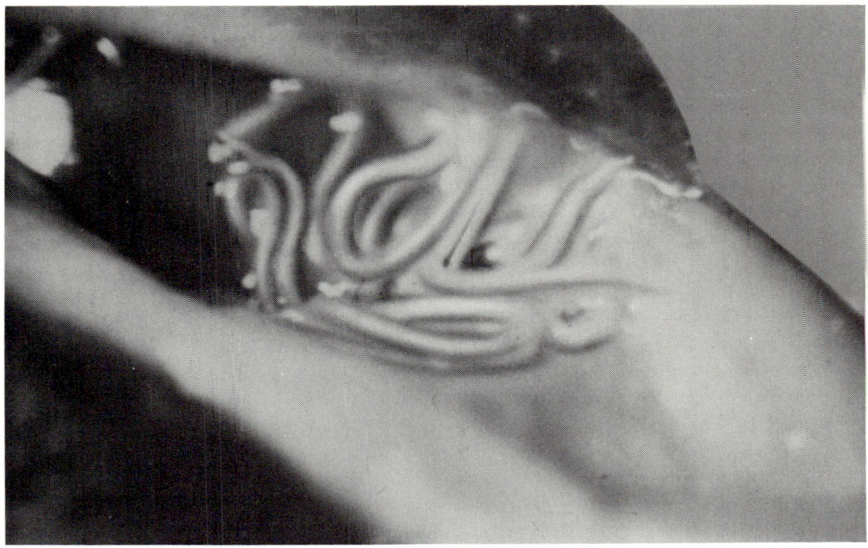

Fig. 5–6. Thelazia on the inner surface of the third eyelid. (Courtesy of Dr. William Zontine, Lancaster, Cal.)

of the lid or skin. Squamous cell carcinoma which is fairly common in the conjunctiva of the horse and cow does occur, but it is rare in the dog. Other tumors of the conjunctiva in the dog, including viral papilloma (Fig. 5–7), hemangioma, hemangiosarcoma and melanocytoma seem to occur more often in the bulbar conjunctiva than in the palpebral conjunctiva. One report suggested solar radiation was involved in the pathogenesis of squamous cell carcinomas, hemangiomas, and hemangiosarcomas of the conjunctiva in a colony of Beagles.[3] We have seen 3 subconjunctival mast cell tumors in the past 3 years, all presented as rapidly growing tumors under the conjunctiva (Plate 4E). The tumors had the gross appearance and consistency of a lipoma. No recurrence was reported in a 6 month or longer follow-up after surgical excision.

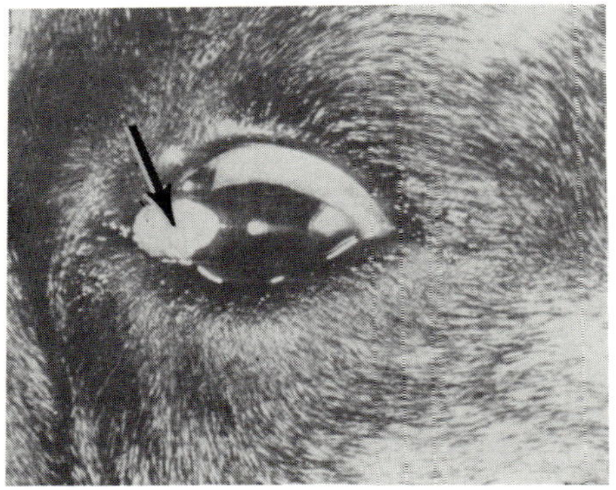

Fig. 5–7. Viral oral papilloma growing on the conjunctival covering of the membrane nictitans. (Courtesy of Dr. Wayne H. Riser, Philadelphia, Pa.)

Treatment. Because of the loose attachment of the bulbar conjunctiva neoplasm limited to the bulbar conjunctiva can be easily excised and the conjunctival wound closed with 6 ō catgut or other absorbable suture. Tumors of the palpebral conjunctiva may require more careful dissection and wound closure.

Conjunctival Flap Surgery

5:55 There are many conventional methods of separating the conjunctiva from the sclera and stretching it over a part or all of the cornea to cover a lesion. It becomes necessary in man to utilize the bulbar conjunctiva as such, but the veterinary surgeon has a real advantage in this respect in that the well-developed third eyelid of the dog can be used. There are few instances in which tra-

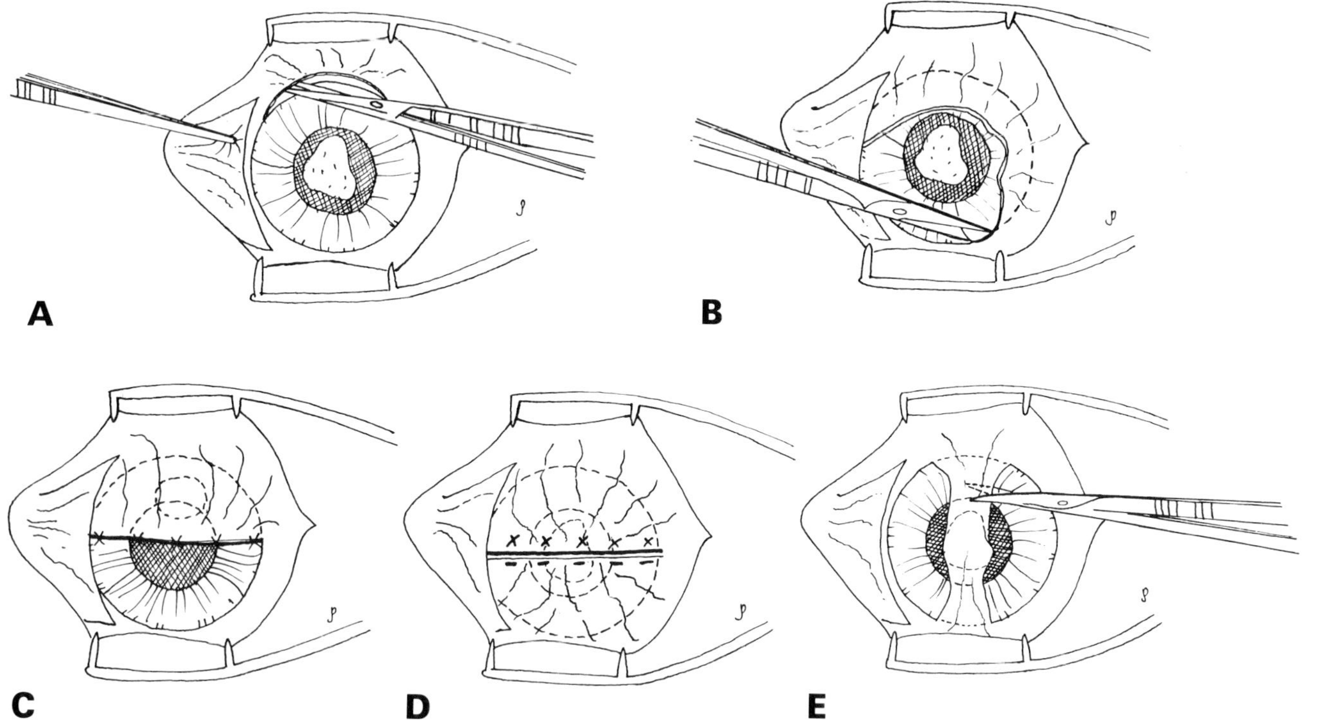

Fig. 5–8. *A.* For preparation of the hood (180 degrees) or complete (360 degrees) bulbar conjunctival flap, the conjunctiva is incised at the limbus. *B.* Continued dissection for the complete bulbar conjunctival flap; the conjunctiva is loosened from the episclera by alternating sharp-blunt action with ophthalmic scissors. *C.* For the hood (180 degrees) bulbar conjunctival flap, 4 to 6 6-0 nonabsorbable simple interrupted sutures anchor the leading margin of the conjunctiva directly to the cornea. *D.* Either 4 to 5 interrupted mattress sutures or a single purse-string 5-0 or 6-0 nonabsorbable suture is used to appose the dorsal and ventral bulbar conjunctiva for the complete bulbar conjunctival flap. *E.* After removal of sutures from the complete bulbar conjunctival flap, the conjunctiva is adherent to the corneal ulcer site. The remaining conjunctiva is transected, leaving a small graft in the corneal defect.

ditional conjunctival flap procedures must be used in the dog, *e.g.* when the third eyelid has been removed, or is an advantage to provide tissue to 'patch' an extensive thinned area of the cornea. Several procedures have been described for use in the dog.[2,7] The complete (360 degree) or the hood (180 degree) flap (Fig. 5–8) may be used, depending on the size and shape of the corneal defect.

If being used as a "patch," the flap should be left in place 3 to 4 weeks before being released or trimmed (Fig. 5–8E).

REFERENCES

1. Bistner, S., et al.: Conjunctival Bacteria, M.V.P., *50*:45, 1969.
2. Bistner, S.I., Aguirre, G.D., Batik, G.: *Atlas of Veterinary Ophthalmic Surgery,* Philadelphia, W.B. Saunders Co., 1977.
3. *Canine Medicine,* 2nd ed., Santa Barbara, American Veterinary Publications, Inc., p. 519, 1959.
4. Castroviejo, R.: Plastic and Reconstructive Surgery of the Conjunctiva, J. Plastic and Recons. Surgery, *24*:9, 1959.
5. Cello, R.M.: The Use of Conjunctival Scrapings in the Diagnosis and Treatment of External Diseases of the Eye, Gaines Vet. Symp., Oct. 24, 1956.
6. Correa, W.M., et al.: Canine Conjunctivitis, J.A.V.M.A., *138*:503, 1961.
7. Gelatt, K.N.: *Veterinary Ophthalmology,* Philadelphia, Lea & Febiger, 1981, pp. 340–341.
8. Helper, L.: Diagnostic Techniques in Conjunctivitis and Keratitis, Vet. Clin. No. Am., *3*:357–365, 1973.
9. Helper, L.C., Blogg, R.: A Modified Third Eyelid Flap Procedure, JAAHA, *19*:955–956, Nov/Dec, 1983.
10. Jones, G.W.: A Preliminary Report of the Flora in Health and Disease of the External Ear and Conjunctival Sac of the Dog, J.A.V.M.A., *127*:443, 1955.
11. Knapp, S.E., et al.: Thelaziasis in Cats and Dogs, J.A.V.M.A., *138*:537, 1961.
12. Magrane, W.G.: An Evaluation of the Use of Antibiotics in Canine Ophthalmology, No. Am. Vet., *32*:169, 1951.
13. Magrane, W.G.: The Clinical Use of Chloromycetin in Canine Ocular Infections, No. Am. Vet., *34*:39, 1953.
14. Olsen, O.W.: *Animal Parasites: Their Biology and Life Cycles,* Minneapolis, Burgess Publishing Co., 1962, p. 296.
15. Peiffer, R.L., Gelatt, K.N., Gwin, R.M.: Inferior Medial Entropion as a Cause of Epiphora and Its Correction in the Dog, J. Canine Practice, 5:27, 1978.
16. Spaeth, E.B.: *Principles and Practice of Ophthalmic Surgery,* 4th ed., Philadelphia, Lea & Febiger, p. 607, 1948.
17. Stone, A.B. and Schrock, J.E.: Bacterial Conjunctivitis in the Dog, J.A.A.H.A., *8*:10–12, 1972.
18. Urban, Marie, Wyman, M., et al.: Conjunctival Flora of Clinically Normal Dogs, J.A.V.M.A., *161*:201–206, 1972.
19. Vaughan, D., Cook, R. and Asbury, T.: *General Ophthalmology,* 3rd ed., Los Altos, Lange Medical Publications, 1962.
20. Verwer, M.A.J. and Gunnink, J.W.: The Occurrence of Bacteria in Chronic Purulent Eye Discharge, J.S.A.P., 9:33, 1968.
21. Duke-Elder, Sir S.: System of Ophthalmology VIII, Part 1&2, St. Louis, C.V. Mosby Co., 1965.

6

DISEASES AND SURGERY OF THE CORNEA AND SCLERA

THE CORNEA

Anatomy

6:1 The cornea is the clear, transparent, anterior segment of the external fibrous tunic of the eyeball. It is almost circular and, like the globe as a whole, it varies in dimensions among breeds. The diameter will vary from 12.5 to 17 mm and there is seldom more than 1 mm difference in the vertical and horizontal meridional measurements. The vertical meridian has the smaller dimension. The radius of curvature is usually about 8 mm. The thickness varies from about .6 to .95 mm.

6:2 (1) The cornea in the dog has but four distinct layers (Fig. 6–1): *epithelium* (0.08 mm thick); *stroma* (substantia propria) (0.5 to 0.6 mm thick); *Descemet's* membrane, which is about four times the thickness of the endothelium; and, *endothelium*, which is just one row of cells. Oda and Fukuda[62] were unable to recognize Bowman's membrane (as in man) by electron microscopic studies of the canine cornea. Other anatomists include a tear (precorneal) film and a basement membrane when counting corneal layers. (2) The tear film (Fig. 6–2), although not visible on histologic examination of a prepared section of the cornea, is extremely important for maintenance of corneal health and transparency. Insufficiency results in corneal and conjunctival inflammation—keratoconjunctivitis sicca (Par. 6:67). The tear film is 6 to 10 microns thick and is comprised of three layers: a superficial lipid layer, produced by the meibomian glands; a middle watery layer produced by the lacrimal gland and gland of the third eyelid (Par. 4:45); and a mucinous layer on the corneal epithelium produced by the goblet cells of the conjunctiva. Whereas the lipid layer is distinct, the mucinous and watery layers are somewhat intermixed.[35] The superficial oily layer helps prevent evaporation of the watery layer, and, because of its high surface tension, retards overflow at the lid margins. The mucoid layer serves to bind the aqueous layer to the cornea. The molecules are thought to be bipolar with a lipophilic end attaching to the corneal epithelium and a hydrophilic end having an affinity for water.

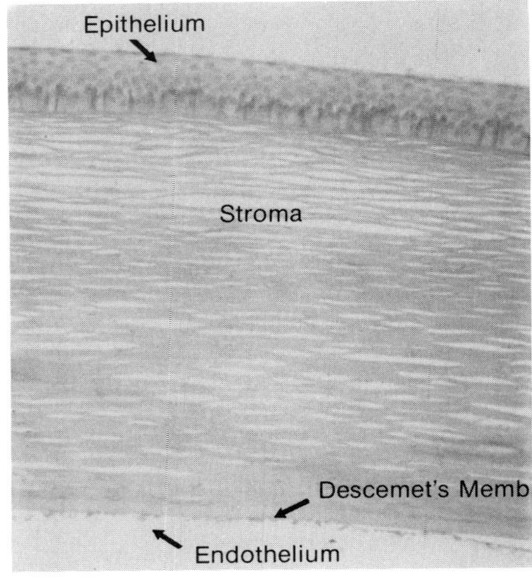

Fig. 6–1. Layers of the cornea 100×. (Courtesy of Dr. A. C. Andersen, Davis, Cal.)

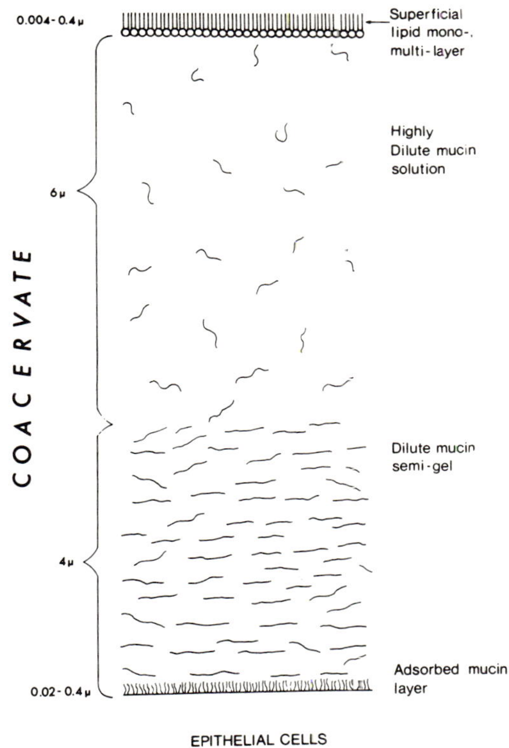

Fig. 6–2. Proposed structure of the pre-corneal tear film.[35]

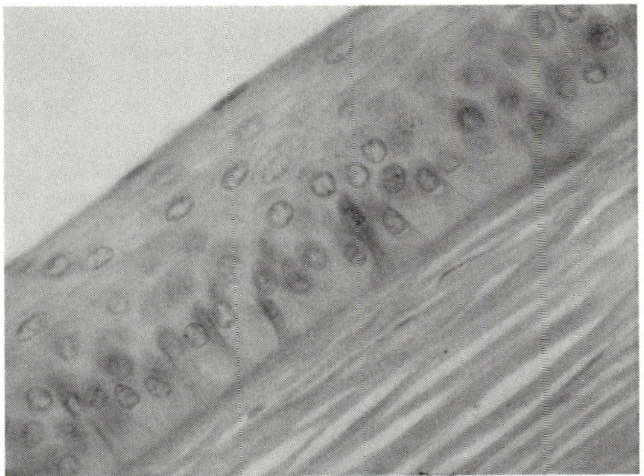

Fig. 6–3. Corneal epithelium 450×. (Courtesy of Dr. A. C. Andersen, Davis, Cal.)

6:3 The *epithelium* has its basal layer of columnar cells surmounted by from two to four layers of polyhedral and four to ten layers of squamous cells (Fig. 6–3). Practically it can be considered a *continuation* of the *bulbar conjunctiva.*

6:4 The *stroma,* comprising 90% of the corneal thickness, consists of connective tissue arranged in lamellae which are broad bands of collagen fibrils extending over the entire width of the cornea and arranged in lamellae parallel to its surface. Keratocytes (corneal fibroblasts), found in the intralamellar spaces, form the stroma by producing the collagen that surrounds them. The fibrils are arranged so precisely that any alteration (*e.g.* edema) that creates a change in this regular arrangement results in loss of transparency. Scar formation following injury or ulceration can occur because the fibrils are not in the proper arrangement. A rich nerve supply enters the middle layer of the stroma, runs forward in a radial fashion to the center of the cornea and terminates as a plexus under the epithelium, with free nerve endings running between the epithelial cells.[18] The collagen fibers of the stroma of the cornea *pass* uninterruptedly *into* the *sclera.* The sclera is composed of interwoven collagen without precise lattice arrangement of the fibrils. This difference accounts for the cornea being transparent and the sclera white and only translucent.

6:5 *Descemet's membrane* is a thin, firm, structureless, transparent, and highly *elastic* layer which is, in reality, a modified basement membrane of the endothelium. It often remains when other layers are destroyed, and then gives rise to a descemetocele (Par. 6:130).

6:6 The *endothelium* consists of a single layer of flat mesothelial cells (4μ thick) covering the inner surface of Descemet's membrane. Both of these layers are *continuous* with the *iris* and *ciliary body.* The term "endothelium," though widely used in ophthalmology, is inaccurate and misleading. There are no endothelial cells in the cornea. The term "mesothelium" or "mesenchymal epithelium" denotes those cells derived from mesoderm and which line body cavities. The cells on the back of the cornea meet these criteria, but ophthalmologists persist in using the former designation.

6:7 The transition area between the cornea and the conjunctiva and sclera is known as the *limbus*. The area is rich in blood vessels and nerve endings and is marked by an oblique line of pigment cells which may, in some normal eyes, extend between the corneal lamellae for some distance beyond the corneoscleral junction.

Physiology

6:8 The cornea is an avascular tissue, receiving its nutrition through a process of dialysis from the perilimbal vessel plexus (Fig. 6–4) and, to a lesser extent, from the aqueous and tears.

6:9 The cornea consists largely of protein, namely, mucin, collagen, elastin, albumin and globulin. Collagen is present in the greatest concentration and is one of the factors involved in wound healing.

6:10 The corneal proteins play an important part in limiting the penetration of acid burns of the cornea. When acid touches the cornea, its proteins are immediately precipitated by the acid. This precipitate in turn acts as a

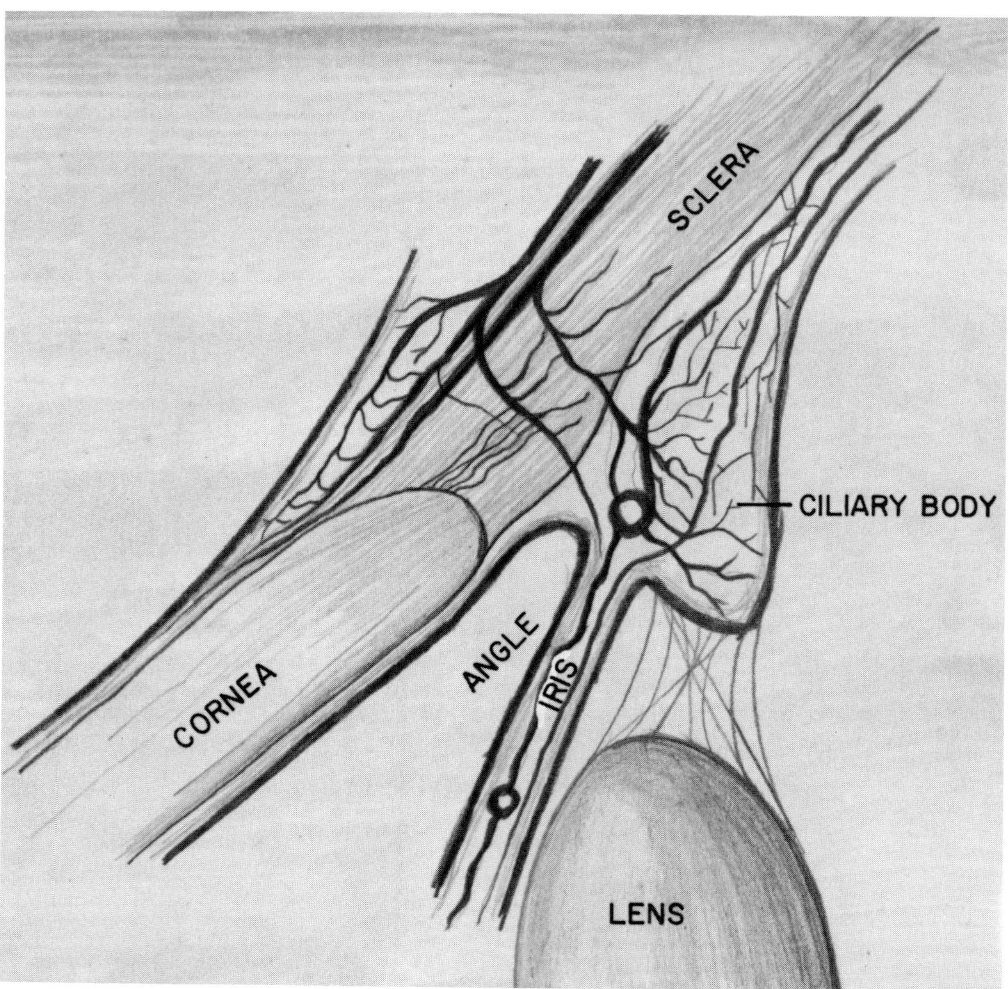

Fig. 6–4. Angle and perilimbal vessel plexus.

barrier to the further penetration of the acid into the deeper structures of the cornea (Fig. 6–5). This phenomenon accounts for the fact that it is possible to use carbolic acid and trichloroacetic acid for cauterizing without danger of perforation. In contrast, alkalies do not form a precipitate with the proteins of the cornea, but rather pass through and in many instances cause irreparable damage.

6:11 Most of the corneal metabolism is carried out by the epithelium. Dietary deficiencies influencing this metabolism include riboflavin, a lack of which will result in vascularizaiton of the cornea. Vitamin A, while more important to the well-being of the retina, is known to have a definite influence on epithelial cells and is of importance also in the metabolism of the cornea. Deficiency results in keratomalacia (Par. 6:110).

6:12 The endothelium and epithelium control the water content of the cornea. Since it is well established that the corneal stroma has a marked affinity for water, it is important that an intact epithelium and endothelium be maintained; otherwise, edema and loss of transparency result. The endothelium is more important than the epithelium in this respect, since it is possible to lose considerable epithelium without showing corneal edema, but minimal loss of endothelium results in demonstrable corneal edema (opacity). This has been demonstrated often in instances of epithelial ulceration, with little or no accompanying edema, versus the severe edema, with resultant opacity, that accompanies injury to the endothelium through disease (Par. 7:43), degeneration, or following intraocular surgery. The endothelium acts, not just as a barrier, but as a "pump" to maintain the relatively dehydrated state of the cornea.

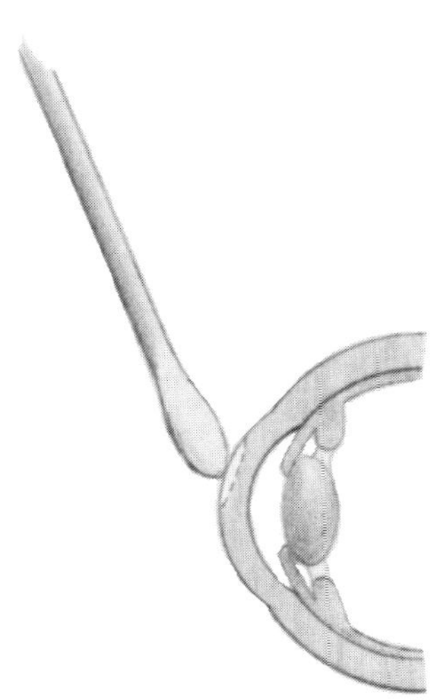

Fig. 6–5. Acid application to cornea with resultant precipitate (dotted line) barring further acid penetration.

6:13 The transparency of the cornea also becomes temporarily impaired when abnormal pressures are applied to it. With the sudden rise of intraocular pressure in acute glaucoma, the cornea becomes cloudy (Par. 9:24). Once this pressure is relieved, the cloudiness disappears.

6:14 To maintain the transparency of the cornea it must be bathed with a fluid having an osmotic pressure higher than interstitial fluid. If the cornea is bathed with a hypotonic solution, it becomes cloudy due to the loss of the osmotic forces acting on the corneal epithelium. When the cornea is cloudy because it is edematous, clearing can be assisted by bathing the eye with a hypertonic solution, such as 10% salt or glycerin solution in order to proceed with ophthalmoscopy or to view the iris and lens.

6:15 The cornea is an extremely sensitive structure, being richly supplied with free nerve endings (Par. 6:4) (Fig. 1–8). An insensitive cornea, in which a reflex is absent while being "feathered" with a wisp of cotton, is a prominent diagnostic sign of glaucoma (Par. 9:26) and neurotrophic keratitis (Par. 6:111). It also has been noted frequently that in those corneal lesions accompanied by extreme photophobia and pain, the lesion is situated in the superficial layers of the cornea and the more severe the photophobia, the more superficial the pathologic process is likely to be. An eye that does not appear to be involved in any way, except for the discomfort shown, will often take a fluorescein stain over a large but very superficial area. It is believed that the pain and photophobia are due largely to vasodilatation taking place in the ciliary body and iris and ciliary spasm. Thus the use of atropine to paralyze the iris sphincter and the ciliary body will alleviate the pain and photophobia (Par. 3:24).

6:16 All of the layers of the cornea are capable of spontaneous regeneration, with the exception of Descemet's, which depends upon the endothelium for regeneration. Epithelial regeneration takes place by sliding or migration of cells, or by multiplication of cells (mitosis). The migratory activity occurs first and almost immediately following an abrasion of the cornea. Cell division follows in 24 to 36 hours. It has been shown, however, that small epithelial defects may be healed entirely without any cell multiplication—simply by cell migration. The rapidity with which these changes occur often has been evident in dogs in which the cornea takes a stain immediately following an abrasion (denoting loss of epithelium), only to exhibit complete regeneration 24 hours later, when a second attempt at staining fails.

6:17 Almost anything used on the cornea will interfere with corneal healing; however, infection will interfere with healing more than any medication used on the cornea. Ointments retard more than solutions of drugs, with the exception of local anesthetics, in which the reverse is true. Powders are still more deleterious in their effect on regeneration. With this information in mind, the careful clinician will then use drugs on the abrasions or ulcers of the cornea only as long as it is necessary to prevent infection or to bring an infection under control. Anesthetic agents should not be used in the daily treatment. Many a stubborn, non-healing ulcer has healed quickly, following cessation of all medication to the eye.

Congenital Anomalies

6:18 *Dermoid.* (Fig. 6–6 and Plate 6A) In this embryological defect, misplaced skin containing hair follicles may involve the cornea alone or both the conjunctiva and cornea (Par. 5:12). The anomaly is noticed by the owner soon after the lid separation takes place.

6:19 Often there are no associated symptoms or corneal lesions noted until the hairs in the dermoid grow longer. If irritative symptoms occur before the puppy reaches an age when an anesthetic can be safely administered and the eye approached surgically, instillation of castor oil or cod liver oil will lubricate and protect the cornea. A superficial keratectomy (Par. 6:167) with complete excision of the dermoid (Fig. 6–6A and B) is usually performed at about three months of age. The use of an antibiotic ointment for several days following surgery is sufficient. The cornea regenerates rapidly and usually with little or no scar.

6:20 *Microcornea* is usually associated with microphthalmos (Par. 8:12), a not uncommon hereditary anomaly in the poodle, miniature schnauzer and collie breeds.

6:21 *Megalophthalmos* (hydrophthalmos, buphthalmia) results from developmental defects of the filtration area of the chamber angle. The extensible sclera and cornea of the puppy are unable to withstand the raised tension and the whole globe becomes enlarged.

6:22 *Corneal dystrophies* are non-inflammatory degenerative lesions of the cornea. They may be congenital or acquired. Waring and McMillan[57] reported a congenital corneal dystrophy in Siberian Huskies. It may occur in one of two forms, superficial or deep. A bilateral axial donut-shaped lesion may vary in severity from just a haze that can be seen only by transillumination or biomicroscopy to diffuse cloudiness that impairs vision. It is most often non-progressive. They concluded

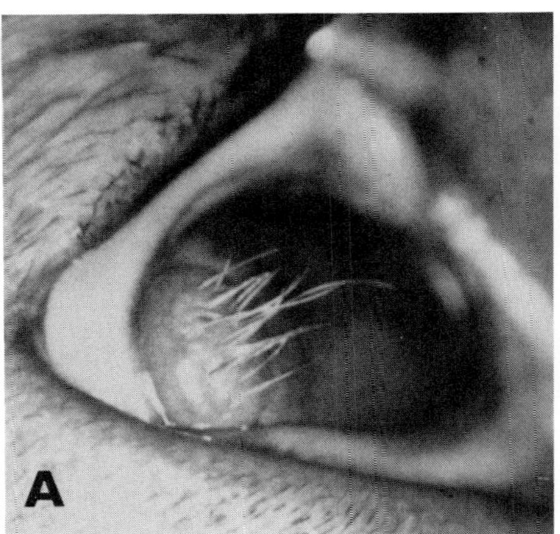

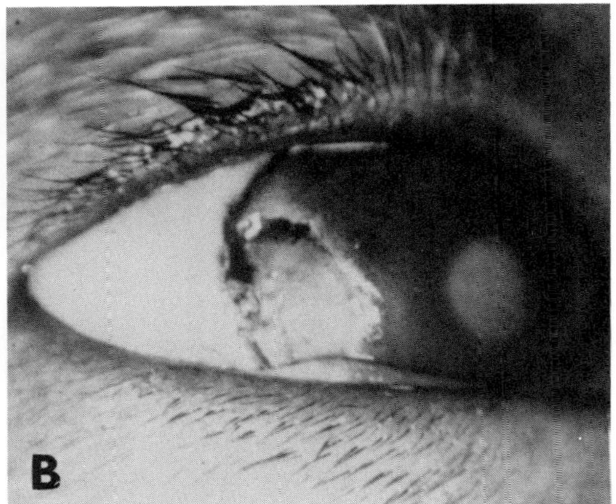

Fig. 6–6. *A.* Corneal dermoid. *B.* Immediately following removal.

it was inherited as a recessive trait with variable expressivity. Dice[20] has reported a corneal dystrophy in the Shetland Sheepdog, and Gwin[28] a posterior polymorphos dystrophy of the American Cocker Spaniel that appears similar to that disease in man. Deep multifocal vesicular or linear opacities were observed. There was no corneal edema. Specular microscopy revealed enlargement and opacity of endothelial cells and a thin, hazy membrane just anterior to the endothelium that obscured the view in some cases.

6:23 Acquired dystrophies are of two types: (1) *superficial* and (2) *endothelial*. In one type of superficial dystrophy, a granular glistening plaque develops during a period of several weeks (Fig. 6–7A). Some cases may follow an ocular inflammatory disease, e.g., pannus, but many cases occur in otherwise normal eyes. In some cases, a blood vessel or two may eventually extend from the limbus to the lesion (Plate 6B). Lesions may appear unilaterally or bilaterally and often progress to involve only a small portion of the cornea, and then remain that size. Some lesions become more dense, while others regress and disappear in 6 to 12 months. In a German Shepherd (Plate 6H), the bilateral corneal dystrophy that developed over a 6-month period was completely gone 1 year later. A viral etiology has been postulated;[41] however, there is not general agreement on the cause.

6:24 Other cases of superficial dystrophies that, in turn, tend to involve the deeper stroma can be attributed to lipid infiltration. Lescure[47] reports loss of corneal transparency from lipid dystrophy (corneal fat) that usually occurs centrally but may be marginal or peripheral. Startup[83] describes primary fatty degeneration (corneal lipidosis) as central opacities that appeared as needle shaped crystals on biomicroscopy. He believes secondary fatty degeneration may result from the transformation of scar tissue. In man, almost all cases of lipid infiltration into the cornea occur in vascularized corneas. There often is no detectable systemic lipid abnormality.[7] A bilateral lipid dystrophy (Fig. 6–7B) was encountered in a 7-year-old male, mixed breed dog with a total serum cholesterol of 1040 mg/100 ml. The dog was presented for euthanasia because of almost complete loss of vision. Superficial keratectomy, performed prior to necropsy revealed the dystrophy was limited to the outer ⅓ of the cornea. Frozen sections stained with oil red O revealed large amounts of lipid material in the superficial portions of the substantia propria of the cornea. Numerous cholesterol clefts were also present in this area. These deposits were attended by a severe reaction.[2]

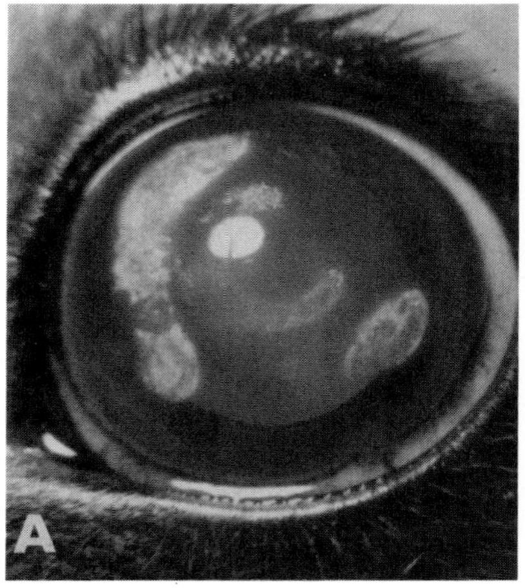

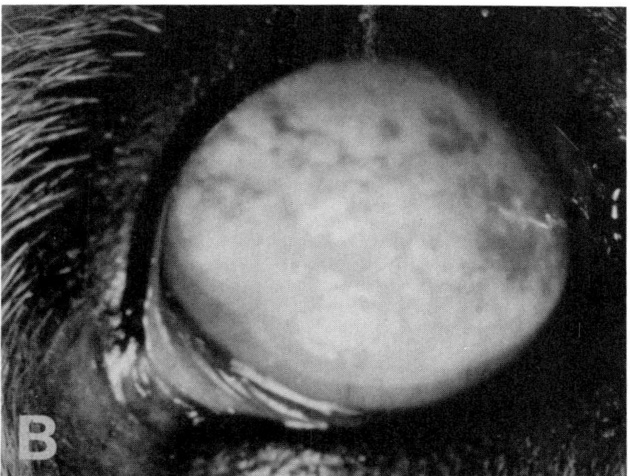

Fig. 6–7. Corneal dystrophies.

6:25 A deposition of lipoid material in the limbal area of older dogs is occasionally seen. This lesion is stationary and no treatment is necessary. It may or may not be comparable to arcus senilis of man. A single case of verticillate corneal dystrophy similar to that rarely found in man has been described.[8] Both corneas showed brown whorl-like pigmented streaks radiating from the center toward the limbus where they joined patches of darker brown pigment.

6:26 *Treatment.* A superficial keratectomy (Par. 6:167) is indicated in those instances in which the lesion is *progressing*, becomes disfiguring, or interferes with vision. The keratectomy should include several millimeters of normal tissue beyond the periphery of the lesion. Regeneration of epithelial and some stromal tissue takes place following surgery, and the cornea remains clear. Except in those cases of associated systemic lipoidosis, return of the lesion to the original or another area of the cornea seldom occurs. On occasion, in long-standing cases, the dystrophy will have invaded the deeper stroma. In these instances some haze may remain following regeneration of the overlying tissue.

6:27 *Endothelial dystrophy* is the second type of acquired corneal dystrophy. It is characterized by a corneal edema in an otherwise normal eye, caused by failure of the endothelial (mesothelial) 'pump' mechanism that normally maintains the relative dehydration of the cornea. The dystrophy may involve the entire cornea or only a portion of the cornea (Plate 9C), if only a portion of the endothelium is degenerate. It occurs in older dogs, especially old Boston Terriers and Chihuahuas. Dogs may have unilateral involvement, but the other eye usually becomes involved within weeks or months.

6:28 In diagnosis, careful examination of the eye to exclude other causes of corneal edema, especially glaucoma, and anterior uveitis, is important. The degree of pupil dilation in response to Mydriacyl* is a valuable aid in evaluation for anterior uveitis, especially if the corneal haze precludes careful examination of the iris. In endothelial dystrophy, dilation should be complete; whereas, if anterior uveitis is present the response to Mydriacyl is reduced.

6:29 *Treatment.* Since endothelial dystrophy is a non-inflammatory degenerative change, corticosteroids and other medications are of no value. Subconjunctival or continued topical steroid therapy is contraindicated, because such treatment may inhibit healing of a corneal injury and enhance bac-

*Tropicamide, Alcon Laboratories, Ft. Worth, Texas

terial infection. A full thickness corneal graft would be the best treatment and has been reported,[29] but it is not commonly done in the dog, and, when done, has not been highly successful. Fortunately, even dogs with bilateral involvement demonstrate less visual impairment than one would expect.

Keratitis

Characteristics of Keratitis

6:30 Of all the species the veterinarian has to care for, the incidence of corneal disease is highest in the dog. Formston[25] believes this may be due to a number of factors, including a higher degree of domestication, a multiplicity of breeds, the extreme vulnerability of the cornea to trauma in certain of the brachycephalic types, the prevalence of lid and cilia anomalies, and the possible influence of virus disease, distemper and hepatitis. The incidence of corneal disease varies among breed. Some are relatively immune to any form while others are most susceptible. The brachycephalic types, *e.g.* Pekingese, pug, Boston terrier, which have prominent eyes, are particularly prone to corneal ulceration with perforation. The boxer exhibits a corneal erosion syndrome. The German shepherd has a chronic superficial keratitis peculiar to the breed. Poodles and dachshunds seem susceptible to an obstinate superficial punctate keratitis accompanied by haze, vascularization and pigmentation. The Boston terrier appears to have senile endothelial dystrophy more than any other breed.

6:31 Inflammation of the cornea generally presents one or more of the following objective signs: (1) loss of transparency, (2) ciliary injection, (3) vascularization, (4) cellular deposits in the aqueous, and (5) ulceration.

6:32 (1) *Loss of transparency* may be partial or complete and may result from (*a*) a change in the water content of the cornea (edema) (Par. 6:12); (*b*) from an inflammatory exudate of one type or another, usually a leukocyte infiltration.

6:33 (2) *Ciliary injection* (Table 5–1). The circumcorneal vessels, which are derived from the anterior ciliary vessels, become engorged in varying degrees. The conjunctival vessels often appear injected too, especially if the keratitis is an extension of a conjunctivitis.

6:34 (3) *Vascularization.*[51] Since the cornea is an avascular tissue (Par. 6:8), in order to increase its defenses against irritants in pathologic conditions, metabolism is increased; first, by an augmentation of the normal circulation, which is evident clinically as a circumcorneal injection; and secondly, by the actual invasion of the cornea itself by new vessels. Circumcorneal injection is the invariable accompaniment of inflammatory or irritative processes in the cornea, and is, essentially, the engorgement of the perilimbal plexus, which is normally not grossly visible.

6:35 Adler[1] concludes that most diseases of the cornea result in its vascularization, and the type of vessels and their location in the cornea are often clues to the nature of the disease process. The diseases which commonly affect *epithelial structures* are accompanied by *superficial vascularization*, the vessels coming across the limbus from the conjunctiva. Those diseases affecting *parenchymatous tissues*, on the other hand, are characterized by *deep vessels*, coming from the anastomosis of the long posterior ciliary arteries and the anterior ciliary arteries. Once the cornea has become vascularized, the vessels remain throughout life. They are frequently empty of blood (ghost vessels) but their presence can always be detected with suitable magnification, and are testimony to the fact that the cornea has been the seat of a previous inflammatory process.

6:36 Once the process of vascularization is understood a more accurate prognosis and the proper choice of treatment can be determined. The two types of vascularization are referred to as *superficial* and *deep*, and from their appearance in the cornea are easily distinguishable one from the other (Plate 6C and D), and remember, as mentioned previously, deep vessels mean deep trouble.

6:37 The superficial vessels run directly under the epithelium and in the superficial stroma and can often be seen as a continuation of vessels in the adjacent bulbar conjunctiva. They are bright red and branch in tree-like fashion (Fig. 6–11).

6:38 The deep vessels, since they are derived from the deep ciliary vessels, disappear from view at the margin of the cornea as they run into the sclera. They are darker purple and appear as long straight lines or form brush-like clumps.

6:39 (4) *Cellular deposits and increased protein in the aqueous*, often referred to as "aqueous cells and flare," are an indication that the neighboring deep parts (iris and ciliary body) are also involved. The turbidity may be slight, or a hypopyon (pus in the anterior chamber) may develop. The pus is an exudation from the iris and ciliary body when these parts participate in the inflammation (Par. 7:43) and does not necessarily imply actual infection within the eye.

6:40 (5) *Ulceration* may be superficial or deep, spreading or stationary. The extent of ulceration is best detected by the use of fluorescein (Par. 2:20) which stains green all ulcerated or abraded parts. Aside from the loss of corneal substance there is nearly always some grayish infiltration immediately surrounding the ulceration.

6:41 *Subjective* symptoms of keratitis include pain, photophobia, lacrimation, and blepharospasm. These symptoms may be slight or pronounced, depending upon the type of keratitis.

Classification of Keratitis

6:42 Diseases of the cornea have been variously classified under the etiology, topical and histologic localization, and clinical and pathologic features of their early or late manifestations. It will always be difficult to type or classify every case of keratitis. Overlapping or concurrent findings tend to obscure the picture. For the sake of simplicity and to render a discussion of therapeutic measures more realistic, the following classification, based on the most salient features at the time of presentation.

A. Superficial without vascularization
   1. Superficial punctate keratitis
   2. Corneal erosion syndrome
   3. Other
B. Superficial with vascularization
   1. Pannus
   2. Exuberant granulation tissue
C. Pigmentary keratitis
D. Interstitial Keratitis
E. Ulcerative Keratitis
   1. simple
   2. deep
   3. serpent or dendritic
   4. nutritional
   5. neuroparalytic
F. Keratoconjunctivitis
   1. Keratoconjunctivitis sicca
   2. Triple "S" syndrome

Superficial Without Vascularization

6:43 A general diagnosis of superficial keratitis is made when the involvement is limited to the epithelium and superficial part of the stroma.

6:44 (1) *Superficial punctate keratitis* may be unilateral, but is often bilateral on presentation. The center of most of the punctate lesions stain with fluorescein. Some lesions seem to be developing, others healing (Plate 9A and B). Some inflammation of the conjunctiva, blepharospasm and epiphora are the usual associated findings. Corneal vascularization may occur in long-standing cases. The etiology is in question. This is not a common disease, but those cases encountered have been unresponsive to medical therapy. With or without topical antibiotics to prevent secondary bacterial infection, some cases appear to be self-limiting after running a course of several months, while others continue with remissions and exacerbations for extended periods. Dachshunds, Shelties and Poodles seem to be affected more than other breeds. Dice[20] suggests that, in the Sheltie, a basement membrane dystrophy may be the underlying cause. Treatment with idoxuridine or other antiviral agents has not been of value. Superficial keratectomy to remove the affected area has been successful in some cases. Long-term judicious use of topical corticosteroids has also been quite helpful.

6:45 (2) *Corneal erosion syndrome* (Plate 7E) could be classified as a type of ulcerative keratitis, but is classified separately, because it has several unique features, and is probably related to a basement membrane defect. This term is used to describe an ulceration occurring most often in older Boxers, but occasionally in other older dogs. The lesion is superficial, has no tendency to deepen, but has an overhanging border, detectable by fluorescein stain. There is no associated conjunctival discharge, other than epiphora. Corneal opacity, or vascularization is not present in the early stages, but may be extensive later (Plate 9H). The ulcer may remain stationary for a long period of time, during which the animal may exhibit marked signs of pain and photophobia. No causative agent has been found. Relapses following healing are common. Often, some weeks or months later, a new area of the cornea becomes involved or the fellow eye may be afflicted. Severin[77] records an incidence of 80% of his total cases appearing in spayed females over 5 years of age, and believes that estrogens are essential for epithelial health and to prevent recurrence. Slatter[78] calls the lesion *superficial corneal erosion* and reports the incidence highest in the Boxer and the Corgi, but reported no sex predilection or value of estrogen. Wyman[91] uses the term *indolent ulcer.* Other terms have also been used for this disease. Magrane originally classified it as a *rodent ulceration.*[50] Roberts[68] describes it as an *indolent type of superficial ulceration.*

6:46 *Corneal erosion syndrome,* as described in man[22,24] seems to be the best descriptive term for this disease. In this clinical condition in man, some cases appear to follow trauma, but in others, it is believed to be dystrophic in nature.[22] The epithelium is apparently able to regenerate normally and

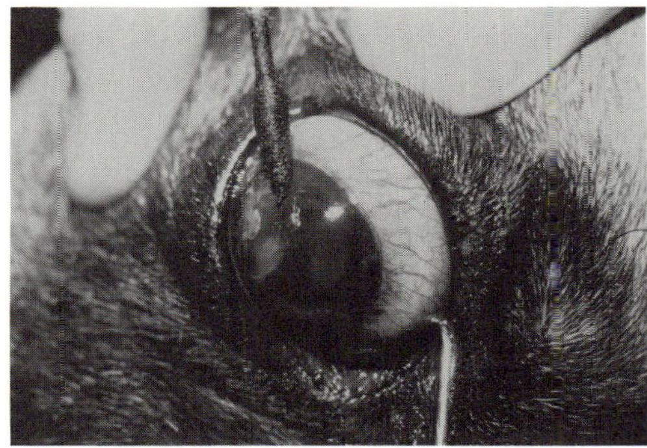

Fig. 6–8. Epithelial erosion: Strong tincture of iodine on a cotton-wound toothpick is used to roll back the loose epithelium.

cover the wound, but, for some reason, fails to regain its normal adhesion to the underlying tissue at least for some time. Electron microscopic studies in man show an absence of the basement membrane in the area of recurrent erosion.[27] An ultrastructural study of epithelial biopsies of a case of non-traumatic origin revealed no infective agents or inflammation, but an absence of hemidesmosomes and a separation of the basement membrane which provided a structural basis for the epithelial erosion.[84] The syndrome in the dog appears to be similar.

6:47 Treatment consists of careful stripping of the overhanging epithelial edge and protecting the cornea to allow newly formed epithelial cells to adhere and fill the defect.

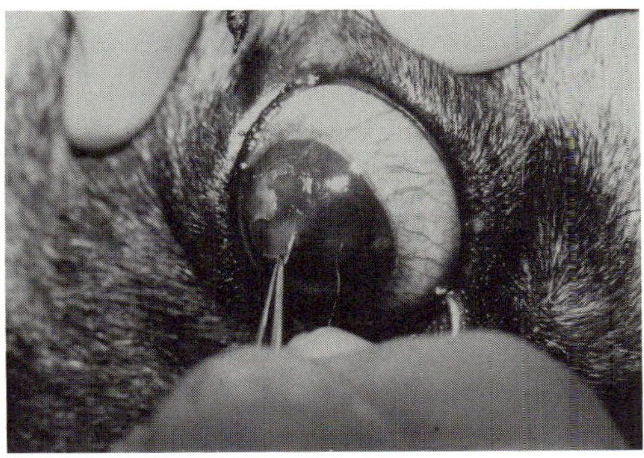

Fig. 6–9. Epithelial erosion: The rolled-back loose epithelium is carefuly stripped off all around the ulcer with a small forceps.

First, stain the area with fluorescein and flush with eye wash. Stain under the overhanging edge will appear brighter green. Next, paint the ulcer from the center forward and push back the overhanging edge with 7% tincture of iodine, on a cotton wound toothpick (Fig. 6–8), then strip the overhanging edge (Figs. 6–9, 6–20) with Bishop Harmon or other small mouse-toothed forceps. Finally, paint the area and surrounding 1 to 2 mm, from the edge toward the center, with the iodine on the toothpick. Dispense antibiotic eye drops to be used only BID and 1% Atropine eye drops to be used daily, if blepharospasm is evident. (The owner should also be advised to keep the dog out of bright light.) Recheck in 3 weeks. If healing but not completely healed, carefully restrip any overhanging edges. If no progress, restrip and put up a third eyelid flap for 3 weeks. Delay the use of topical steroids for reduction of vascularization for at least 3 weeks after epithelialization is complete.

6:48 (3) Other causes of superficial keratitis without vascularization include any factor that will produce corneal irritation. Since vascularization and pigmentation are a normal response to long-term stress, in the absence of these alterations, look for *recent* changes, such as mechanical or chemical irritants, decreased tear production, exophthalmos with poor lid closure, or any other factors that would increase corneal stress.

Superficial with Vascularization

6:49 (1) *Pannus* is subepithelial vascularization of the cornea. This term has been adopted to describe a specific disease occurring most commonly in the German Shepherd. The term *atypical pannus* has also been applied to a vascularizing corneal disease occurring in breeds other than the German Shepherd.[49] Other authors who have described the lesion in the German Shepherd have variously classified it as chronic superficial keratitis, pterygium, pseudopterygium, corneal metoplasia or degenerative pannus. It seems unfortunate that the term pannus and, especially, degenerative pannus, are used for this specific disease, because pannus is a general term for vascularization from any cause. Degenerative pannus, in human ophthalmology, is used to describe vascularization following other eye diseases, such as trachoma and glaucoma. Uberreiter, who first described the disease, called it chronic superficial keratitis, probably a more appropriate name.

6:50 The lesion begins as a grayish haze at the limbus. In most instances, it affects both eyes and begins on the temporal side (9:00 o'clock position on the right eye; 3:00 o'clock position on the left eye) (Plate 6E). The film, with accompanying blood vessels and pigment continues to spread over the cornea until it is eventually covered, with blindness resulting (Plate 8C). In early cases biomicroscopy (Par. 2:6) reveals white infiltrates and "peppery" translucent deposits preceding the grossly observable lesion into what appears to be clear corneal tissue. Histologic examination of biopsied lesions reveals that these cloudy and translucent areas are subepithelial infiltration by plasma cells, lymphocytes, and small mononuclear cells.

6:51 Chronic superficial keratitis takes several forms. The spread on the cornea may be slow and otherwise symptom free, or it may assume an inflammatory form in which a rapid "cobblestone" build-up is noted on the cornea, and in which the conjunctiva, including the third eyelid (Par. 4:57) is obviously a part of the inflammation (Plate 6F). An accompanying catarrhal discharge can be expected in this form.

6:52 *Etiology.* The cause is unknown. Überreiter[85,87] was unable to incriminate a bacterial component or effect an inoculation in healthy controls. Environmental conditions do not seem to be of primary importance because the disease is encountered throughout the United States and many parts of the world in those dogs confined to the home as well as those in a constant outside exposure. Several authors think that ultraviolet radiation from sunlight is a potentiating factor and makes the disease more difficult to control.[80] There is apparently no genetic factor involved.[72] The disease is most likely immune-mediated. Dogs affected with chronic superficial keratitis and clinically normal dogs were tested for cellular hypersensitivity using the leukocyte migration inhibition technique to three ocular antigens. Affected dogs had statistically significant increases in hypersensitivity cellular responses against corneal antigens.[44] In another study[5] patterns indicative of an allergic phenomenon led to the examination of serum proteins in German shepherds. Affected dogs lacked evidence of the immunoglobulin IgG_d which may decrease the eye's ability to tolerate environmental changes.

6:53 *Treatment.* Therapy is primarily directed toward suppression of the immune response. Destruction or removal of the lesion is simple enough, but constant steroid therapy is necessary in most cases to prevent return of the lesion. Lamellar corneal grafts to replace removed diseased tissue, and the use of autologous or homologous conjunctival grafts have been used in an unsuccessful attempt to prevent return of the lesion. X-ray and beta-ray irradiation have been given a thorough trial and found to be wanting. Early pannus often responds well to irradiation initially, only to recur. Small repeated doses and single massive doses of beta-ray irradiation have been tried and the results do not differ appreciably, with a temporary remission only resulting. Pure carbolic-acid cauterization of a pannus area has proved to be a more rapid and satisfactory means of destroying the metaplastic tissue than either x-ray or beta radiation. The diseased tissue will slough from the underlying stroma and regeneration will readily take place, but relapse and return of the pannus will occur later unless steroid therapy is continued.

6:54 The use of cryotherapy to slough the vascularized or pigmented surface of the cornea has also been proposed.[36] It offers no advantage over older methods proposed to slough the corneal surface, is less precise than superficial keratectomy and does not replace the need for continued steroid therapy to prevent recurrence.

6:55 It remains, then, that the use of steroids should supersede the other choices in initiating therapy. The subconjunctival method (Par. 3:61) is the preferred treatment and is *especially* valuable in the inflammatory type mentoned (Par. 6:51). Ten mg of a repositol type steroid to each eye will cause regression of the lesion and clearing of the cornea of all but some residual haze and pigment. Concurrent and follow-up instillation of steroid-antibiotic combinations in drop or ointment form twice a day will ordinarily prevent a relapse and return of the disease. In the summer many individuals suffer a "flare-up" of the lesion despite continued topical steroid therapy. In these instances another subconjunctival injection will reverse the process. Occasionally a patient responds well to a change of the steroid preparation. The reason for this remains obscure.

6:56 A superficial keratectomy (Par. 6:167) is the quickest way of removing the lesion. Ordinarily, however, this procedure is reserved for removal of areas of pigment, corneal dystrophy or other opacity, if sight is not satisfactory after the inflammation and vascularization are controlled with steroids. Following the keratectomy, the underlying stroma will be found to be clear, and a blind animal will have vision restored (Fig. 6–37C). Following regeneration of the corneal epithelium, previously mentioned steroid therapy is commenced.

6:57 *Complications* that can occur during prolonged antibiotic-steroid therapy include keratoconjunctivitis and corneal ulceration caused by bacteria not sensitive to the antibiotics being used, or by fungi. Allergy to the antibiotic, characterized as a conjunctivitis, is also infrequently encountered. These complications are usually evidenced by conjunctivitis with mucoid to mucopurulent ocular discharge. A "flare-up" of the keratitis, or ulcers detected by fluorescein staining may be present. Sensitivity to light, blepharospasm and other signs of ocular discomfort, not usually seen with *pannus*, are also often noted by the owner. In such instances, corneal and conjunctival scrapings and swabs should be collected for identification of bacteria and fungi, by culture and by direct examination (Par. 5:20–24). Treatment should be instituted as indicated by culture and sensitivity results. The steroid should be discontinued until ulcers are healed. A different antibiotic steroid combination should be selected if allergy to the antibiotic is suspected. Other complications include corneal dystrophy (Par. 6:23), epithelial inclusion, cysts and corneal bullae.

6:58 In conclusion it must be emphasized that there is *no need* for a German shepherd to be blinded by pannus. Constant usually twice a day instillation of a steroid is mandatory. An occasional subconjunctival injection may be necessary. Peritomy, chemical cautery, radiation or surgery need not be used until the results of a subconjunctival steroid injection have been noted. A keratectomy is performed only when chronicity and impaired vision due to melanin deposition are not reversible with steroids.

6:59 (2) *Exuberant granulation tissue* (Plate 6G) builds up on the cornea as the result of injury or ulceration. Superficial vessels can be seen extending from the conjunctiva, across the cornea to the area of granulation. Granulation tissue should not be confused with either chronic superficial keratitis pannus or simple superficial vascularization (Fig. 6–10).

6:60 *Treatment* consists of a subconjunctival steroid injection (Par. 3:63), cutting the blood vessels at the limbus (Fig. 6–12), with follow-up topical steroid therapy. Depending upon the amount of granulation tissue, the cornea will clear appreciably within a few days to several weeks. If the superficial vascularization and granulation tissue is not extensive, the steroid injection will suffice. If there is a prominent "build-up" on the cornea (Plate 6G), cutting the blood vessels with cautery at the limbus will hasten resolution. Since subconjunctival and topical steroids are quite effective and cutting blood vessels requires general anesthesia, this procedure is usually reserved for cases being anesthetized for other treatment.

6:61 By dividing the blood vessels, using either heat or electrocoagulation, the source of blood supply to the granulation areas is destroyed at its origin where it arises in the bulbar conjunctiva (Fig. 6–12). Without the support of these vessels, the granulation tissue will disappear, and the cornea will regain its transparency. Each vessel leading from the conjunctiva to the corneal granulation tissue is touched with the cautery just back of the limbus. A steroid preparation may be used afterward to expedite the dissipation of the vessels and granulation tissue. *Caution*—so long as an ulcerated or abraded area stains, it is best to delay cutting of vessels or steroids until the healing process is nearly complete. Vascularization should never be discouraged until it has accomplished its purpose.

6:62 (3) *Other.* Superficial vascularization of the cornea will occur in response to any continued corneal stress caused by foreign bodies, distichiasis, lid neoplasms, chronic keratoconjunctivitis, keratoconjunctivitis sicca, and exposure keratitis. Treatment should be directed at eliminating the cause. Diet deficiencies, especially lack of riboflavin, may result in superficial vascularization. The cornea clears quickly following correction of the diet and the administration of riboflavin (15 mg daily). Vascularization produced by nutritional deficiency is uncommon today, but its possibility must be considered when no other cause is determined, especially if other signs of poor nutrition are evident.

6:63 (4) *Bullous keratitis* (Plate 7A). In bullous keratopathy tiny vacuoles in or under the epithelium coalesce to form vesicles and edema in the superficial corneal tissues. These vesicles are also known as bullae. The area involved becomes very edematous and the blister-like epithelium may rupture leaving an ulcer.

6:64 *Etiology.* The condition usually occurs

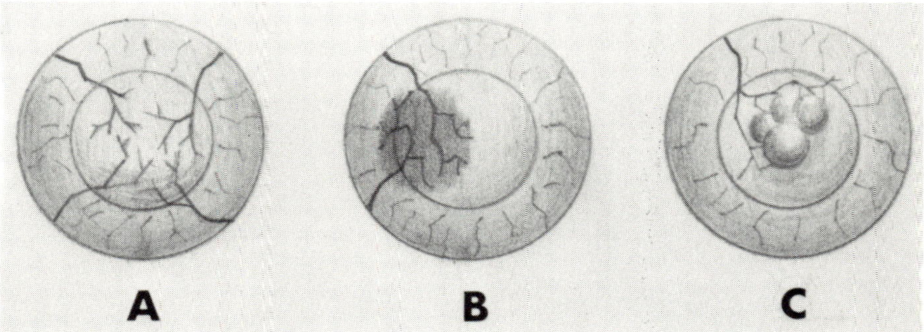

Fig. 6–10. *A.* Superficial vascularization (vessels only). *B.* Pannus. Subepithelial cellular infiltration accompanied by superficial vascularization. *C.* Exuberant granulation tissue. Superficial vessels "feeding" granulation.

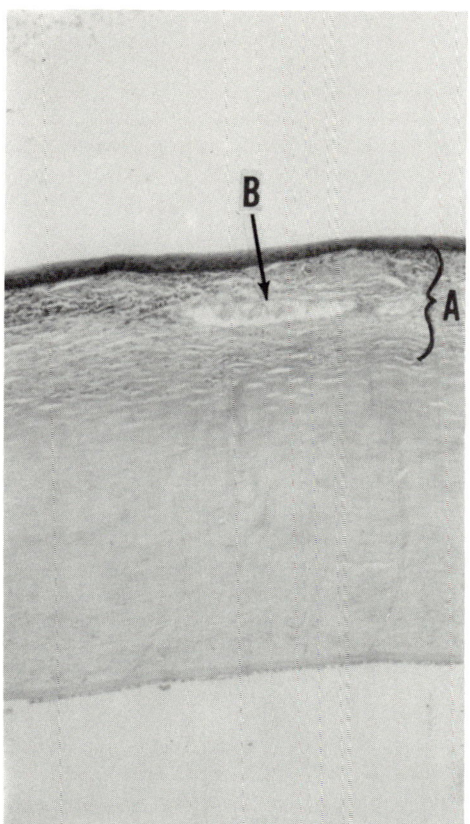

Fig. 6–11. Photomicrograph of pannus. *A.* Area of infiltration. *B.* Blood vessel.

in corneas that are edematous from some other cause, such as endothelial dystrophy or continued elevated intraocular pressure.

6:65 *Treatment.* The underlying cause should be treated if possible. Hypertonic solutions (5% NaCl eye drops) are commonly used but of limited value. Preventing infection with topical antibiotics and the use of a third eyelid flap as a pressure bandage are most helpful. Use of steroids is absolutely contraindicated.

6:66 *Epithelial Inclusion Cysts.* Benign, raised, solitary masses described histologically as epithelial inclusion cysts have been reported in the dog.[73] They appear as a well-delineated cyst or bullous area. Excision by superficial keratectomy followed by topical antibiotics until re-epithelialization occurs is the indicated treatment.

6:67 (5) *Keratoconjunctivitis sicca* (KCS) (dry eye) is characterized by discomfort, blepharospasm and *photophobia* of one or both eyes and a loss of the usual glistening appearance of the cornea. The disease is caused by an insufficiency of tear secretion. The lacrimal gland and the gland of the third eyelid no longer produce the tear film which is so important to the well-being of the cornea (Par. 4:4). Any breed may be affected; however, the incidence appears to be much higher in some breeds. In an analysis of 754 cases of KCS presented at Colleges of Veterinary Medicine, English Bulldogs were at

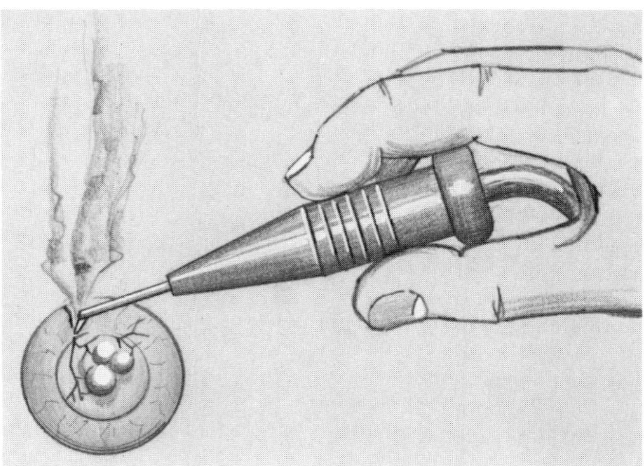

Fig. 6–12. Destruction of blood supply to granulation area by means of electrocoagulation.

greatest risk followed by West Highland White terriers (Table 6–1).[33]

6:68 The conjunctiva becomes red, thickened, and velvety (Par. 5:47), a sticky, ropy secretion invariably accompanies the condition. These findings often lead the clinician wrongly to assume that a chronic bacterial conjunctivitis is responsible. Although a bacterial component may be present, it is usually secondary. Corneal vascularization, pigmentation and/or ulcerations may occur. Upon fluorescein staining the cornea may take a very light stain over its entire surface. (Par. 2:20) This is most evident when viewed with suitable magnification. A *dry nostril* on the affected side (Fig. 6–13) may be present if the watery nasal secretion has also diminished (Par. 6:70). This seems to occur most often in unilateral cases in which injury or other causes for neurologic dysfunction underlies the disease.

6:69 The Schirmer tear test* should be employed. The test paper is folded across its width at the notch and the folded portion is placed in the lower conjunctival cul-de-sac in the vicinity of the temporal third (Fig. 2–15).

Table 6–1. Relative Risk for KCS

Breed	No. of Dogs	Relative Risk
English bulldog	56	12.5
West Highland white terrier	14	5.5
Pug	19	4.5
Yorkshire terrier	12	3.3
Cocker spaniel	81	3.2
Pekingese	28	2.4
Schnauzer (miniature)	26	2.2
English springer spaniel	10	2.1
Scottish terrier	10	1.9
Chihuahua	31	1.7
Fox terrier	13	1.5
Boston terrier	12	1.4
Dachshund	70	1.4
Poodle (miniature and toy)	111	1.4
All breeds combined	754	1
Beagle	14	0.6
Mixed breed	79	0.4
German shepherd	14	0.2

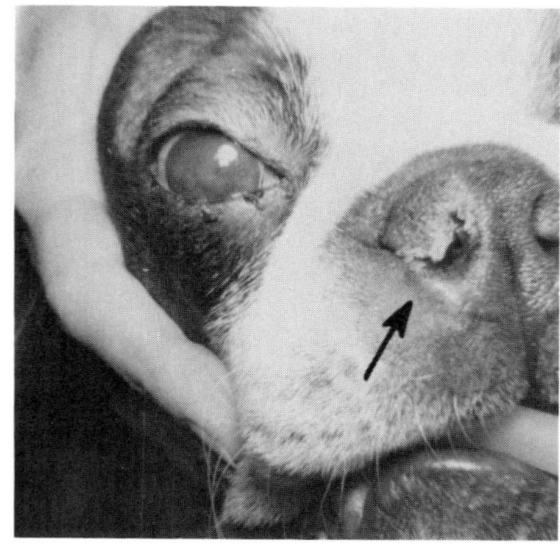

Fig. 6–13. Keratoconjunctivitis sicca. Note associated dry nostril on affected side.

*Cooper Labs., Inc., Wayne, N.J., 07470.

The paper is allowed to remain in place for 1 minute with the eyelid held closed. Following removal the moistened portion is measured from the notch on the mm scale provided. Rubin's study[71] showed Schirmer tear test values varied from 5 to 35 mm per minute with a mean value of 19.8 mm (100 dogs). Under 9 mm for 1 minute indicates less than normal tear production although readings below this figure may be recorded without definite signs of the disease being present. Owners should be notified of the low secretion and alerted to watch for signs of KCS. The following scale is helpful: 15 and over = normal; 9–15 = borderline; below 9 = diagnostic of hyposecretion.

6:70 *Etiology.* The causes for cessation of or insufficient lacrimal secretion are varied and often remain obscure. The following have been recorded: (*a*) *Canine distemper.* Upon recovery from the systemic disease the lacrimal function may return with a resultant clearing of the discharge and return of corneal luster or the KCS may be permanent. (*b*) *Injuries* to the head may damage the glands directly, or may damage the enervation to the glands and lower or stop tear production. A dry nostril (Fig. 6–12) is not uncommon in these cases. (*c*) A chronic *blepharitis/conjunctivitis* syndrome (Par. 5:39) may, in turn, affect the function of the glands either temporarily or permanently. (*d*) *Senility* in itself may be a factor. (*e*) *Congenital* absence of or malfunction of the secreting glands has been encountered in several breeds (Yorkshire terriers, Chihuahuas, Miniature pinschers). There may be an associated microphthalmia. (*f*) *Intoxications* having a direct action on the secretory cells of the lacrimal gland, *e.g.* belladonna poisoning and botulism. (*g*) *Drug induced.* Phenazopyridine, used in some drug combinations for cystitis, is capable of causing a reduction in tear flow resulting in keratitis sicca. The mode of action of the drug is unknown, but the effect appears to be dose related.[79] Sulfonamides have also been incriminated.[60] (*h*) *Hypothyroidism* has been suggested as a possible cause or aggravating factor.[64] Kaswan et al.[38–40] suggest that keratoconjunctivitis sicca (KCS) and hypothyroidism occur concurrently as symptoms of an (*i*) *underlying autoimmune disease* in some breeds. In an immunologic evaluation of 62 dogs with KCS, 40% had concurrent problems indicative of underlying autoimmune disease. The evaluation also showed English Bulldogs, West Highland Whites, and the Shih Tzu breeds to be at high risk. (*j*) *Surgically induced* (Par. 4:59) removal of the lacrimal gland and the gland of the third eyelid always produces KCS. Removal of either gland alone can produce KCS, if the production of tears by the remaining gland is below normal. (*k*) Vitamin A deficiency is a cause in man, but unlikely in the dog, unless on a severely deficient diet.

6:71 *Treatment* (Medical). Artificial tear therapy (Par. 3:94) with or without the addition of antibiotics must be continued until the secreting function returns, as in the case of distemper, or, indefinitely in those conditions mentioned in which permanent loss of function is evident. Commercial preparations of artificial tears (hydroxyethylcellulose and other related solutions) are available under various trade names. If there is no ulceration but the usual conjunctival inflammation and corneal vascularization is present, a repositol steroid is injected subconjunctivally (Par. 3:65). A topical antibiotic-steroid ointment is also used twice a day.

6:72 Pilocarpine can be used as adjunctive therapy providing there are some cells present capable of secreting tears.[3,70] The best results are obtained when the Schirmer tear test strip shows at least several mm of wetting. Even then it is often necessary to continue pilocarpine for 3 to 4 weeks before improvement can be expected. I have been pleased to see complete return of function following the use of oral pilocarpine administration and frequent topical instillation of the antibiotic-steroid and lubricating drops. Ordinarily, the 4% ophthalmic drops of pilocarpine are prescribed for large dogs. The dose is 1 drop of 4% pilocarpine in the food, twice a day per 10 pounds body weight. One per cent can be used in the toy breeds at 1 drop per 2½ pounds. Side effects from excess dosage include excess salivation, vomiting, diarrhea, and tachycardia. If excess salivation occurs, the dose is cut in half and raised 1 drop each meal until the prescribed dose or maximum tolerated level is reached. A response to treatment is evident in rechecks of the Schirmer tear test value and appearance of the eye. Dependent upon this response, the oral pilocarpine may be stopped or continued as needed. The same applies to topical instillations.

6:73 Assessment of thyroid function should be considered and hypothyroidism treated if present. Although thyroid therapy did not result in improvement of KCS in one study,[64] such treatment will aid the general health of the dog.

6:74 *Surgical.* If, after 1 month of medical therapy, there is still inadequate tear production, transposition of the parotid duct (Fig. 1–9) should be considered if the vision and integrity of the globe are to be preserved. There is a close similarity between lacrimal and parotid secretions. By providing the conjunctival and corneal surfaces with a constant source of lubrication via the salivary secretion, the eye will be maintained in a good state. A return of vision can be expected in eyes blinded by vascularization and pigmentation. Totally blind dogs which have undergone bilateral transposition surgery will again resume all of their old activities. Unquestionably, the results attending this procedure are most dramatic and gratifying.[75] *Caution:* Some cases of keratoconjunctivitis sicca are the consequence of a broader disease with an accompanying loss of salivary function. This function should be checked before surgery is decided upon.

6:75 *Technique.* Several methods have been described.[6,11,26,44] All have for their purpose the release of the parotid salivary duct and its papilla (Fig. 6–14) and their transposition to the palpebral fissure. Instruments required: eye speculum, probe, handles and

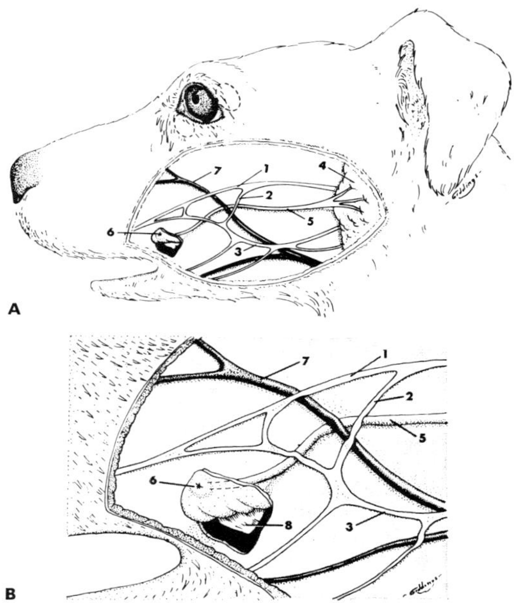

Fig. 6–14. Cutaway drawing of the face (A) and enlargement of the area where the parotid duct enters the mouth (B). Facial muscles have been omitted to illustrate the essential features. 1, Dorsal buccal nerve; 2, anastomosis of dorsal buccal and ventral buccal nerves; 3, ventral buccal nerve; 4, parotid salivary gland; 5, parotid duct; 6, papilla of parotid duct; 7, facial vein; 8, upper carnassial tooth. (Bojrab, *Current Techniques in Small Animal Surgery,* courtesy of Lea & Febiger.)

#64 Beaver blade and #15 BP blade, Allis forceps (2), mosquito forceps (2), eye tissue forceps, Calibri forceps, tenotomy scissors, muscle hook, long-nose hemostat, eye needle forceps and large needle forceps.

1. The patient is placed in lateral recumbency and the side of the face is closely clipped and prepared.

2. The upper lip is retracted and the papilla is located (above the carnassial tooth) (Fig. 6–15A).

3. A very fine, round end probe is lubricated (antibiotic eye ointment) and carefully passed up the duct until resistance is met. Fine monofilament stainless steel suture (3 Ō or smaller), doubled over a paper clip and then twisted in a bone drill to produce a blunt end can be used. Probes aid in the identification and subsequent dissection. The rigidity accomplished by probe insertion facilitates

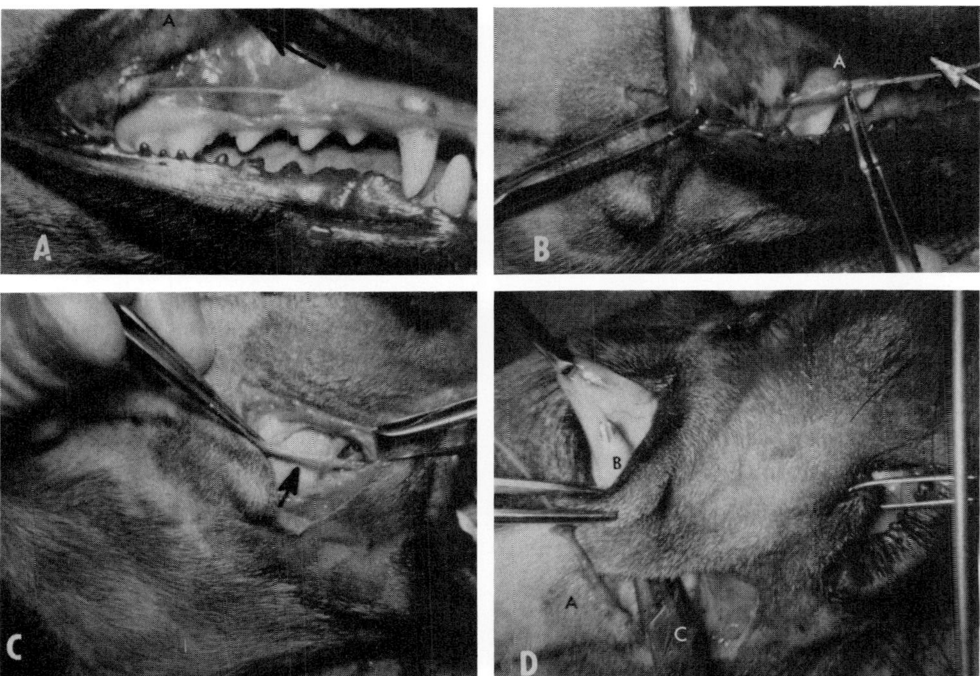

Fig. 6–15. Transposition of parotid duct. *A*. Papilla *(A)*. Probe (arrow) in place in parotid duct. *B*. Papilla and duct *(A)* dissected free. Probe (arrow). *C*. Exposed parotid duct (arrow) with buccal nerve underneath. *D*. Tunneling with a hemostat. Parotid duct with probe in place *(A)*. Base of membrane nictitans *(B)*. Hemostat *(C)*.

the dissection. *Caution*—avoid the use of parenteral atropine preoperatively until after the probe is inserted into the duct.

4. A circular incision is made around the papilla with the tenotomy scissors. The "plug" should be about 6 mm diameter and should be slightly eliptical temporally to allow grasping this tag with the mouse-toothed mosquito forceps.

5. Using the probe as a guide, the papilla and the duct are dissected free from the buccal side (Fig. 6–15B). The dissection through the mouth incision should free the duct as far back as possible.

6. The skin incision is made along the line of the parotid duct. The skin is undermined and reflected dorsally to expose the dorsal and ventral buccal nerves and facial vein. The parotid duct can be felt (probe inside) and seen coursing across the belly of the masseter muscle. The anterior portion lies under the nerves and vein (Fig. 6–15C).

7. The duct is stripped from its bed posteriorly for a distance sufficient to allow its easy extension to the conjunctival cul-de-sac. An assistant can elevate the duct with the muscle hook while the surgeon proceeds to dissect with tenotomy scissors and eye tissue forceps. Undue pressure on the wall of the duct that would compress it against the probe should be avoided.

8. The duct is undermined in the region of the nerves and facial vein and the dissection continued to meet the previously released buccal aspect.

9. Following complete release of the duct, the duct is gently slid back on the probe until the wire is visible. The wire is then cut with heavy blunt scissors, and the cut end protruding from the papilla is bent at a 180° angle to prevent it from entering further into the duct.

10. A hemostat is used to "tunnel" under the skin with the points "tenting" the pal-

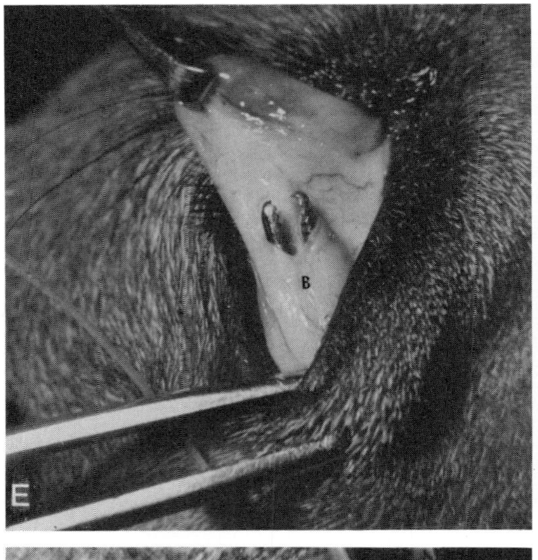

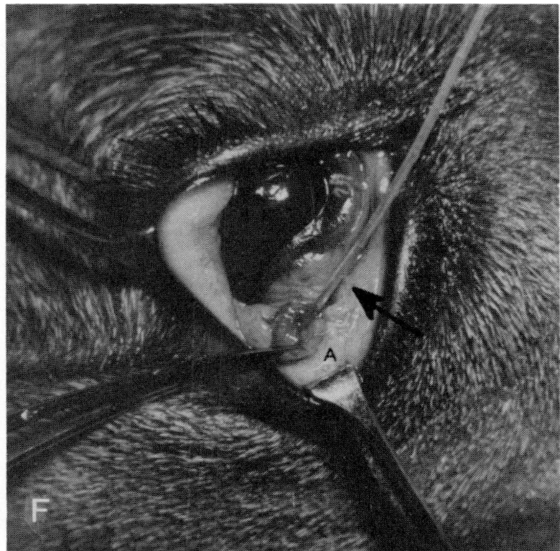

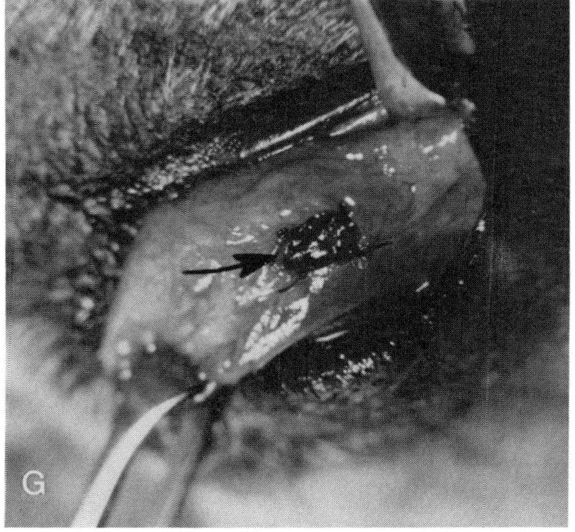

Fig. 6–15. *Continued.* *E.* Closeup of the gland of the third eyelid. Hemostat emerging at base *(B)*. *F.* Papilla *(A)* with probe (arrow) in place at base of membrane nictitans just prior to suturing. *G.* Close-up. Papilla of duct sutured into place (arrow).

pebral conjunctiva at the base of the membrane nictitans (Fig. 6–15D). The membrane nictitans is held perpendicularly. An incision is made between the spread of the forceps allowing them to come through and complete the tunneling (Fig. 6–15E). There is no need for a canthotomy. A small mosquito forceps is placed between the jaws of the forceps and drawn down through the conjunctival incision until visible in the face incision.

11. A Ō catgut suture is placed through the elliptical tag of mucosa on the papilla. This suture is grasped with the mosquito forceps and gently pulled up through the tunnel as the probe and duct are directed into the tunnel to emerge at the base of the membrane nictitans (Fig. 6–15F). Care must be exercised that the duct is not twisted.

12. The papilla is sutured in place with 6-Ō chromic catgut fixed on Atrolac needles (Fig. 6–15G). Sutures are placed opposite each other in the superior, inferior, medial and lateral aspects. Two more supporting sutures may be placed to insure good closure. The probe is not withdrawn until the appositional sutures are in place.

13. The skin closure is completed with 3 Ō or 4 Ō silk or nylon which is also used to close the incision in the mouth.

6:76 *Postoperative care.* The area may be

bandaged for 24 hours to minimize swelling. One to two drops of atropine on a finger can be touched to the dog's tongue to stimulate salivation twice a day for 3 to 4 days. The bitter taste is effective. An antibiotic steroid ophthalmic ointment is applied to the eye twice a day for 10 days. The skin sutures are usually removed on the tenth day. Failures can occur. These may be attributed to one of several causes.

6:77 The cause in most cases is occlusion of the duct due to stenosis or compression at the point where it crosses the orbital rim, just below the conjunctival sac. In these cases, the duct gradually dilates to about 2 to 3 times its normal diameter and remains turgid, but does not rupture. Correction has been accomplished by removing the stenotic area, as long as a year after occlusion.[13]

Pigmentary Keratitis

6:78 A special classification is accorded so-called pigmentary keratitis (keratitis pigmentosa) (corneal melanosis) because of its prevalence. Actually, the condition as such does qualify under the heading of superficial keratitis since usually only this portion of the cornea is involved. Neither should pigmentary keratitis be thought of as a disease entity in itself since it almost invariably is *secondary* to another disease process.

6:79 Roberts' study[69] indicated that practically all pigment in the cornea is melanin and that pigmentation of the superficial cornea originates in the germinal epithelium and, to a limited extent, from the limbus (Par. 6:7). The germinal epithelium has the same embryological origin as that of the conjunctiva, where pigment is found naturally (Par. 5:4). In another study[10] microscopic examination of pigmented corneas from dogs revealed melanocytes in the corneal epithelium, superficial stroma, and adjacent to the superficial vessels. This finding suggests that pigmentary keratitis in the dog develops as a result of migration of limbal melanocytes accompanying corneal neovascularization.

6:80 Michaelson[58] conducted experiments which are important to the understanding of pigmentary keratitis in the dog. He found that when an artificial lesion is made in the cornea of the rabbit, there is, besides an intrusion of the new blood vessels from the limbus, a proliferation or "sliding" of the conjunctival epithelial cells *including* pigment cells into the cornea. This report indicates that proliferation of the limbal melanoblasts into the cornea is apparently, under certain circumstances, a constant reaction to an experimental lesion of the cornea in the rabbit, that the proliferation has certain features in common with the vascular proliferation and occurs at the same time, and that both proliferations are probably due to the same stimulus. As pointed out earlier (Par. 6:7), the limbal area of the dog is similarly marked by a line of pigment.

6:81 In the final analysis, it appears that melanosis of the cornea is a result of migration of conjunctival melanocytes and melanin from the limbus rather than activation of vestigal corneal melanocytes.

6:82 *Etiology.* There are four possible reasons for the deposition of melanin in the cornea.

6:83 1. *Stress.* Melanin from the bulbar conjunctiva and limbal area enters the cornea in the presence of a stress factor. Distichiasis (Par. 4:32) ranks as a primary exciting factor. The rubbing of lashes on the bulbar conjunctiva and cornea of the protruding eye, especially in the Pekingese and pug breeds, causes the migration of the pigment onto the cornea. Long hairs arising from the prominent nasal folds are also a direct cause for pigment deposition in the medial aspect of the cornea. However, there are some Pekingese and pug blood lines that show a congenital predisposition to corneal pigment desposition at an early age. In these, an irritant factor is not apparent. I have observed a decreased blinking in many of these cases, and perhaps, decreased corneal sensitivity. Although the Schirmer tear test is within normal range, I think the stress causing the melanosis in these cases is due to poor tear film distribution.

Some owners also report that the dogs sleep with their eyes open. Treatment consists of continued use of steroid antibiotic drops once or twice a day to inhibit keratitis and melanosis, with instructions to the owner to report any 'cloudy' areas which might indicate ulceration. The goal is to use enough steroid to reduce keratitis and melanosis, but not enough to prevent healing in case of corneal injury. Entropion, chronic purulent conjunctivitis, keratitis sicca (Plate 10F), and pannus also predispose to the migration of the pigment, regardless of breed.

6:84 2. *Following and accompanying superficial vascularization*, as noted also by Roberts[69] and Michaelson.[58] Actually, vascularization, whether it be deep or superficial, is also the result of an exciting stress factor (inflammation), which in turn results in the migration of pigment.

6:85 3. *As a sequela to deep (interstitial) keratitis* (Fig. 6–16). When interstitial keratitis (Par. 6:96) is not recognized as such and is allowed to run its course without the proper treatment, there is often a residual pigment deposition. This, in most instances, is melanin, but hemosiderin deposition resulting from a breakdown of blood vessels in the cornea also may be a contributing factor.

6:86 4. *Migration of uveal pigment* (Fig. 6–17). Following corneal perforation and iris prolapse, an anterior synechia between iris and cornea often results. It is then that uveal pigment migrates through and along the natural nerve and vessel openings and deposits itself in the corneal stroma and on the surface.

6:87 *Treatment.* Since stress or an exciting factor of some sort is usually responsible for the presence of corneal pigment, the first consideration is to determine and eliminate the cause. It is incongruous to persist in the removal of the unwanted pigment only to see its return because of a failure to recognize the cause for its presence. The pattern of corneal pigmentation may assist in the determination of the etiology, *i.e.*, may be adjacent to the irritant.

6:88 If distichiasis or trichiasis is the exciting factor, the lashes must be removed (Par. 4:35). Long hairs arising from prominent nasal folds must, of course, be kept trimmed to prevent their reaching the cornea. Better still, surgical removal of the redundant folds offers a more satisfactory and permament

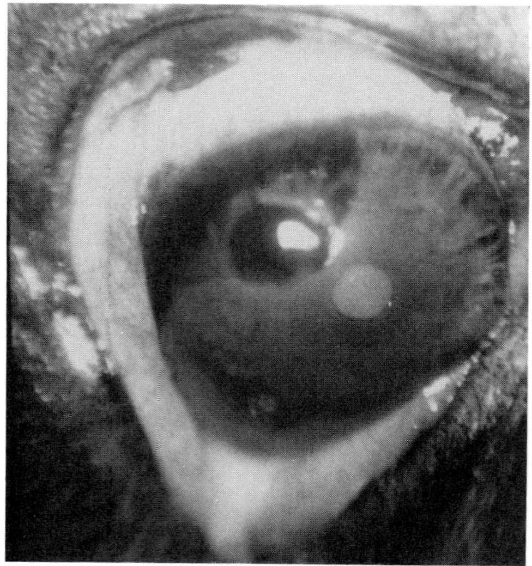

Fig. 6–16. Pigmentary keratitis as a sequel to interstitial keratitis.

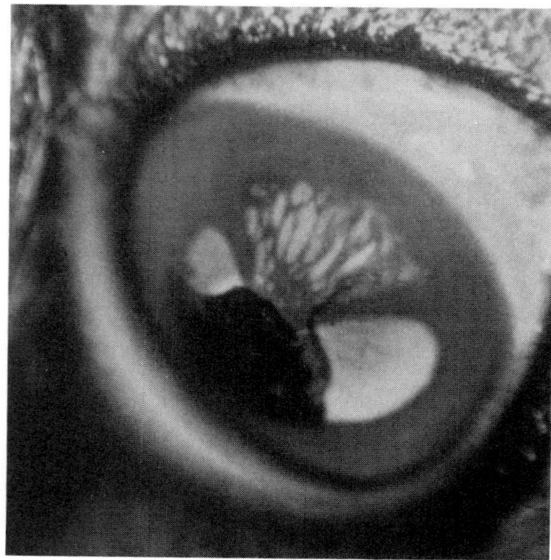

Fig. 6–17. Migration of uveal pigment with deposition on the cornea.

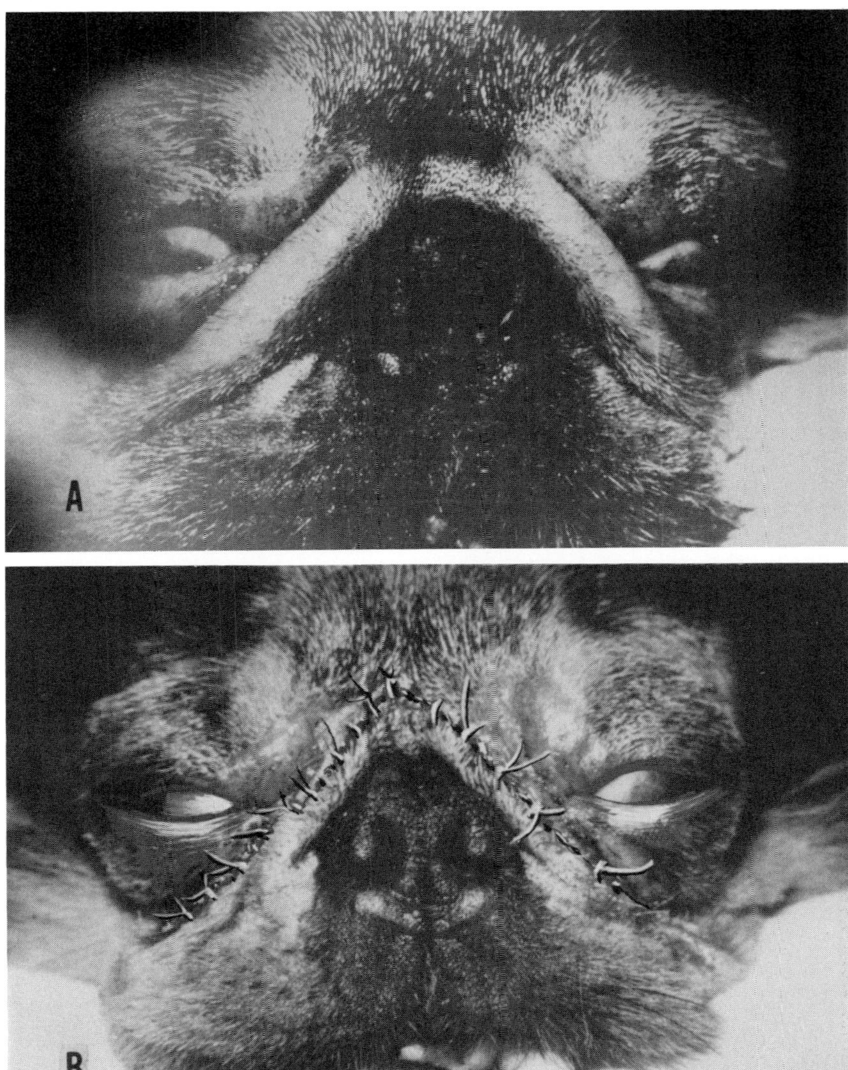

Fig. 6–18. *A.* Nasal folds prepared for surgical removal. *B.* Surgery completed.

method of eliminating this source of irritation. As a bonus, this procedure is also of benefit in those instances in which there is an accompanying chafing dermatitis.

6:89 The surgical procedure is performed simply by preparing the site through close clipping and the usual skin preparation (Fig. 6–18). The exposed ridges are excised at their bases, flush with the surrounding skin, with heavy surgical scissors. The incisions will ordinarily meet above the nose as an inverted V. Interrupted or mattress sutures complete the procedure (Fig. 6–18B).

6:90 Surgical correction of entropion (Par. 4:19) is necessary to prevent further excitation of pigment from that cause. *Warning:* Many Pugs and Pekingese have melanosis of the medial aspect of the cornea, due to the stress of medial entropion or trichiasis with no history of previous active corneal disease. As these dogs get older, some develop corneal stress and active conjunctival or corneal disease and progression of melanin due to low tear production or poor tear film distribution. Correction of the medial canthus entropion or trichiasis will not solve the problem in these dogs. It is important to conduct a complete evaluation before deciding on treatment. In cases of chronic purulent conjunctivitis (Par. 5:34), the pigment migration cannot be controlled until all inflammation and discharge are cleared from the eye. Control of pannus (Par. 6:49) by one of the means previously described is also essential to the control of the accompanying pigmentation.

6:91 It can be quite definitely stated that proper and prompt handling of interstitial keratitis is the best deterrent to the type of pigmentary keratitis which often follows.

6:92 Following the elimination of the exciting cause, little attention need be paid the pigment unless the pupillary area is occluded and vision impaired. Even then, in the absence of further irritation, much of the pigment will eventually dissipate with restoration of vision. If pigment must be removed to restore vision after the underlying causes of corneal inflammation are treated, a superficial keratectomy is the most accurate method (Par. 6:167) (Figs. 6–36, 6–38), and is preferred. Other methods of pigment removal include scraping it from the cornea with, for example, a #64 blade or sloughing it off with phenol cauterization. Cutting (Par. 6:61) (Fig. 6–12) of any accompanying trunk vessels at the limbus may also be indicated. *Caution: In exophthalmic breeds, superficial keratectomy or even corneal scraping or cautery to remove pigment may result in corneal perforation, unless a third eyelid flap is used to protect the cornea for 2 weeks while healing occurs.*

6:93 Radiation in itself has been given a thorough trial[15] and found to be helpful, but also lacking in many respects. Essentially, radiation therapy is just another destructive device which, through its latent action, causes dissipation of pigment. This same objective can be attained far more readily by keratectomy.

6:94 Following removal of the pigment and the associated superficial layers, the eye is treated as though an ulcerative keratitis were present. Atropine drops for alleviation of pain and topical antibiotics to prevent infection are used for the first 5 or 6 days. Thereafter, a steroid-antibiotic preparation is used to effect clearing.

6:95 *Again, unless the pigment is interfering with vision, or needs to be removed for other reasons, it is best left alone.* Uveal pigment deposited in and on the cornea should never be attacked surgically since it is possible to disrupt the "patch" between iris and cornea, and thereby produce a leaking anterior chamber or lost eye.

Deep (Interstitial) Keratitis

6:96 Interstitial keratitis is characterized by deep vascularization and opacity throughout the layers of the cornea (Plate 6D). The condition is an *indication of deep-seated trouble,* with diffuse cellular infiltration and edema allied with inflammation of the iris and ciliary body (uveal tract). The cellular infiltration may be so extensive that the entire cornea has a diffusely opaque appearance like ground glass. Vascularization may be scant or so intense that the cornea has a reddish appearance. The deep short vessels radiate evenly from the limbus toward the center and may escape detection in the early stage of the disease. Later they become more prominent and progress in a brush-like pattern toward the center, but do not always reach to the center. The vascularization may confine itself to segments, but more often involves the whole circumference of the cornea. Occasionally a few superficial vessels will be noted extending over the limbus from the swollen conjunctiva toward the center of the cornea.

6:97 Because of the dense corneal opacity, often the iris cannot be seen and studied. In these instances it must be assumed that the keratitis is merely a part of a uveitis, participation of the uveal tract being hidden by the opaque cornea.

6:98 *Etiology.* Causes of interstitial keratitis include: (1) focal infections, *e.g.* tonsils, teeth, prostate, sinuses, endogenous toxin; (2) specific diseases, *e.g.* distemper, hepatitis, toxoplasmosis or systemic fungus diseases (blastomycosis, cryptococcosis, coccidiomycosis); (3) wound or ocular surgery; (4) severe ulcerative keratitis; and (5) post-vaccinal (hepatitis) antigen-antibody reaction. I have seen severe anterior uveitis and interstitial keratitis with heartworm infestation. Any possible cause for the underlying uveitis must be considered. It is often difficult, if not impossible, to determine the exact cause, and considerable time must be spent in taking history, in a general physical examination, and in utilization of laboratory procedures.

6:99 *Treatment.* Since the appearance of the cornea and the type of vascularization denote involvement of the uveal tract, treatment must be directed toward that structure. Again, the cause should first be determined and treated as such, if possible. Heat (Par. 3:72) in the form of hot moist compresses to the closed lids decreases pain and improves the circulation of the eye. Subconjunctival steroid injections (Par. 3:63) are most helpful in alleviating the corneal inflammation and opacity (edema). Because of the posterior segment involvement, systemic steroids (Par. 3:63) often must also be used to achieve the best results. Subconjunctival and systemic steroids should not be given if systemic fungus disease is suspected.

6:100 X-ray radiation was used for its palliative effect and for the discouragement of vascularization,[52] but is no longer important to the treatment of the disease since the advent of the steroids.

6:101 Paracentesis (Par. 6:163) may be used to collect material from the anterior chamber for direct microscopic examination and for culture. Vitreocentesis (Par. 11:16) (Fig. 11–3) is even better if posterior or segment involvement is present or suspected.

6:102 *Complications and Sequelae.* If proper treatment has not been instigated or has been delayed, a secondary glaucoma sometimes occurs as a result of the uveitis. Some corneal haze and deep corneal vessels may remain permanently. Often this is only discernible with good magnification. Pigmentation of the cornea as a sequela has been discussed (Par. 6:85).

Ulcerative Keratitis

6:103 Ulceration is the most common corneal disease encountered. Ulcerative keratitis denotes loss of substance of the cornea with or without accompanying corneal edema. The extent and degree of involvement are best determined by the use of fluorescein dye (Par. 2:20). The subjective symptoms of pain, photophobia, lacrimation and blepharospasm may be slight or pronounced. The extent of the ulcerative process usually does not seem to correspond to the degree of injury. In fact, superficial abrasions, detectable only by close examination or fluorescein staining, often produce more profound signs than deeper more obvious injuries. This corresponds with the observation that a great majority of corneal nerve endings are in the corneal epithelium (Par. 6:15).

6:104 *Etiology.* Causes of loss of corneal substance include: injury (with subsequent infection), bacterial, fungal infections, nutritional, and *unknown.* Catcott and Griesemer[17] concluded that ulcerative keratitis is readily produced only when infectious organisms are introduced into an abraded surface. A marked pathogenicity of *Pseudomonas aeruginosa* for the canine cornea has been shown in their experiments. The incidence of corneal ulceration due to fungi has been increasing as a result of fungal overgrowth from long-term antibiotic-steroid therapy (Par. 6:55). *Candida* or *Aspergillus* are the usual findings.[31] In suspected cases appropriate diagnostic procedures, including attempts to demonstrate fungi by smears and cultures, should be employed. Material for such studies should be obtained by scraping the cornea since simple swabbing may yield nothing even though the infection is obvious.

6:105 As is true with so many diseases of the eye, breed and strain incidence is of significance. The prominent eyes of the Pekingese, pug and Boston terrier breeds apparently predispose to injury and infection. Also, the eyes in these breeds are often less responsive to treatment. Smythe[82] appropriately states that "corneal insufficiency is undoubtedly hereditary in certain breeding strains and it is noticeable how frequently corneal ulceration appears in some kennels and how infrequently in others, even when the conditions of feeding and management are equal."

6:106 Classification. Corneal ulcers may be classified in many ways, but for descriptive purposes the following is offered.

6:107 1. *Simple ulcer.* In this type the lesion remains small and superficial, with no tendency to spread or perforate. A simple nick or abrasion may be responsible. In most instances epithelial regeneration is rapid and complete in a few days if not infected.

6:108 2. *Deep ulcer* (Plate 7B). The tendency is to involve the deeper layers and may cause perforation if untreated. The progress of this type of ulceration is rapid insofar as depth is concerned, but may or may not spread over the cornea. Symptoms are marked, infection is commonly present, and the anterior uvea may be involved, with pus in the anterior chamber (hypopyon).

6:109 3. *Serpent or dendritic ulcer* (branching like a tree) (Plate 7C), usually associated with a systemic virus infection is not as common in the dog as in the cat. The tendency is for the ulceration to spread, branch, and involve the deeper layers.

6:110 4. *Nutritional ulcer* (Plate 7D). The term *keratomalacia* is used to denote corneal ulceration due to an avitaminosis A, which, in turn, is due to lack of ingestion of vitamin A or to lack of its absorption from the gastrointestinal tract and proper utilization by the body. The entire cornea is dull and lusterless (mildly edematous) and the ulcer, while superficial, may involve a large area. The lesion really results from an erosion since the cornea becomes soft. The condition is not common to the dog, but it is important that the cause be recognized since there will be no response to other than vitamin A therapy.

6:111 5. *Neuroparalytic* (neurotrophic) (Plate 9G). This type of keratitis is produced by a fifth (trigeminal) nerve lesion which interrupts sensation and the trophic impulses to the epithelial cells. The cause of sensory loss is varied but acute trauma is usually responsible. Signs include a dry, lusterless, *insensitive* cornea and an exposure keratitis with ulceration. The condition may be confused with keratitis sicca. As an aid to diagnosis the sensitiveness of the cornea should be compared to the fellow eye (Par. 2:21).

6:112 *Treatment of Ulcerative Keratitis.* Treatment of ulceration in general should embody methods which are aimed at control of the infection and hastening of the repair processes. Elimination of a possible cause, of course, must always be considered. Any corneal friction, *e.g.* entropion, distichiasis, foreign bodies, may be directly responsible for the ulceration.

6:113 Ulcerative keratitis cases often need to be hospitalized, especially if thought to be infected. If treated on an out-patient basis, it is important that a re-examination be made in not to exceed forty-eight hours. Re-staining will indicate the progress of healing.

6:114 Cauterization (Par. 3:16) of most ulcers is important to the sterilization of the area, thus paving the way for regeneration. Strong (7%) tincture of iodine offers an efficient mode of disinfecting and cauterizing ulcers. A piece of cotton is wound tightly on the end of a toothpick, dipped into the iodine and then exposed to the air for a few seconds to rid the applicator of the excess. It is now brushed upon the ulcer, especially at its infiltrated margins (Fig. 6–19). This procedure can usually be accomplished under topical anesthesia.

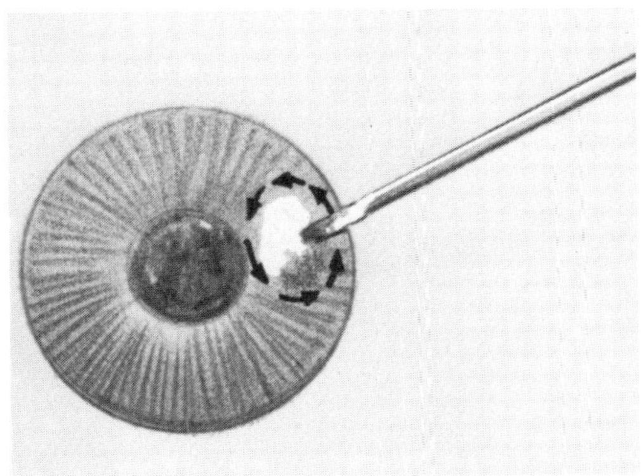

Fig. 6–19. Iodine cauterization of corneal ulcer using a cotton-wound toothpick.

6:115 Use of the antibiotic preparations (Par. 3:45) by topical instillation should be preceded by cleansing of the conjunctival sac (Par. 3:48). Systemic use of chloramphenicol (Par. 3:44) and/or chemotherapy (Par. 3:50) may be indicated in deep ulceration associated with hypopyon. The sodium succinate form of chloramphenicol 25 to 37.5 mg has also been used by subconjunctival injection (Fig. 3–2) in this type of ulceration. Other antibiotics that may be administered by subconjunctival injection are: neomycin 10 to 100 mg; bacitracin 5,000 U; penicillin G crystalline 100,000 to 500,000 U, and gentamicin 10 mg. (Par. 3:46). When using potentially nephrotoxic drugs, such as neomycin or gentamicin, one must not exceed the daily systemic dose. Five days of oral chloramphenicol, at 75 to 100 mg/pound/day, in divided dose, should be used in all cases of corneal injury due to a scratch, and in other cases in which corneal penetration is evident or suspected.

6:116 A unique corneal response to trauma or ulceration is the elaboration of collagenase by the injured epithelial cell. Some bacteria and fungi, especially *Pseudomonas*, produce large amounts of proteolytic enzymes, including collagenase. The significant corneal response to the collagenase is stromal dissolution (melting) of the cornea. Prevention of stromal loss and corneal perforation is thought to be achieved with the use of collagenase inhibitors.* A disadvantage to their use is a lack of stability and the necessity for frequent instillations. Considerable controversy exists as to the efficacy of this type of therapy. Collagenase inhibitors as adjuncts to antibiotic therapy were evaluated in experimentally induced *Pseudomonas* keratitis in rabbits. Neither the combination of a chelating agent and polymixin B nor that of cysteine and polymixin B was more effective than the polymixin B alone. Proponents of the use of collagenase inhibitors suggest that pseudomonas produces proteolytic enzymes besides collagenase, invalidating this study as proof that collagenase inhibitors are not of value.

6:117 Clinical impressions indicate that the use of an ulcer mix containing a collagenase inhibitor (Par. 3:51–3:52) and the frequent application inherent in its use, is very beneficial in treating melting ulcers.

6:118 Almost anything used on the cornea tends to retard corneal regeneration; however, destruction of the corneal stroma by infection is of utmost concern. Whereas appropriate antibiotic ointments used twice a day, or drops used 4 times a day, are adequate *to prevent infection*, ointments 4 times a day or, preferably, drops used hourly are needed *to treat an infected ulcer.* If pseudomonas infection is indicated by purulent discharge, appearance of the ulcer, or corneal scrapings, gentomycin or tobramycin, topically, with or without concurrent subconjunctival injection (Par. 3:46) should be used until results of culture and antibiotic sensitivity are available. Frequency and intensity of medication should be reduced as one gains control over the infection (Par. 6:17). The *criteria* for *control* include: clearing of the discharges, filling in of the lesion (less staining), and relief from subjective symptoms.

6:119 Topical anesthetics have long been popular for affording pain relief in corneal injury or ulceration. Extensive research has established that topical application of most anesthetics inhibits mitosis in the intact ep-

*Acetylcystine (20%). Mucomyst, Mead Johnson Laboratories, Evansville, Ind.

ithelium, migration of epithelial cells over injured areas, and cell division in the regenerating epithelium. In addition, use of topical anesthetics may predispose to further corneal damage (Par. 3:38). Generally, therefore, an atropine instillation, once daily, will more adequately serve the purpose of relieving the discomfort caused by iris and ciliary spasm associated with corneal abrasion or ulceration (Par. 3:24) and is preferred over the use of anesthetics.

6:120 The use of topical steroids is definitely contraindicated in abrasions or in corneal ulcers in which a bacterial or mycotic contamination is present or is apt to develop. Corticosteroids retard healing and increase the activity of collagenase. Admittedly, steroids will decrease pain and minimize inflammatory response in corneal injuries, but this fosters a false sense of security. Sufficient evidence (Par. 3:56) has been gathered to emphasize the fact that many eyes have been lost because the detrimental effects of steroids were not appreciated. Steroids should only be used if needed, for relief of associated inflammatory symptoms when epithelialization is complete.

6:121 *Bandaging* (Par. 3:81) is helpful, but only occasionally necessary. The use of a third eyelid flap (Par. 4:63) is one of the better means of promoting healing in chronic ulceration. Scleral contact lenses have been advocated as a means of covering the involved site and encouraging healing.[76] Loss of lenses was a problem in a recent study.[59]

6:122 A superficial keratectomy (Fig. 6–35) will often hasten healing of a chronic, stagnant, ulcerative process with accompanying vascularization, granulation, and pigmentation (Plate 7G).

6:123 *Specific treatment* for the types of ulceration described varies with each case but, in general, the following may be applicable. (Please read the discussion of treatment in general (Par. 6:112–6:121) before proceeding with specific therapy.)

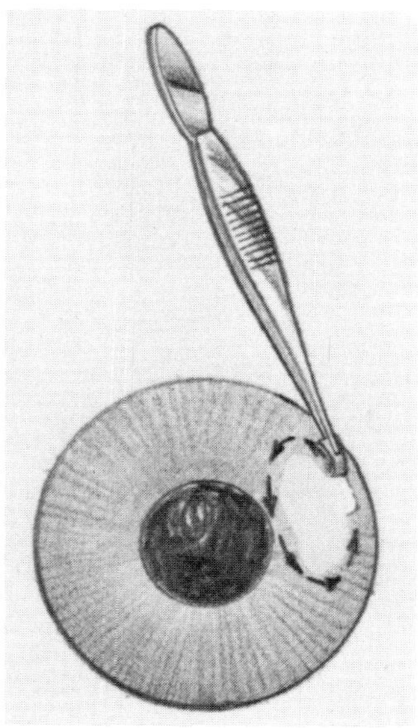

Fig. 6–20. Stripping of overhanging epithelium in corneal erosion.

6:124

1. *Simple ulcer*
   - (*a*) Iodine cautery
   - (*b*) Atropine
   - (*c*) Topical antibiotic
     (For corneal erosion syndrome see Par. 6:47)

6:125

2. *Deep ulcer*
   - (*a*) Clean discharges
   - (*b*) Iodine cautery
   - (*c*) Atropine
   - (*d*) Antibiotic therapy
     (topical, subconjunctival, systemic)
   - (*e*) Collagenase inhibitor
   - (*f*) Vitamins (oral or parenteral)
   - (*g*) Possible third eyelid flap

6:126

3. *Dendritic ulcer*
   - (*a*) Clean discharges
   - (*b*) Iodine cautery
   - (*c*) Atropine
   - (*d*) Antibiotics
   - (*e*) Collagenase inhibitor

(*f*) Vitamins
(*g*) Possible third eyelid flap

6:127
4. *Nutritional ulcer*
(*a*) Vitamin A
(*b*) Topical treatment as needed

6:128
5. *Neuroparalytic (neurotrophic)*
(*a*) Artificial tears
(*b*) Antibiotic therapy (topical)
(*c*) Protective tarsorrhaphy or conjunctival flap.

Acquired Deformities of the Cornea (Fig. 6–21)

6:129 Protrusions or acquired deformities of the cornea may result from injury or ulcerative keratitis. They include: (1) descemetocele, (2) iris prolapse, (3) staphyloma, and (4) ectasia.

6:130 A *descemetocele* occurs when an ulceration proceeds down to Descemet's membrane (Fig. 6–22) and is warning that an iris prolapse is imminent. Occasionally the corneal defect, in association with a descemetocele or iris prolapse, will appear healed only to rupture some weeks or months later. Aqueous will escape and the anterior chamber will become shallow. Following this pressure relief, the wound will again seal with a filling of the chamber. This "weak patch" is thus subject to recurrent rupture.

6:131 *Treatment.* Impending rupture of a descemetocele or rupture itself is a serious consequence, but need not equate to loss of the eye. Goals of treatment should include identification and vigorous treatment of infection, if present, dilation of the pupil with atropine and repair of the rupture or weak area of the cornea. A lamellar homograft (Par. 6:184) (Fig. 6–40) gives the strongest support. This requires adequate magnification, proper instrumentation and corneal suture material. The next strongest repair can be accomplished by a 360 degree conjunctival flap (Fig. 5–8). The simplest technique which is often quite satisfactory is a third eyelid flap (Par. 4:63) (Fig. 4–24) kept in place for 18 to 21 days. With any treatment, it is extremely important to avoid vigorous restraint during examination or anesthesia, in order to avoid rupturing the descemetocele. Rapid decompression of the eye results in more intraocular inflammation and even hemorrhage. Such complication does not spell disaster, but should be avoided if possible. Application of the appropriate antibiotic drops hourly or ointment four times a day to the surface of the flap or graft is essential if infection is suspected. Atropine should be applied twice a day to keep the pupil dilated and reduce pain.

6:132 An *iris prolapse* (Plate 8A and Fig. 6–23) is associated with loss of aqueous humor and temporary collapse of the anterior chamber. When a portion of the iris becomes entangled in the wound or protrudes beyond and adheres to the edges, the anterior chamber re-forms. When the iris does not protrude beyond the normal curvature of the cornea, it becomes adherent either to the back of the cornea or fills in the space. When final healing is accomplished, an *adherent leukoma results.*

6:133 *Treatment.* If the iris protrudes beyond the cornea, this portion is disengaged from the wound and snipped off flush with the cornea (Fig. 6–24). The corneal wound is sutured, and a protective third eyelid flap is then brought into place in the manner described (Par. 4:63) and aftercare is the same as that for descemetocele (Par. 6:131). An iris that does not protrude (impending prolapse) but is incarcerated within the corneal stroma is best not disturbed. Again, a supportive third eyelid flap is indicated to prevent progression of the prolapse. In case of a large iris prolapse with complete loss of the anterior chamber, suturing of the cornea (Fig. 6–29) or a keratoplasty (Par. 6:184) (Fig. 6–40), and reforming of the anterior chamber should be accomplished after cutting off the prolapsed iris. In cases of massive iris prolapse, complicated by intraocular infection, the eye should be enucleated.

6:134 A *staphyloma* is a bulging cicatrix lined by prolapsed iris. In other words, it is

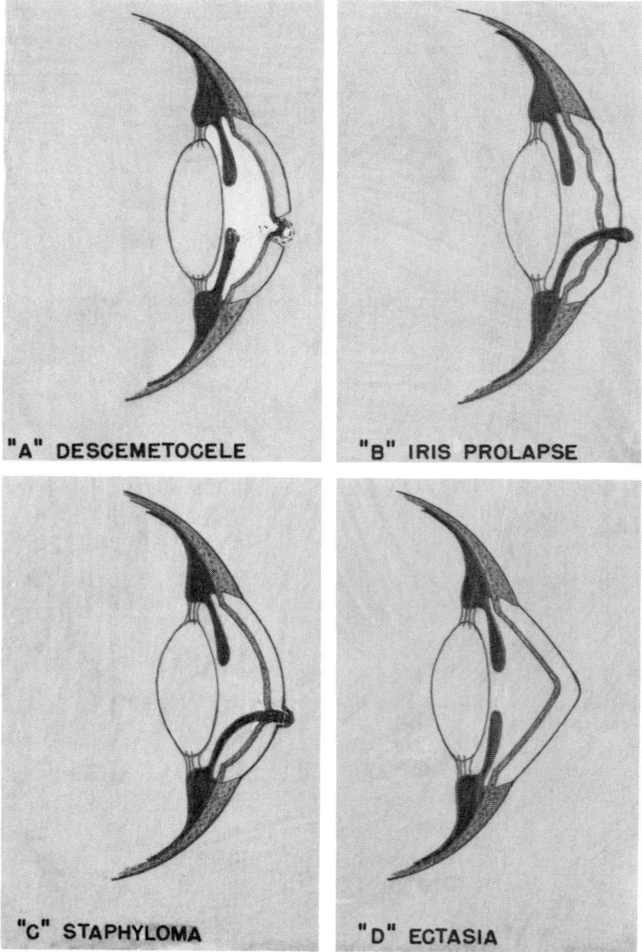

Fig. 6–21. Acquired deformities of the cornea.

a protruding iris prolapse over which a fibrin film and layer of epithelium have formed. This in turn helps to create a seal between the iris and surrounding cornea. In this condition the cornea, in the prolapsed area, has been partially or nearly entirely destroyed.

6:135 *Treatment.* If the area is small and there remains a considerable portion of normal or near normal cornea, the prolapsed portion is snipped off. Or, if it is evident that a small prolapsed portion and the surrounding cornea are and have been strongly adhered for some time, it is best left alone. If a massive prolapse is present and the eye is blind, it should be enucleated.

6:136 *Ectasia* (keratectasia) is a protrusion of the cornea alone resulting from chronic inflammatory changes with subsequent thinning. It may be due to softening of the cornea following interstitial keratitis. The bulging portion is opaque and conical (keratoconus). When the condition is fully developed, treatment is of no avail.

6:137 In ectasia, the center of the cornea is thinned, and the cornea is weakened. A more common cause of a conical shape to the cornea is severe corneal edema and central thickening associated with endothelial dystrophy (Par. 6:27) or inflammatory decompensation

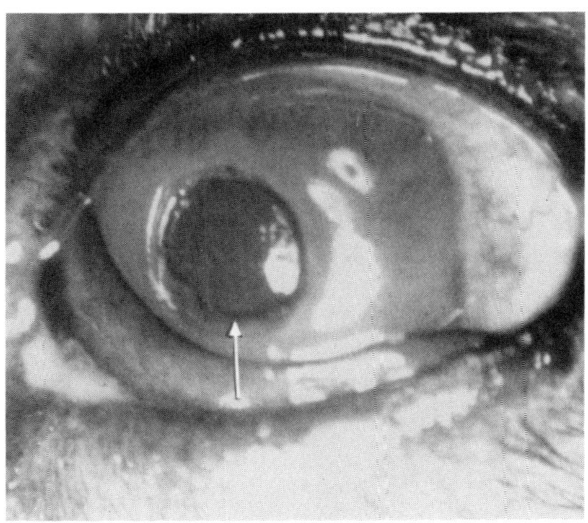

Fig. 6–22. Descemetocele.

(Par. 7:35). In these cases, the cornea is not weakened; however, bullae formation with subsequent ulceration may occur as a complication.

Tumors of the Cornea

6:138 Neoplasms of the cornea rarely occur and almost always represent secondary extensions of lesions which are primary to some other part of the eye, *e.g.* the uveal tract (Par. 7:81). A primary epithelioma of the cornea was reported in a ten-year-old shepherd.[48] The growth was on the nasal margin of the cornea and was successfully removed without recurrence. Dermoid tumors have been discussed under congenital anomalies of the cornea (Par. 6:18). Corneal epithelial inclusion cysts have been reported.[73] These raised, solitary corneal masses are limited to the superficial layers of the cornea. They are easily removed by keratectomy. Limbal melanocytomas (Par. 6:201) may also extend into the cornea. An area of corneal dystrophy is often present along the leading edge (Plate 10H).

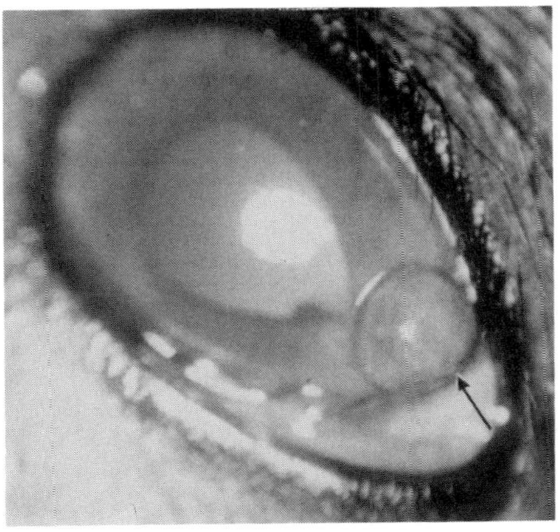

Fig. 6–23. Iris prolapse as a result of perforating injury to the cornea. Note the change in the shape of the pupil.

Foreign Bodies of the Cornea (Plate 10E)

6:139 Foreign bodies, consisting of splinters (Fig. 6–25), thorns, awns, flakes of paint (Fig. 6–26) or metal, etc., may adhere or become embedded in the cornea causing pain, lacrimation and photophobia. A shotgun pellet may penetrate a cornea but usually becomes embedded in the posterior part of the globe or in the retrobulbar area. If the presence of a foreign body goes unnoticed or it is not removed, ulceration and/or edema and vascularization of the cornea may result. Excessive granulation tissue formation on the cornea may cover an embedded splinter (Plate 8B).

6:140 *Treatment.* When the foreign body is superficial, it can usually be removed under topical anesthesia in one of several ways. Useful instruments for this purpose include: an eyedropper to suck it from the surface; the point of a hypodermic needle or pointed blade to lift it from the cornea; or, eye splinter or dressing forceps to withdraw it.

6:141 When it is more firmly attached or has penetrated into the corneal stroma, it must be lifted or dug out with a spud (Fig. 6–27) or curette (Fig. 6–28). Deeply embedded splinters with a covering of epithelium must be "cut down on." Under general anesthesia, an incision is made over the splinter with a No. 15 B.P. or No. 64 Beaver blade. It may then be removed by lifting. Care must be taken not to perforate the cornea. Aftercare consists of a drop of atropine once a day and an antibiotic or sulfacetamide solution several times a day until reepithelialization is complete.

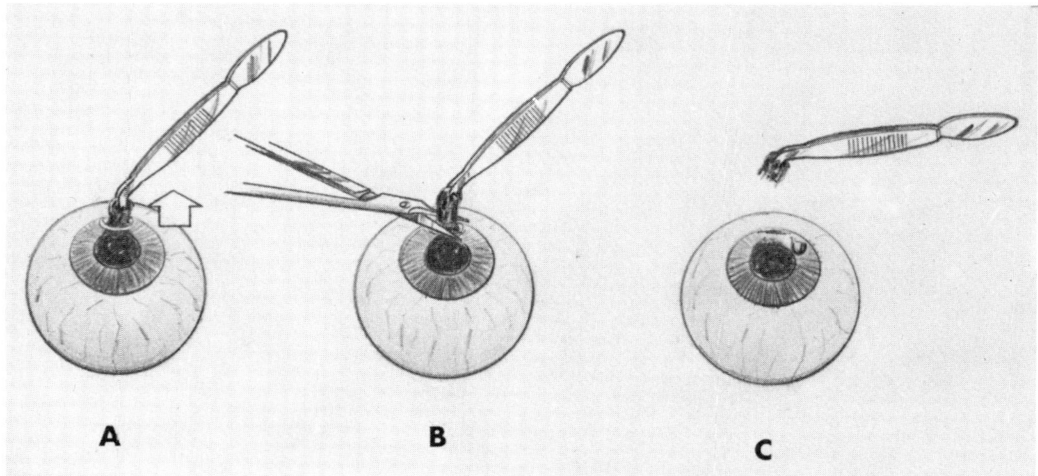

Fig. 6–24. Surgical correction of iris prolapse. *A*. Prolapsed portion disengaged from the opening. *B*. Prolapsed portion snipped off flush with the cornea. *C*. Appearance immediately following extirpation of the iris prolapse.

Wounds of the Cornea (Plate 10G)

6:142 Wounds may be non-penetrating or penetrating. Non-penetrating wounds and abrasions, though painful, heal readily (Par. 6:16) unless infected. Treatment consists of a drop of atropine once a day and an antibiotic or sulfacetamide solution several times a day until re-epithelialization is complete.

6:143 Penetrating wounds of the cornea are subject to prolapse of the iris or injury to the deeper parts. If the perforating wound is limited to the cornea, the treatment then depends upon the extent of the laceration. Small corneal perforations seal readily with quick reformation of the anterior chamber. The use

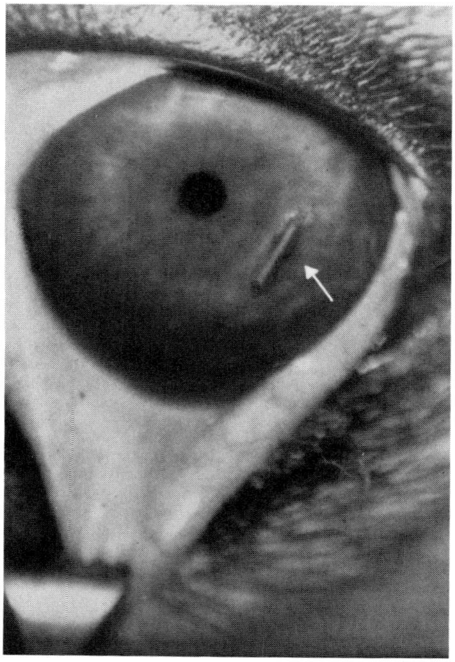

Fig. 6–25. Splinter embedded in cornea.

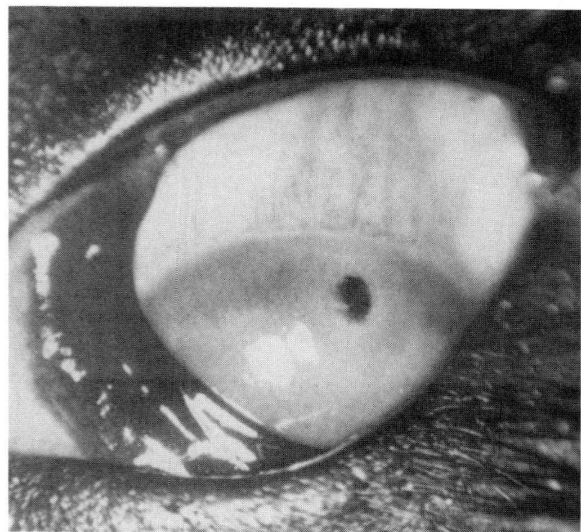

Fig. 6–26. Paint flake embedded in cornea.

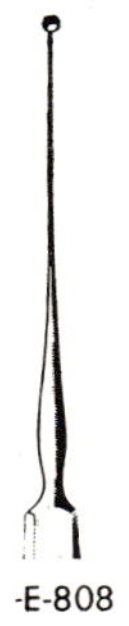

Fig. 6–27. Foreign body spud.

of a third-eyelid flap (Par. 4:60) and/or bandaging (Par. 3:89) following instillation of atropine and an antibiotic will immobilize the globe until a good seal is effected. Systemic chloramphenicol (6:115) should always be given in cases of cat scratch or other corneal penetration in which infection might be introduced. Deep stromal edema along the track of a wound is often a clue to corneal penetration. If penetration is even just suspected, give chloramphenicol at 25 mg/pound, 3 times a day, for a minimum of 5 days, in addition to topical atropine and chloromycetin.

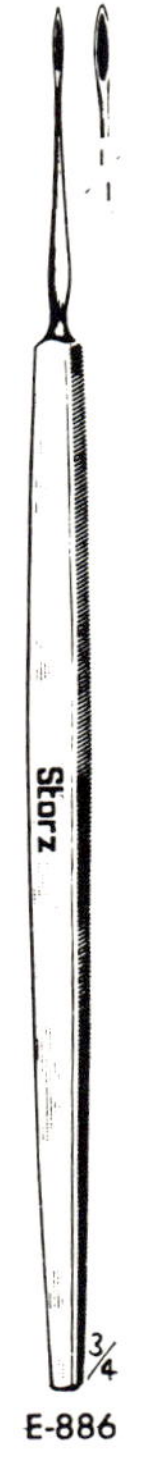

Fig. 6–28. Foreign body curette.

6:144 Extensive lacerations with collapse of the anterior chamber require the careful placement of corneal sutures. If iris protrudes through the wound, it is safer to excise it (Par. 6:132) as no iris or foreign material should remain between the wound edges.

6:145 *Technique. (a)* The anterior chamber should be cleansed of easily removed clots or debris. This may be accomplished by careful irrigating with sterile saline solution or balanced salt solution (BSS), using a lacrimal needle and syringe or irrigator. If the clot cannot be removed in this manner, sterile cellulose (Weckcell) sponge spears may be used to roll the clot on. Removal of all clots and fibrin is not essential. They will be absorbed in 10 to 14 days. Further damage and perhaps renewed bleeding can be caused by flushing or manipulation to remove clots. *(b)* Interrupted sutures of 8-0 silk* or other suitable suture are placed so that they do not penetrate through the entire thickness of the cornea (Fig. 6–29A). This type placement prevents "wicking" from the anterior chamber. Colibri forceps or a special corneal forceps† that prevents needle penetration (Fig. 6–30) is used to grasp the corneal edges about 1 to 2 mm from the edge. The sutures must oppose the edges radially to avoid buckling. As many sutures are placed as are necessary to make the wound leak-proof. They are tied firmly but with care that sloughing of the corneal tissue will not occur. *(c)* An infusion of an air bubble is made to reform the anterior chamber, prevent formation of anterior synechiae, and to check the snugness of the suture line (Fig. 6–29B). *(d)* Following topical instillation of atropine and an antibiotic the lids may be sutured (Fig. 9–15) and a bandage applied. If bandaging is not feasible, a supportive third eyelid flap (Par. 4:63) may be used.

*8-0 silk, 1767 G. Ethicon, Somerville, N.Y.
†Lawton Co., Inc., 435 4th Ave., New York, N.Y.

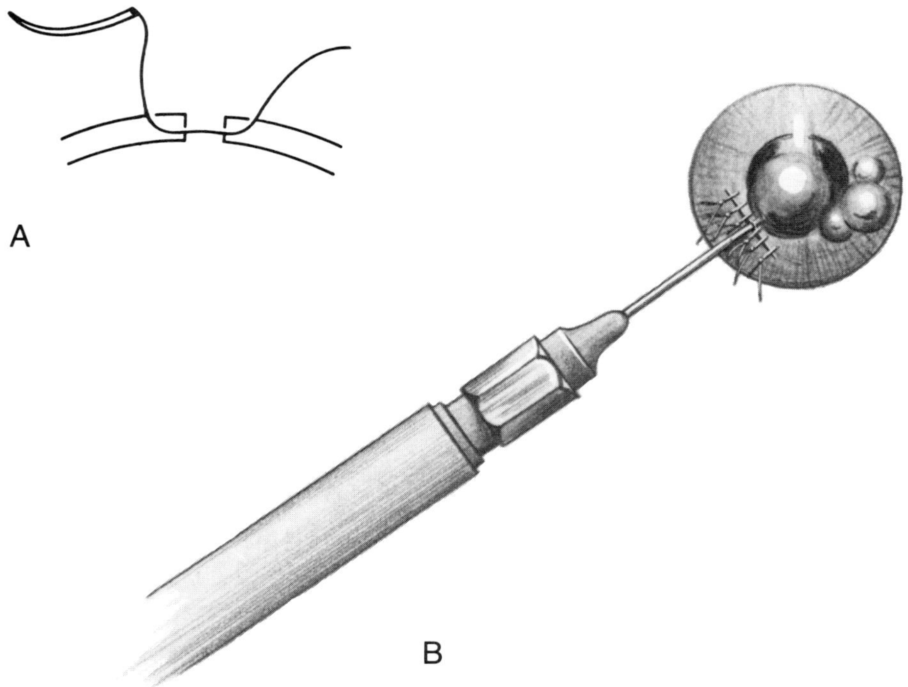

Fig. 6–29. Corneal wound repair. *A*. Proper suture placement. *B*. Reformation of the anterior chamber by infusion of air bubbles. Lacrimal cannula and hypodermic syringe.

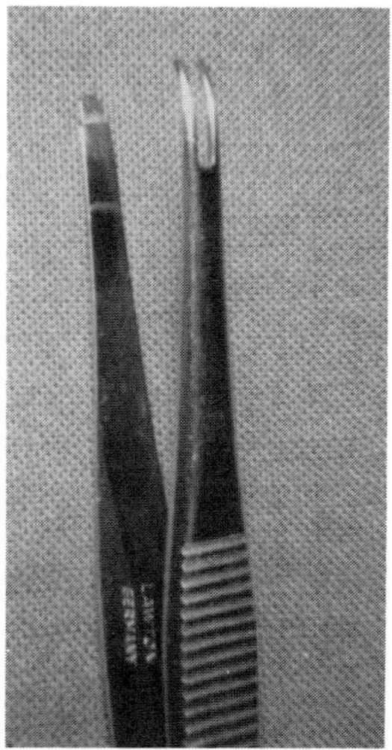

Fig. 6–30. Special corneal forceps.

6:146 Aftercare again should include atropine and a topical antibiotic. The corneal sutures are removed in 2 to 3 weeks. Subconjunctival chloramphenicol, 37.5 mg–50 mg, after surgery, followed by oral chloramphenicol, 75 mg–100 mg/pound/day in divided doses should be given if infection is considered likely.

6:147 Repair of corneal lacerations constitutes major surgery. Good results cannot be expected unless the proper instruments and suture material are used and unless the operator has attained proficiency in microsurgery and exercises good judgment in the aftercare.

6:148 The experimental use of adhesives in eye surgery has been given considerable recognition in the last few years. Various adhesives of the cyanoacrylate group are being used on an investigational basis as an adjunct to corneal sutures, and in some instances, as a total replacement for sutures.[43,55,65] When they become generally available, their usefulness to the general practitioner appears promising. They are relatively easy to apply, are known to successfully seal fairly large lacerations, and use of newer derivatives is resulting in a minimum of scarring and neovascularization of the cornea.

Burns of the Cornea

6:149 Corneal burns produce pronounced subjective symptoms and, if neglected, may result in irreparable damage and loss of vision (Par. 3:18). Alkaline burns from detergents and soaps used in bathing are the most common types encountered (Plate 7F).

6:150 Regardless of whether the corneal burn is caused by lime, plaster, or chemicals, the eye and conjunctival folds should be immediately and copiously irrigated with normal saline solution or tap water as a first aid measure at home. Instillation of atropine for pain relief (Par. 3:24) and soothing preparations such as methylcellulose drops (Par. 3:94) usually suffice. An antibiotic to prevent secondary infection may be warranted.

6:151 Thermal and ultraviolet burns are treated symptomatically. Inhalation anesthesia burns (cone administration) are best prevented by protecting the cornea with a bland ointment or castor oil (Par. 3:93). General anesthesia also causes a temporary reduction of tear production[88] that implies a need for corneal protection.

Opacities of the Cornea

6:152 Lack of transparency of the cornea may result from anything that disrupts the precise arrangement of the corneal fibrils (Par. 6:4). The causes include edema, inflammation, ulceration, or injury. Adhesions to the endothelium interfere with the ability of endothelial cells to "pump" fluid out of the cornea, resulting in corneal edema and opacity (Plate 9E,F). A small segment or the entire cornea may lose transparency. These opacities may be transient or permanent. Transient opacities are usually associated with healing of superficial ulceration and injury and in superficial punctate keratitis (Par. 6:44). Permanent, dense opacities and scarring will be found in corneal dystrophies (Par. 6:22), and in the condition spoken of as adherent leukoma (Plate 9E), or, in any case where the corneal stroma is replaced in the healing process. When the severe corneal edema associated with deep keratitis (Par. 6:96) subsides, the cornea will have a faint cloudiness throughout. The opacity and edema associated with bullous keratitis (Plate 7A) may clear with treatment, but a residual haze often remains. Loss of transparency associated with glaucoma is usually transient. The cornea clears rapidly once the pressure is normalized but, if the increase has been of long duration, streaks remain (Par. 9:25).

6:153 According to density, a corneal opacity is called *nebula* (Fig. 6–31A) when faint and cloud-like; *macula* (Fig. 6–31B) when more pronounced and discernible as a gray spot in daylight; and *leukoma* (Fig. 6–31C) when dense and white.

6:154 *Treatment.* Topical steroids are helpful in hastening corneal clearing once an ulcer is healed. The opacity associated with corneal dystrophy is easily removed by performing a superficial keratectomy (Par. 6:166). Leukomatous scars are best left alone. Opacity associated with deep keratitis can be minimized by using steroids by subconjunctival injection and topically.

SURGICAL PROCEDURES OF THE CORNEA

Fixation of the Globe

6:155 Often the clinician is prone to neglect performing a relatively simple procedure involving the cornea and associated perilimbal conjunctival structures because he has found it exceedingly difficult to fix the globe in a proper manner. The elasticity of the bulbar conjunctiva in all breeds, the natural reces-

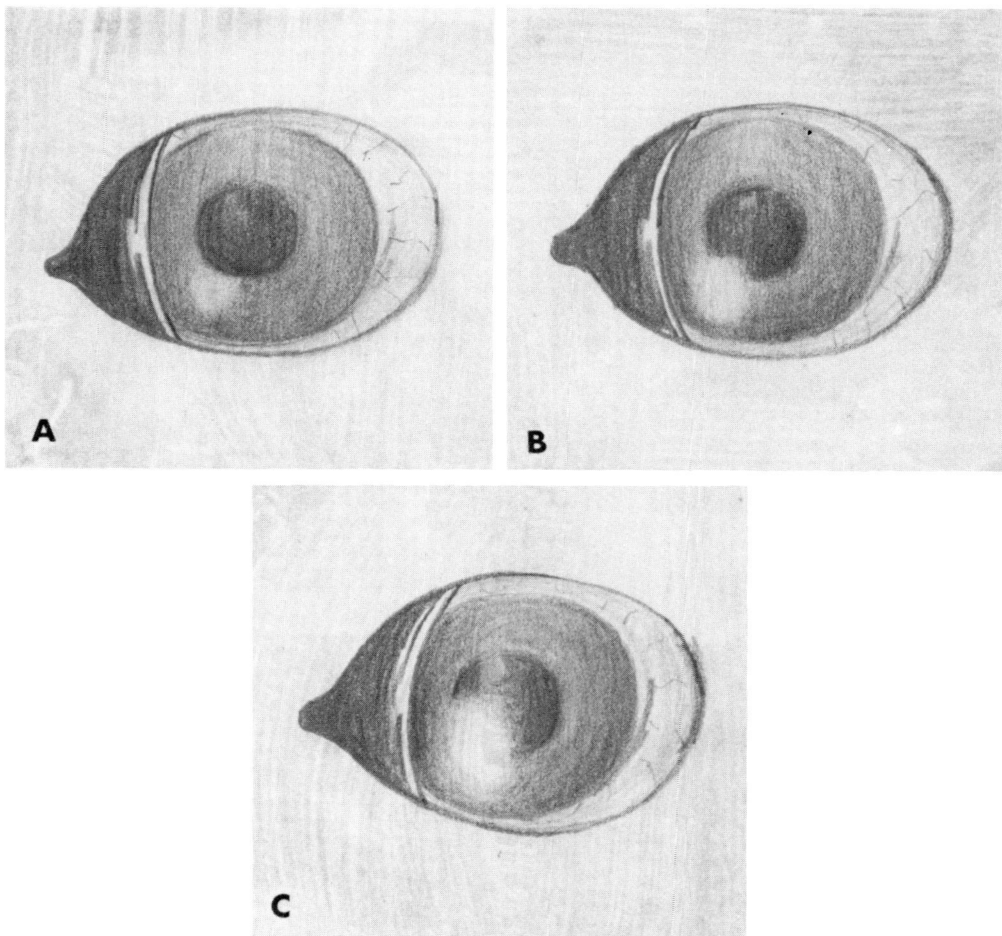

Fig. 6–31. Corneal opacities according to density. *A.* Nebula. *B.* Macula. *C.* Leukoma.

sion of the globe in others, and the tendency for the eye to "roll back" under general anesthesia certainly contribute to this difficulty. Regardless of these facts, with proper instruments and a little practice, the eyeball can be fixed in any position to facilitate the performance of the desired procedure.

6:156 Instruments used are: a medium muscle (strabismus) hook, rat-toothed mosquito forceps, and eye fixation forceps (Fig. 6–32). With the use of the muscle hook it is possible to proptose a globe intentionally in order to start a superficial keratectomy properly. This smooths and renders taut the bulbar conjunctiva and minimizes hemorrhage in the vascular perilimbal area during the actual keratectomy procedure. The eyes of Pekingese, pugs, Bostons, boxers, German shepherds, and cockers can be proptosed easily to facilitate the reaching of an area, and to smooth out the conjunctival folds when making incisions down to the sclera. In other breeds, or when the palpebral fissure is small, a canthotomy (Par. 4:11) is first performed.

6:157 In the proptosing of a globe the muscle hook is introduced from the lateral canthus, and is inserted between the membrane nictitans, and the globe (Fig. 6–33). Then,

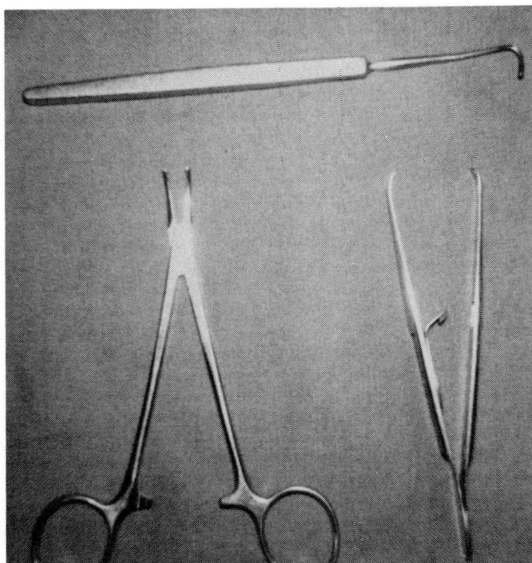

Fig. 6–32. Instruments used for fixation of the globe. Muscle hook, curved rat-toothed mosquito forceps, and fixation forceps (Graefe-spring catch)

with pressure exerted in a lifting manner the globe is lifted up and out against the upper lid. By spreading the lids with the other hand, the eye will proptose a reasonable distance beyond the lid margins. It can be fixed in this position by having an assistant continue to exert pressure with the hook and/or the rat-toothed mosquito forceps (Figs. 6–34, 6–37) or with the index finger (Fig. 6–36). Once the dissection of, for example, a pannus lesion or dermoid is well under way, the globe may be allowed to retract as the fixation forceps on the diseased tissue will suffice to control the eye for the continuation of the surgery.

6:158 There is no danger to the eye attending the proptosing procedure as the extraocular muscles allow for this "play" (Par. 1:20). However, proptosing of a globe should *never* precede or be used to fix the eye in an intraocular operative procedure, or when the cornea is weakened by an ulcer or injury.

6:159 The muscle hook is also used to rotate the eye in any desired direction. A slow, steady pressure is exerted to bring any aspect of the anterior portion of the eye into view. This facilitates cutting of blood vessels at the limbus (Par. 6:61), or the use of the beta-ray applicator at the limbus (Fig. 3–4), and exposes the inferior aspect of the globe so that it might be grasped and held with rat-toothed mosquito forceps in preparation for, for example, superficial keratectomy (Par. 6:167).

6:160 Rat-toothed mosquito forceps will bite well into the bulbar conjunctiva and underlying episcleral tissue. This fixation alone or in conjunction with the eye fixation forceps placed on another part of the globe will be sufficient to start the preparation of the conjunctival flap used in glaucoma and cataract surgery. Once a good flap is prepared, usually the fixation instruments can be released.

6:161 Stay sutures placed in either or both the body of the superior and inferior recti muscles can be used for globe fixation. This type of fixation is best suited to the human eye which has better extraocular muscle development. Vierheller[89] places a bridle suture in or around the superior rectus muscle in intraocular procedures. The eye must be rolled downward. A small ½ circle needle is dipped through the conjunctiva about 12 mm back of the limbus so that a loop of fine stitching material may be drawn around the muscle. The ends of the bridle suture are then clipped to the drape under gentle traction.

6:162 Überreiter[86] reported use of stay sutures in this manner. The upper eyelid is pulled upward by means of a lid retractor; the tendon of the superior rectus muscle is grasped through the conjunctiva with a muscle forceps and a stay suture is inserted beneath it with the aid of a full-curved needle. Similarly, a second stay suture is put into the interior surface of the membrane nictitans.

PARACENTESIS

6:163 Paracentesis of the anterior chamber has been used in treatment of deep corneal ulcers, removal of blood or hypopyon and to promote formation of plasmoid aqueous, which has a higher antibody titer.[16] With the

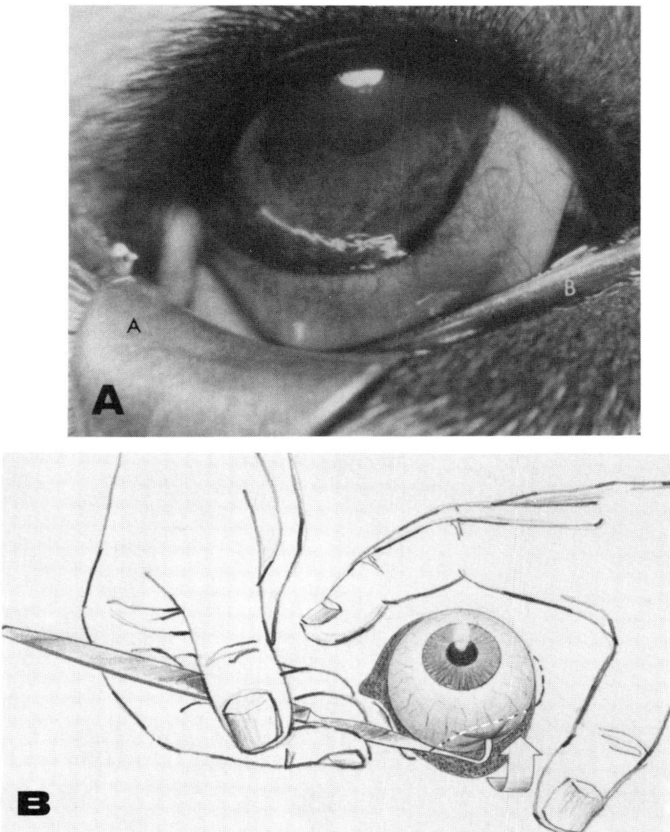

Fig. 6–33. Preliminary step for proptosing of the globe. *A*. Muscle hook in position under the globe (A) lid retractor; (B) muscle hook. *B*. "Cut-away" view.

advent of newer antibacterial and antiinflammatory agents, the use of paracentesis is limited primarily to infrequent collection of samples for diagnostic purposes and decompression of the anterior chamber to facilitate repair of a descemetocele.

6:164 *Technique*. Paracentesis can be accomplished by inserting a 22- to 25-gauge needle on a 3-ml syringe, through the conjunctiva, just back of the limbus, and then through the limbus into the anterior chamber. Immobilization of the globe with a mosquito forceps (Fig. 6–5), facilitates the procedure. If the paracentesis is to collect material for diagnostic purposes, it is advisable to use a 22-gauge needle, and to replace the volume withdrawn with air, to reestablish the intraocular pressure, thus reducing the chance of intraocular hemorrhage in an already inflamed eye. Injection of air is easily accomplished by having 1 to 1½ ml of air in the syringe prior to inserting the needle. Tipping the syringe down to allow the air to rise after the sample is withdrawn, allows injection of the air. Pinching the episcleral tissue with a Bishop Harmon forceps placed across the needle is helpful in preventing leakage of air as the needle is withdrawn.

6:165 Paracentesis of an already inflamed eye should be performed only if, after careful consideration, one decides that the information to be gained outweighs the risk of general anesthesia and increased inflammation produced by the procedure. Vitreocentesis (Par. 11:16) is more likely to reveal the causative

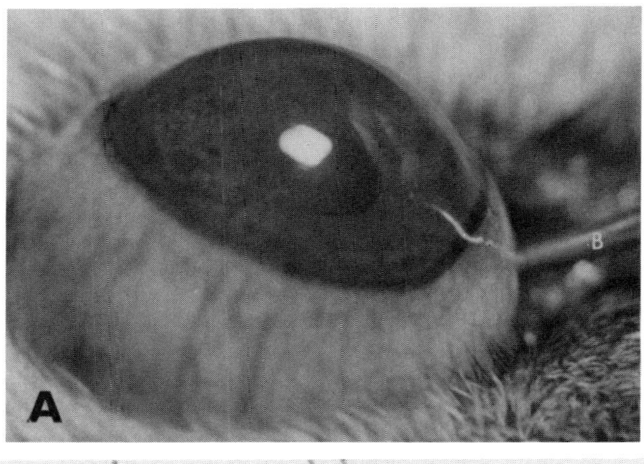

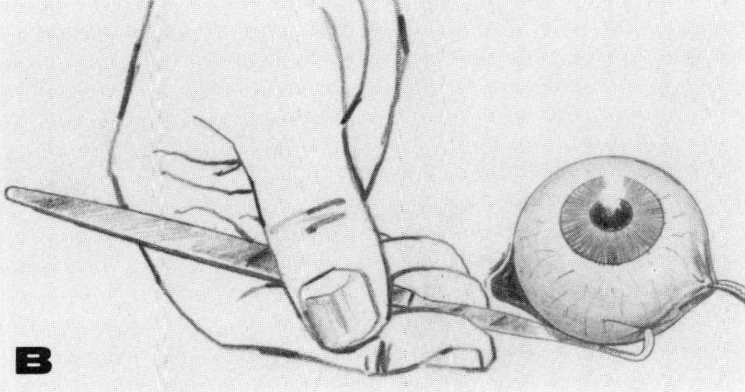

Fig. 6–34. The proptosed eye. *A*. Muscle hook holding the globe (B) muscle hook. *B*. "Cut-away" view and additional fixation with rat-toothed mosquito forceps.

agent in panophthalmitis or endophthalmitis, such as caused by blastomycosis.

Superficial Keratectomy

6:166 Removal of the superficial corneal layers is indicated for dermoids (Par. 6:19), advanced pannus (Par. 6:56), dystrophy (Par. 6:26), hyperplasia (Par. 5:44), superficial stagnant or recurrent ulceration and superficial scarring not associated with adherent leukoma.

6:167 The lamellar structure of the cornea (Par. 6:4) allows for a keratectomy at any level. The following method is considered the safest, most practical way of removing the pathological tissue at a corneal level which will generally result in finding a clear stroma underneath, but leaves enough of the corneal stroma to preclude penetration or rupture of the eyeball.

6:168 *Technique* (Fig. 6–35). Instruments required are: No. 64 Beaver blade or No. 15 B.P. blade; blunt tip, thin bladed tenotomy or strabismus scissors; eye tissue forceps; and fixation forceps. The eye is first proptosed and immobilized to facilitate the procedure (Par. 6:157).

6:169 An incision is made through the conjunctiva and Tenon's capsule down to the sclera (Fig. 6–35A). The incision site is usually 1 to 2 mm from the limbus but is made at whatever distance from the limbus may be required to include any accompanying conjunctival pathology. Having reached the scleral level, the operator now has a landmark and the proper level for the dissection.

6:170 The resection of the lesion is done in

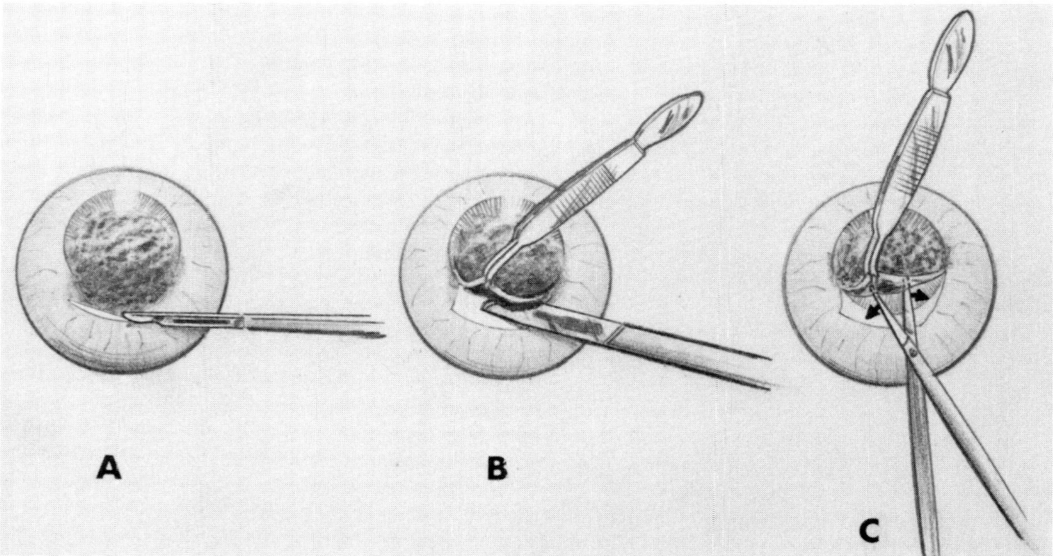

Fig. 6–35. Superficial keratectomy. *A.* Initial perpendicular knife incision to the sclera. *B.* Flat knife incision through the limbal area. *C.* Scissors used in spread fashion to separate lesion from clear cornea.

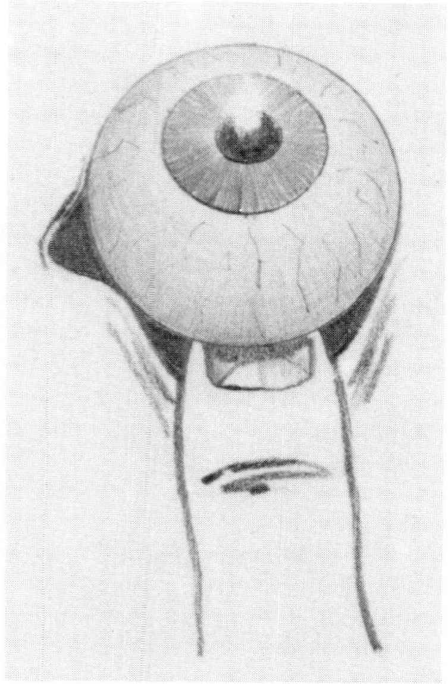

Fig. 6–36. Proptosed eye fixed with index finger.

the manner of skinning an animal (Fig. 6:36B). The stroke of the blade is parallel with the line of cleavage and slight pressure is exerted with the flat of the knife against the scleral and, then, the corneal surface. In the dissection to the limbus, the back edge of the point may be used. Upon reaching the limbus the sharp edge, held flat to the surface, must be used to shave through this very adherent structure (Par. 5:1). Upon reaching the cornea the rest of the peeling off advances quickly and easily. With a firm grip on the portion to be removed the proptosed eye may be allowed to return to the orbit. First, however, it is well to touch the bleeding points on the scleral side with either the electrocoagulator (Par. 3:84) or with a muscle hook that has been heated over an alcohol lamp.

6:171 The eye speculum is inserted for better exposure and the dissection is continued using either the back of the blade and/or the scissors in spread fashion (Fig. 6–35C). The scissors are also used to snip through this limbal margin, one blade on the corneal and the other on the scleral side. Irrigation with sterile saline solution is necessary to keep the

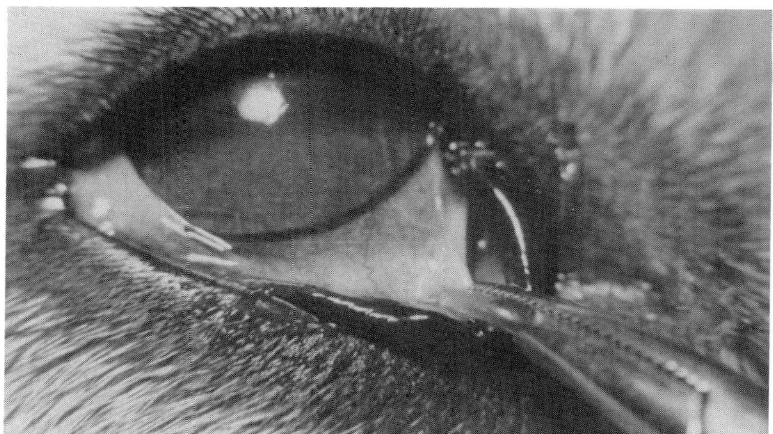

Fig. 6–37. Rat-toothed mosquito forceps being used for positioning and fixation of the globe.

structures moist and to wash away the blood and debris.

6:172 Finally, when the resection has reached normal tissue, the scissors are used to cut the lesion from its base. Ordinarily, about one-third of the corneal thickness has been removed (Fig. 6–38).

6:173 If one has made the original incision deep enough, the iris and pupillary margin are readily made out. Should this not be true and the corneal tissue is not clear, then either the incision has not reached the proper level or the scar or lesion involves the deeper layers of the cornea and cannot be successfully removed. If the proper level has been reached (scleral landmark), it is seldom that a deeper opacity (Par. 6:47) will be encountered in the dog's cornea. In any event, a further level beyond this should not be sought since there is danger of perforating the cornea.

6:174 If the lesion is limited to one segment of the cornea, it is not necessary to peel off the entire surface. Only the lesion and clear cornea a few millimeters beyond should be removed. The remaining healthy corneal tissue is instrumental in hastening healing of the area from which the lesion was excised (Par. 6:16). When the incision is made away from the limbus, the operator no longer has a scleral landmark or "backstop." A "feel" for the proper depth is acquired through practice. Following the incision into clear cornea, fluorescein stain is used to outline the length and depth of initial cut.

6:175 If the entire top layer needs to be removed, healing will take longer and will be accompanied by considerable vascularization and granulation. Beta radiation at the completion of surgery has been used to prevent too rapid an invasion of vessels and granulation tissue (Fig. 3–5), but is not essential. Approximately 1500 r.e.p. administered at each area of the excised limbus will allow re-epithelialization to take place in a more orderly fashion. Now topical and even subconjunctival sutures are used after re-epithelialization is complete, 6–8 days after surgery, to reduced neovascularity.

6:176 *Aftercare.* Following surgical procedure a drop of atropine and an antibiotic are instilled. The eye or eyes are bandaged (Figs. 6–39, 3–6), and a protective collar is placed (Fig. 4–6A). *Caution:* A third eyelid flap (Par. 4:63) should be applied to protect the cornea during healing of grossly exophthalmic eyes. Ordinarily the bandage is removed the next day and the eye is treated "open" with atropine and the antibiotic. There is certainly no contraindication to daily bandage changes and the advantages have been enumerated (Par. 3:90). However, if both eyes have been

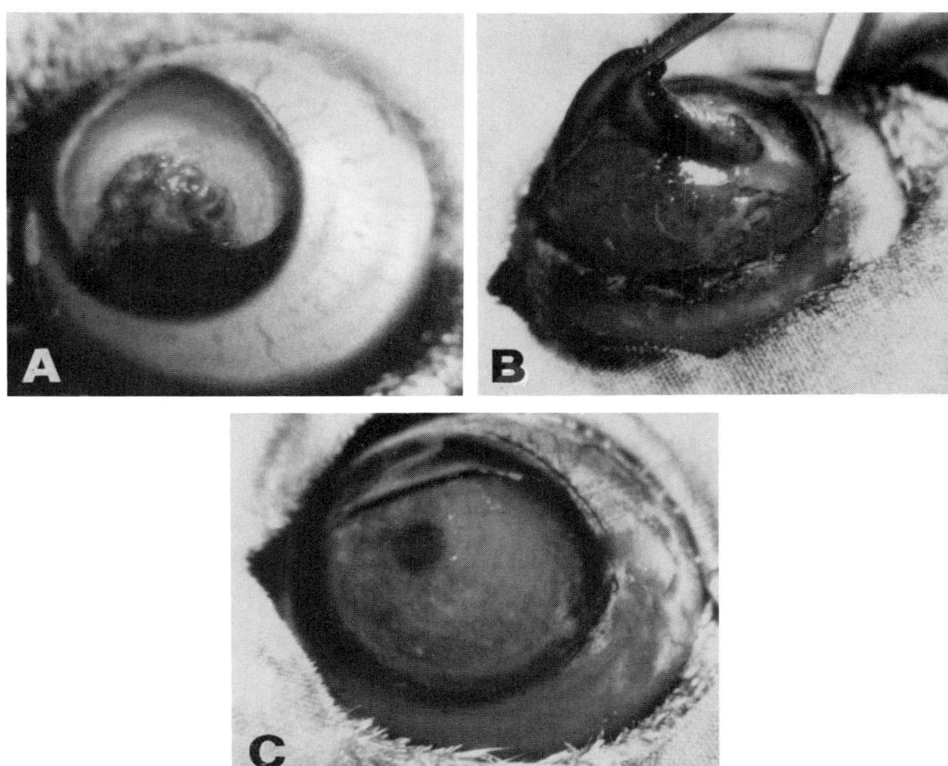

Fig. 6–38. *A*. Eye afflicted with heavy pannus proptosed in preparation for superficial keratectomy. *B*. Halfway through surgery. Note clear stroma under lesion being removed. *C*. Surgery completed. Note line of demarcation between normal intact cornea (upper one third) and area from which lesion was removed.

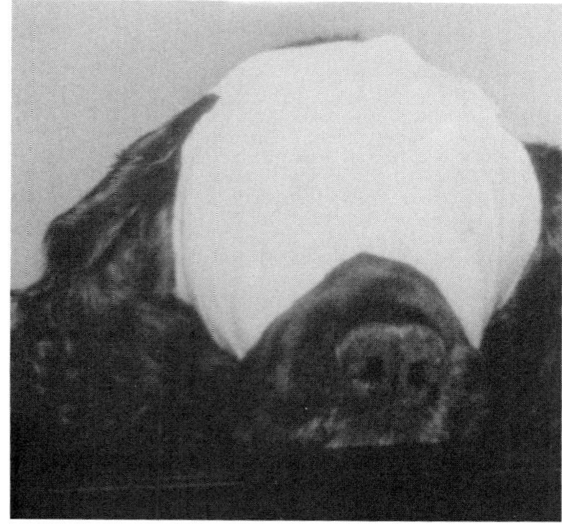

Fig. 6–39. Binocular bandage.

operated on and are covered, there is the problem of ambulation. On the second or third day, when the cornea begins to epithelialize, it assumes a light milky hue and may give rise to fear that the operation has not been successful. At about the sixth postoperative day the cornea will appear somewhat more cloudy but is now re-epithelialized to the point that a topical steroid-antibiotic preparation can be started. The atropine is stopped. If excessive vascularization and granulation are noted, subconjunctival steroid injections (Par. 3:63) are indicated. The patient can usually be discharged on about the tenth postoperative day with the steroid-antibiotic preparation being used for only another week or so (pannus excepted) (Par. 6:55). The cornea will be healthy and clear in from 2 to 4 weeks following surgery.

6:177 In a study[32] on the effect of superficial keratectomy on the thickness of the dog's normal cornea, I found that the thickness increased up to 220% of its original thickness during the first 2 weeks after keratectomy. This appeared to be due to edema. Topical and subconjunctival steroids were used postoperatively. Subsequent measurements of the cornea revealed a lack of complete stromal regeneration. The thickness was only about 75% of the original thickness, 6 months after the keratectomy, indicating that, although reepithelialization takes place rapidly (6 to 8 days), stromal regeneration is a slow process, if indeed it does occur.

6:178 It is not necessary to employ lamellar grafts to fill the corneal defect left by the excision. In fact, in several instances when a lamellar graft was used on one eye and the second left to heal naturally, the best end result was achieved in the second eye.

Corneal Grafts (Keratoplasty)

6:179 A few papers[12,21,45,55,67] have been written on the use of partial (lamellar) and total (penetrating) corneal grafts in the dog. These investigators have concerned themselves primarily with the development of techniques using normal corneas. Consequently, the indications for keratoplasty procedures for the dog have not been well established. It is apparent, however, that there would be few indications for the use of grafts in the dog as compared to man. Visual requirements differ. Astigmatism, and other aberrations caused by changes in the corneal curvature and thickness, that would require correction in man, seem to cause no noticeable visual impairment for the dog.

6:180 Of even more significance is the fact that the simple superficial keratectomy procedure (Par. 6:156) for the purpose of removing pannus lesions, dermoids, dystrophic areas, hyperplasia and superficial scars from the cornea is followed by natural corneal regeneration, thus negating the need for replacement grafts. As pointed out (Par. 6:178) the use of lamellar grafts may well complicate rather than help achieve satisfactory healing.

6:181 To establish indications for corneal transplantation in the dog, based on results obtained, an accurate selection of cases is important since the graft may become involved in any concurrent pathology. For example, removal of a pigmented area from the cornea with the purpose of replacing that defect with a graft is destined to failure unless the cause of the pigmentation is eliminated and its reentry to the graft prevented.

6:182 Mueller and Formston[61] summarized their investigation as follows: "Corneal grafting in the dog presents many problems which are unknown in human corneal surgery and techniques giving a high success rate in man will not necessarily present an equally high number of good results in dogs. Experimental techniques which have given inferior results in the normal eye are likely to be disastrous when tried on the diseased cornea and conservative treatment might well be more successful than major corneal surgery."

6:183 Corneal and scleral grafts have been reported to be successful in cases of extensive corneal ulcers and for other corneal repairs.[42,63] A successful full-thickness corneal transplant for treatment of endothelial dystrophy has also been reported, but is not commonly utilized.[29]

8:184 *Lamellar homografts* are helpful and their use may be imperative in those instances in which a fistulous corneal lesion fails to fill in (Plate 7H). In cases of this type a descemetocele is present which will "seal over" for a period, only to rupture with leakage of aqueous. This process then repeats itself over and over. We have found a homologous lamellar graft procedure, described by McLaughlin[56] to be beneficial for treating leaking descemetoceles, strengthening areas of impending corneal rupture, or repairing areas of corneal rupture and iris prolapse not amenable to suturing.

6:185 The procedure is as follows: After induction of general anesthesia and standard preparation for intraocular surgery, a lateral canthotomy is performed to facilitate exposure. The remainder of the surgery is done with the aid of an operating microscope. In Figure 6–40A, the circle represents the corneal defect. Two parallel incisions are made extending from the limbus past the defect (Fig. 6–40B), using a #64 Beaver blade (Fig. 3–16). The distance separating these incisions is 2 to 3 mm greater than the diameter of the corneal defect. The incisions are made to a depth of approximately one-half the corneal thickness. An incision is made joining the two parallel incisions and a one-half thickness keratectomy is performed, using a #69 Beaver blade, undermining the corneal tissue (graft) to the limbus. The graft is left attached at the limbus until the recipient site (graft bed) is prepared. The graft is made 0.5 to 1 mm larger in length and width than the graft bed to compensate for the slight contraction of the graft after its removal from the cornea. Edematous or disrupted corneal tissue in the area of the defect is removed by keratectomy, creating a half thickness "bed" to receive the graft in the area of the defect (Fig. 6–40B). The graft is freed from the limbus, positioned in the graft bed and sutured, using either a continuous or interrupted pattern (Fig. 6–40C) and using 8 or 9 Ō nylon or polygalactin 910* suture.

6:186 Postoperativē care consists of using antibiotic and 1% atropine ointments topically twice a day until the donor site is epithelialized, as evidenced by negative fluorescein dye retention, after which antibiotic-steroid combination ointment and atropine are used. After 30 days, topical treatment is discontinued and a subconjunctival injection of 4 to 8 mg triamcinolone acetonide (Par. 3:65) is performed, if indicated, to reduce any corneal vascularization.

6:187 Keratoplasty procedures can be classified as higly specialized surgery. The indi-

*Vicryl. Ethicon, Inc. Somerville, NJ 08876

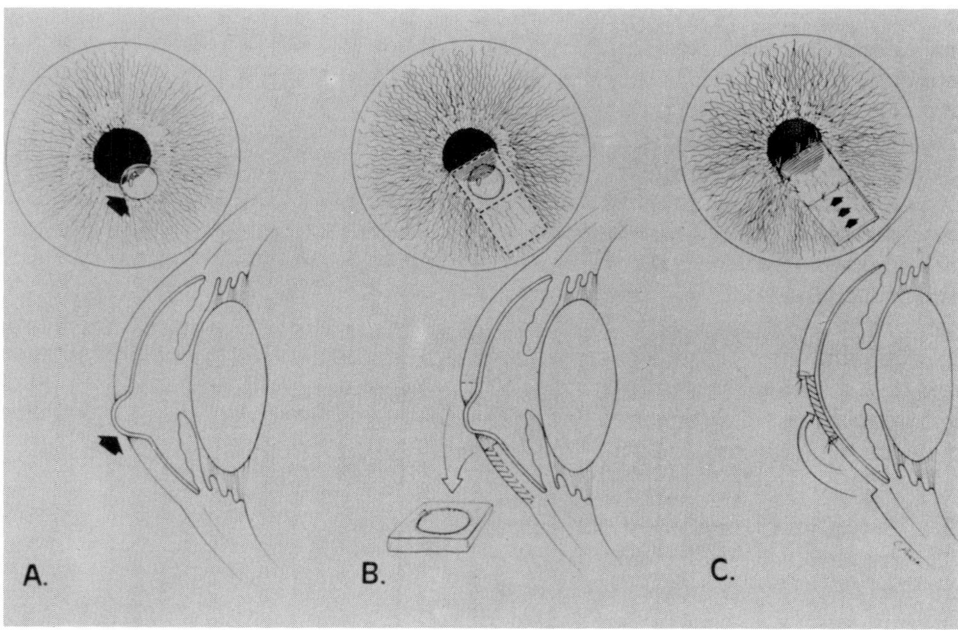

Fig. 6–40. *A*. Diagram representing a descemetocele. *B*. Preparation of the graft bed and graft. The graft tissue (crosshatched) is undermined, but left attached at the limbus until after the diseased tissue around the defect (stippled) area is removed. C. The partial-thickness, autogenous graft is positioned and sutured using a continuous or interrupted pattern.

cations are few, the instrument requirements and surgical astuteness are absolute. Enlisting the aid of a medical or veterinary ophthalmologist skilled in this field is obligatory.

THE SCLERA

Anatomy and Physiology

6:188 The sclera is the tunic which, with the cornea, forms the external fibrous layer of the eyeball and serves to maintain the form of the globe (Par. 1:14). The structure of the sclera is made up of a laminated pattern of fibrous tissue and elastic fibers. An outstanding feature of the dog's eye is the variation in thickness.[66] At the equator it is thin (0.28 mm), while in the ciliary region, it is much thicker (1.0 mm or more) and it has a well-developed venous plexus. Around the optic nerve the sclera is again thicker (0.8 mm).

6:189 The histologic structure of the sclera is similar to the cornea. There are, however, more elastic irregularly arranged fibers, a greater state of hydration, and the sclera contains blood vessels and lymphatics. The theory explaining the difference between the cornea being transparent and the sclera white is based on the arrangement of the collagen fibrils of the lamellae. The fibrils of the cornea are in a regular lattice arrangement equidistant from one another whereas the sclera is composed of interwoven collagen without precise lattice arrangement. Transparency is dependent on this precise arrangement (Par. 6:4).

6:190 The sclera is punctured at several points for the passage of nerves and blood vessels. The head of the optic nerve is situated in the posterior wall and may be central, or it may be lateral or medial to the posterior pole. The part through which the nerve passes is known as the *lamina cribrosa*. Prince[66] points out that there is not an actual hole in the sclera. The scleral fibers separate and reduce in number until they form a fine screen through which the optic nerve fibers pass. The limbal area of the sclera is pigmented laterally and medially, but not dorsally and ventrally.

6:191 Surrounding the sclera is the quite vascular episclera (Par. 1:16) which unites in the limbal area with the conjunctiva and sclera. Its main function is to provide nutrition to the outer parts of the almost avascular sclera.

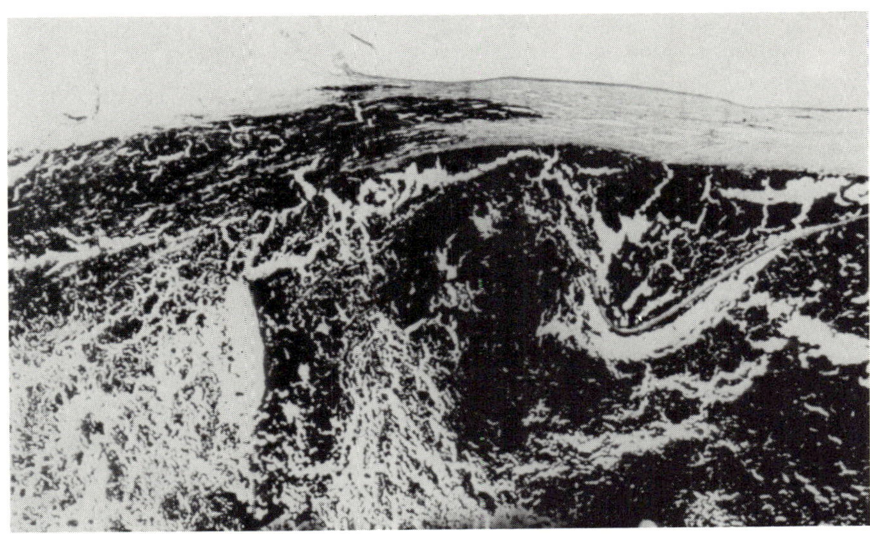

Fig. 6–41. Scleral invasion of an intraocular melanoma.

Diseases

6:192 Affections of the sclera include inflammation, staphyloma, injuries, and extension of intraocular tumors (Fig. 6–41). All occur infrequently.

6:193 *Episcleritis* (Plate 8D) is a localized inflammatory lesion involving primarily the perilimbal area. The area is somewhat engorged, is nodular in appearance and feel, is immovable, and looks suspiciously neoplastic. The conjunctiva can be moved over it freely. Usually only one eye is involved. The course is chronic and there is a tendency for it to recur.

6:194 In man episcleritis is a disease of systemic origin. In the dog we have seldom been albe to determine a specific cause, although a particular hypersensitivity is believed to play a role. Steroid therapy consisting of subconjunctival injections (Par. 3:65) and a follow-up with drops or ointment will allay the process and keep it under control. As mentioned, relapses are common and continual use of steroid preparations may be necessary. A transient periodic episcleritis lasting for a few hours to a few days has been observed in several instances.

6:195 *Nodular fasciitis* is a benign, nodular proliferation of fibroblasts and vascular tissue involving the superficial fascia.[75] The disease resembles nodular episcleritis and must also be differentiated from a number of other benign and malignant fibrous connective tissue lesions. Several cases have been reported.[9,46] In these instances the lesions continued to enlarge and infiltrate the cornea is spite of corticosteroid therapy. Excision was required to effect recovery. A diagnosis of nodular fasciitis was based on the histologic features of nodular proliferation of capillaries, histiocytes and fibroblasts with arrangement both in parallel bundles and haphazardly.

6:196 *Sclerouveitis* has been described[23] as a rather well-defined clinical and histopathologic entity in dogs which appears to be associated with a basic systemic autoimmune phenomenon and sets this disease apart from other scleral and uveal disorders. The clinical features include: a mass in the anterior superior sclera with progressive invasion of the adjacent sclera and underlying uveal tract; eventual involvement of both eyes; outward signs of remission with corticosteroid therapy which, then, diminishes quickly with subsequent secondary complications such as glaucoma and loss of the eye. Treatment with a systemic cyclophosphamide and prednisone combination has been encouraging.

6:197 *Staphyloma* (Plate 10D) or ectasia of the sclera occurs when the wall has been weakened by the buphthalmos of chronic glaucoma (Par. 9:35) (Plate 16E). In these instances the scleral wall becomes uniformly thin, takes on a "blue" appearance because of the underlying uveal tissue showing through, and may bulge in the weakened sections. Penetrating wounds and poor closure following a scleral incision into the anterior chamber in, for example, glaucoma and cataract surgery, also predispose to a localized staphyloma. A congenital posterior ectasia of the sclera is found in the collie breed as part of collie eye anomaly (Par. 11:84).

6:198 Treatment of sclera ectasia depends upon the cause. Glaucomatous eyes that have reached this stage are good candidates for an intraocular prosthesis. If the bulging is due to wounds or poor surgical closure, a repair may be made by incision, debridement (including excision of uveal tissue caught in the wound), tight suturing with catgut or 6–0 mersilene and accurate replacement of the episcleral tissues including Tenon's capsule and the conjunctiva. The aftercare is similar to that described for wounds of the cornea (Par. 6:146).

6:199 *Injuries* usually occur as the result of bites and punctures from sharp objects or shotgun pellets. Penetrating wounds of the sclera, which result in loss of vitreous or are associated with an intraocular hemorrhage, usually end up in loss of the globe because of a subsequent panophthalmitis, or, the eyeball will become shrunken and fibrotic (phthisis bulbi).

6:200 An attempt should be made to preserve an eye by suturing the scleral and conjunctival wounds after excision of the prolapsed vitreous and uveal tissue. Small clean wounds often heal without reaction and merely require ceansing and the use of topical antibiotics. Radiographs of the head region are helpful in determining the presence and location of suspected pellets or foreign bodies, although they are usually allowed to remain if intraocular or in the orbit. Most penetrating foreign bodies, *e.g.*, glass, pellets, and many plastics, are inert and are well tolerated by the eye.[74] The relative infrequency with which they are encountered and the expertise and equipment needed for their removal do not justify further discussion.

6:201 *Tumors.* Tumors involving the sclera are not common; however, two distinct syndromes involving proliferative melanosis have been reported. The first, an epibulbar melanocytoma, (Plate 10A), is seen primarily in German shepherds. It is a subconjunctival, raised melanotic mass at the limbus, and often extending into the cornea. A band of corneal dystrophy is often present along the eroding border. Removal by superficial keratectomy-sclerectomy, in which about one-third thickness of the cornea and sclera is removed, in my experience, is most often curative, even if the underlying sclera is infiltrated with pigment. Histologically, the lesion has been variously classified as a melanocytoma, malignant melanoma and melanoma spindle type A with a low degree of malignancy. It is important to recognize this tumor and differentiate it from a tumor of the uveal tract (Plate 8G) that has extended into the sclera (Fig. 6–41). In the former, the eye and sight can be saved; in the latter, it should be treated by enucleation or exenervation of the orbit to prevent metastasis (Par. 7:94). The second syndrome occurs in older Cairn terriers.[19] These dogs may have multiple black, slightly elevated masses on the sclera (Plate 10B). These masses are a part of a generalized pigment proliferation in the eyes that often results in glaucoma. No satisfactory treatment, other than palliative to control the intraocular pressure, has been found.

REFERENCES

1. Adler, F.H.: *Physiology of the Eye*, 2nd ed., St. Louis, The C.V. Mosby, Co., p. 41, 1953.
2. A.F.I.P. Accession 1303901.
3. Aguirre, G.D., Rubin, L.F., and Harvey, C.E.: Keratoconjunctivitis Sicca in Dogs, J.A.V.M.A., 9:1566–1578, 1971.
4. Allen, J.H.: *May's Diseases of the Eye*, 24th ed., Baltimore, The Williams & Wilkins Co., 1968.
5. Anderson, L.K., et al.: *Serum Immunoglobulin Changes Associated with Canine Keratitis*, Proc. Am. C. Vet. Ophth. (5th), Dallas, Texas, 1974.
6. Baker, G.J. and Formston, C.: An Evaluation of Transplantation of the Parotid Duct, J.S.A.P., 9:261, 1968.
7. Baum, J.L.: Cholesterol Keratopathy, A.J.O., *67*:372, 1969.
8. Barnett, K.S. and Grimes, T.D.: Verticillate Corneal Dystrophy in a Dog, J.S.A.P., *12*:297–299, 1971.
9. Bellhorn, R.W. and Henkind, P.: Ocular Nodular Fasciitis in a Dog, J.A.V.M.A., *150*:212, 1967.
10. Bellhorn, R.W. and Henkind, P.: Superficial Pigmentary Keratitis in the Dog, J.A.V.M.A., *149*:173, 1966.
11. Bennett, J.E.: The Management of Total Xerophthalmia, Arch. Ophth., *81*:667, 1969.
12. Bernis, W.O.: Partial Penetrating Keratoplasty in Dogs, South-western Vet., *15*:30–43, 1961.
13. Betts, D.M., Helper, L.C.: The Surgical Correction of Parotid Duct Transposition Failures, JAAHA *13*:(6), 695–700.
14. Campbell, L.H., et al.: Chronic Superficial Keratitis in Dogs: Detection of Cellular Hypersensitivity, Am. J. Vet. Res., *36*:669–671, 1975.
15. Candlin, F.T., Catcott, E.J. and Magrane, W.G.: Beta-ray and X-ray Therapy in Diseases of the Eye, No. Am. Vet., *36*:295, 1955.
16. *Canine Surgery*, 4th ed., Santa Barbara, American Veterinary Publications, Inc., p. 332, 1957.
17. Catcott, E.J. and Griesemer, R.A.: A Study of Corneal Healing in the Dog, Am. J. Vet. Res., *15*:265, 1954.
18. Cello, R.M.: The Pathology of Corneal Disease, A.A.H.A. Seminar, Los Angeles, 1962.
19. Covitz, D., Barthold, S., Ditters, R., et al.: Pigmentary Glaucoma in the Cairn Terrier, Transactions, ACVO, 1984, 246, 247.
20. Dice, Paul: Corneal Dystrophy in the Shetland Sheepdog. Trans ACVO, pp. 241–242, 1984.
21. Dice, P.F., Severin, G.A., and Lumb, W.V.: Experimental Autogenous and Homologous Corneal Transplantation in the Dog, J.A.A.H.A., 9:245–251, 1973.
22. Duke-Elder, S.: *System of Ophthalmology: Vol. VIII: Diseases of the Outer Eye: Part II: Cornea and Sclera*, St. Louis, The C.V. Mosby Co., 1965.
23. Fischer, C.A.: *Sclerouveitis in Dogs*, Proc. Am. C. Vet. Ophth., 1972.
24. Flynn, M.A. and Esterly, D.: Bilateral Recurrent Erosion of Cornea, A.J.O., *62*:964, 1966.

25. Formston, C.: Keratitis in Animals, *Aspects of Comparative Ophthalmology*, London, Pergamon Press, 1966.
26. Gelatt, K.N.: Treatment of Canine Keratoconjunctivitis Sicca by Parotid Duct Transposition. J. Am. An. Hosp. Assoc., 6:1–11, 1970.
27. Goldman, J.N., et al.: The Basement Membrane of the Human Cornea in Recurrent Epithelial Erosion Syndrome, Trans. Am. Acad. Ophth., *73*:471, 1969.
28. Gwin, R.M., Cunningham, D.E., Shaver, R.P.: Posterior Polymorphous Dystrophy of the Cornea of Cocker Spaniels: Preliminary Clinical and Specular Microsopic Findings, Trans ACVO, 154–164, 1983.
29. Gwin, R.M., Polack, F.M., Warren, J.K., et al.: Primary Canine Corneal Endothelial Cell Dystrophy: Specular Microscopic Evaluation, Diagnosis and Therapy, JAAHA, *18*:no. 3, 471–480, 1982.
30. Gundersen, M.T. and Liebman, S.D.: Effect of Local Anesthetics on Regeneration of Corneal Epithelium, Arch. Ophth., *31*:29, 1944.
31. Haggerty, T.E. and Zimmerman, L.E.: Mycotic Keratitis, So. Med. J., *2*:153–159, 1958.
32. Helper, L.C.: *Effect of Superficial Keratectomy on the Thickness of the Dog's Cornea*, Proc. Am. C. Vet. Ophth., 1973.
33. Helper, L.C.: Keratoconjunctivitis sicca in Dogs. Transactions, Am Acad. Ophthal. and Otolaryngol. *81*:624–628, 1976.
34. Hogan, M.J. and Zimmerman, L.E.: *Ophthalmic Pathology*, 2nd ed., Philadelphia, W.B. Saunders Co. p. 311, 1962.
35. Holly, F., Lemp, M.A., Dohlman, C.H.: Surface Chemistry of the Tear Film and Dry Eye Syndromes (Monograph), Dept of Corneal Research, Retina Foundation, Boston, MA.
36. Holmberg, D.L., Scheifer, H.B., Parent, J.: The Cryosurgical Treatment of Pigmentary Keratitis in Dogs, An Experimental and Clinical Study, Vet. Surg., *15*:no. 1, 1–4, 1986.
37. Jensen, E.C.: Experimental Corneal Transplantation in the Dog, J.A.V.M.A., *142*:11–21, 1963.
38. Kaswan, R.L., Martin, C.L., Dawl, D.L., et al.: Immunological Evaluation of Sixty-two Dogs with Keratoconjunctivitis sicca, AJVR, *46*:no. 2, 376, 1985.
39. Kaswan, R.L., Martin, C.L., Chapman, W.L.: Keratoconjunctivitis sicca: Histopathologic Study of Nictitating Membrane and Lacrimal Glands from 28 Dogs, AJVR, *45*:no. 1, 112, 1984.
40. Kaswan, R.L., Martin, C.L., Dawe, D.L.: Rheumatoid Factor Determination in 50 Dogs with Keratoconjunctivitis sicca, JAVMA, *183*:no. 10, 1073, 1983.
41. Keller, W.F., et al.: *Experimentally Produced Canine Herpetic Keratitis*, Proc. Am. C. Vet. Ophth. (3rd), Dallas, Texas, 1972.
42. Keller, W.F., Blanchard, G.L., and Kuhns, E.L.: The Clinical Application of Homologous Corneal and Scleral Grafts in the Dog, J.A.A.H.A., *9*:265–269, 1973.
43. Kublin, K.S. and Refojo, M.F.: Closure of Ocular Lacerations with an Adhesive, J.A.V.M.A., *156*:313, 1970.
44. Lavignette, A.M.: Keratoconjunctivitis Sicca in a Dog Treated by Transposition of the Parotid Salivary Duct, J.A.V.M.A., *148*:778, 1966.
45. Lavignette, A.M.: Lamellar Keratoplasty in the Dog, Sm. An. Clinician, *2*:183–197, 1962.
46. Lavignette, A.M. and Carlton, W.W.: A Case of Ocular Nodular Fasciitis in a Dog, J.A.A.H.A., *10*:503–506, 1974.
47. Lescure, M. l'Agrere F.: La Cornee du Chien Pathologic et Therapeutique Acts, Actes de la Conference Nationale des Veterinares Specialistes de Petits Animaux, 1st trimestre, p. 10, 1964.
48. Lettow, E., et al.: Epithelioma der Cornea bei einem Hund, Berliner and Münchener Tierärztliche Wochenschrift, *12*:248, 1964.
49. Magrane, W.G.: *Canine Ophthalmology (3rd Ed)*, Philadelphia, Lea & Febiger, p. 118, 1977.
50. Magrane, W.G.: Keratitis, Upjohn Veterinary Scope. *1*:11, 1956.
51. Magrane, W.G.: Vascularization—Its Significance in Diseases of the Cornea, J.A.V.M.A., *126*:208, 1955.
52. Magrane, W.G.: X-ray Therapy in Interstitial and Pigmentary Keratitis, No. Am. Vet., *29*:582, 1948.
53. Martin, C.L.: Canine Epibulbar Melanocytomas and Their Management, JAAHA, *17*:83–90, Jan/Feb 1981.
54. Martin, C.L., Kaswan, R.: Distemper Associated Keratoconjunctivitis sicca, JAAHA, *21*:355–359, May/Jun, 1985.
55. McEntyre, J.M.: Experimental Penetrating Keratoplasty in the Dog, Arch. Ophth., *80*:372, 1968.
56. McLaughlin, S.A., Brightman, A.H., Brogdon, J.D., et al.: Autogenous Partial-thickness Corneal Grafting in the Dog, Trans ACVO, 146–155, 1984.
57. Waring, G.O., McMillan, Alan, Reveles, P.: Inheritance of Crystalline Corneal Dystrophy in Siberian Huskies, JAAHA, *22*:655–658, 1986.
58. Michaelson, I.C.: Proliferation of Limbal Melanoblasts into the Cornea in Response to the Corneal Lesion, Brit. J. Ophth., *36*:657, 1952.
59. Morgan, R.V., Bachrach, A., Ogilvie, G.K.: An Evaluation of Soft Contact Lens Usage in the Dog and Cat, JAAHA, *20*:885–887, Nov/Dec, 1984.
60. Morgan, R.V., Bachrach, A.: Keratoconjunctivitis sicca Associated with Sulfonamide Therapy in Dogs, J.A.V.M.A., *180*:432–434, 1982.
61. Mueller, F.O. and Formston, C.: Keratoplasty in the Dog, Res. Vet. Sci., *10*:168, 1969.
62. Oda, Y. and Fukuda, S.: Electron Microscopic Studies on the Animals' Cornea, J. Electronmicroscopy, *11*:183–184, 1962.
63. Parshall, C.J.: Lamellar Corneal-Scleral Transposition, J.A.A.H.A., *9*:270–277, 1973.
64. Peruccio, C.: Incidence of Hypothyroidism in Dogs Affected by Keratoconjunctivitis sicca, Proceedings of American Society of Veterinary Ophthalmology and International Society of Veterinary Ophthalmology, April, 47, 48, 1982.
65. Peruccio, Claudio, Bosio, P., Cornaglia, E.: Indications and Limits of Cyanoacrylate Tissue Adhesive in Corneal Ulcers and Perforations, Trans. ACVO, 1983, 135–153.
66. Prince, J.H., Diesem, C.D., Eglitis, I. and Ruskell, G.L.: *Anatomy and Histology of the Eye and Orbit in Domestic Animals*, Springfield, Charles C Thomas, 1960.

COLOR PLATES

Plate 1. Some normal variations of the fundus

A. Fundus drawing. Adult dog.
B. Normal disc and tapetum lucidum. Courtesy: Dr. F.F. Lescure, de l'École Nationale Véterinaire de Toulouse.
C. Normal disc in the tapetum nigrum.
D. Fundus of a nine-month-old beagle. The optic disc is circular and surrounded by a pigmented ring.
E. Fundus of an eight-month-old beagle. Myelinated nerve fibers extending into the retina obscure the margins of the optic disc.
F. Fundus of a seven-month-old beagle. The veins join in the center of the optic disc.
G. Variation in arteriolar pattern. Tortuous vessels in contrast to straight vessels usually seen.
(D to G. Courtesy: Rubin, L.: *Atlas of Veterinary Ophthalmoscopy.* Lea & Febiger, Philadelphia, 1974.)

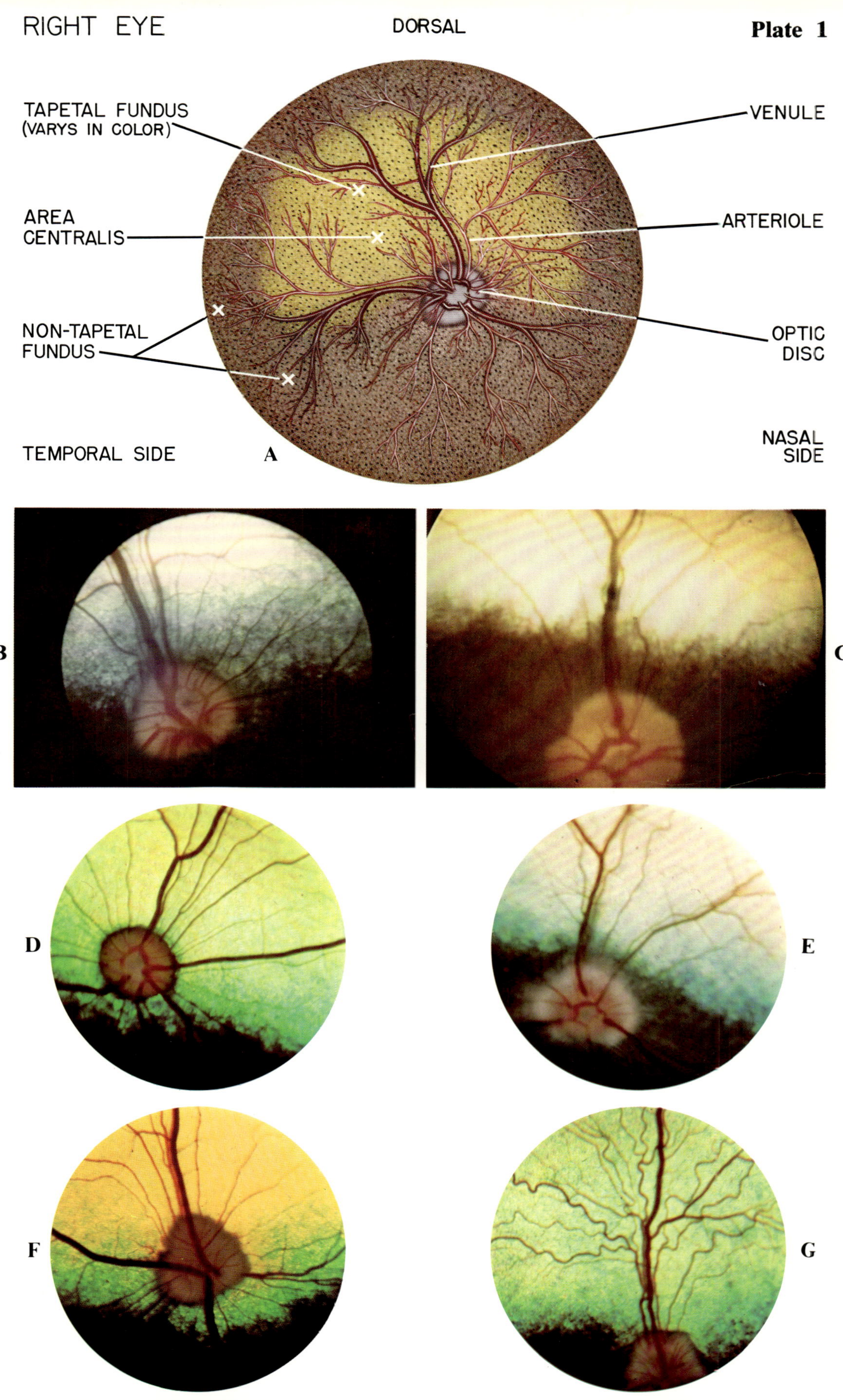
RIGHT EYE
DORSAL
TAPETAL FUNDUS
(VARYS IN COLOR)
VENULE
AREA
CENTRALIS
ARTERIOLE
NON-TAPETAL
FUNDUS
OPTIC
DISC
TEMPORAL SIDE
A
NASAL
SIDE
B
C
D
E
F
G

Plate 2

A. Entropion.
B. Ectropion.
C. Distichiasis with corneal damage.
D. Eversion of the membrane nictitans.
E. Elevation of the third eyelid.
F. Blepharitis.
G. Prolapse of the nictitans gland.
H. Foreign body embedded in inner surface of the membrane nictitans with resultant corneal damage. (Courtesy: Dr. M. Wyman, Ohio State University.)

Plate 2

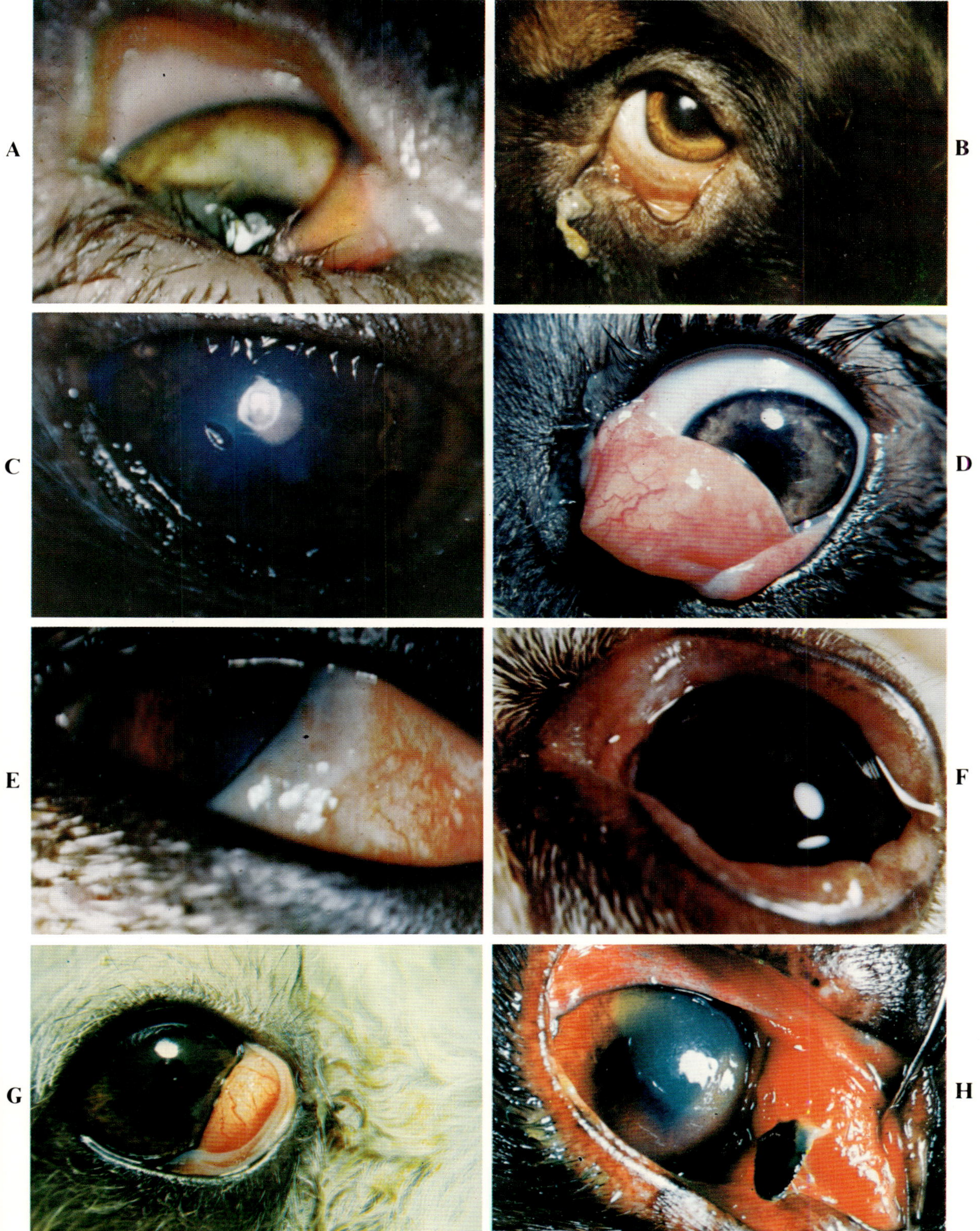

Plate 3

A. Plasma cell infiltration of the membrane nictitans. (Courtesy: Dr. G. Teichert, Berlin, West Germany.)

B. Chronic keratoconjunctivitis resulting from removal of the membrane nictitans. Note small tag (temporal) remaining.

C. Histiocytoma of lid and conjunctiva.

D. Lymphoma of the membrane nictitans and conjunctiva. (Courtesy: Dr. M. Wyman, Ohio State University.)

E. Symblepharon involving the lid and conjunctiva. (Courtesy: Dr. G. Severin, Colorado State University.)

F. Dacryocystitis. Exudate being flushed from the lacrimal sac and canaliculi with a lacrimal needle and saline solution.

G. Tarsorrhaphy. *L,* adhesion between upper and lower lid and area for eventual severance.

H. Meibomian cyst (internal chalazion).

Plate 3

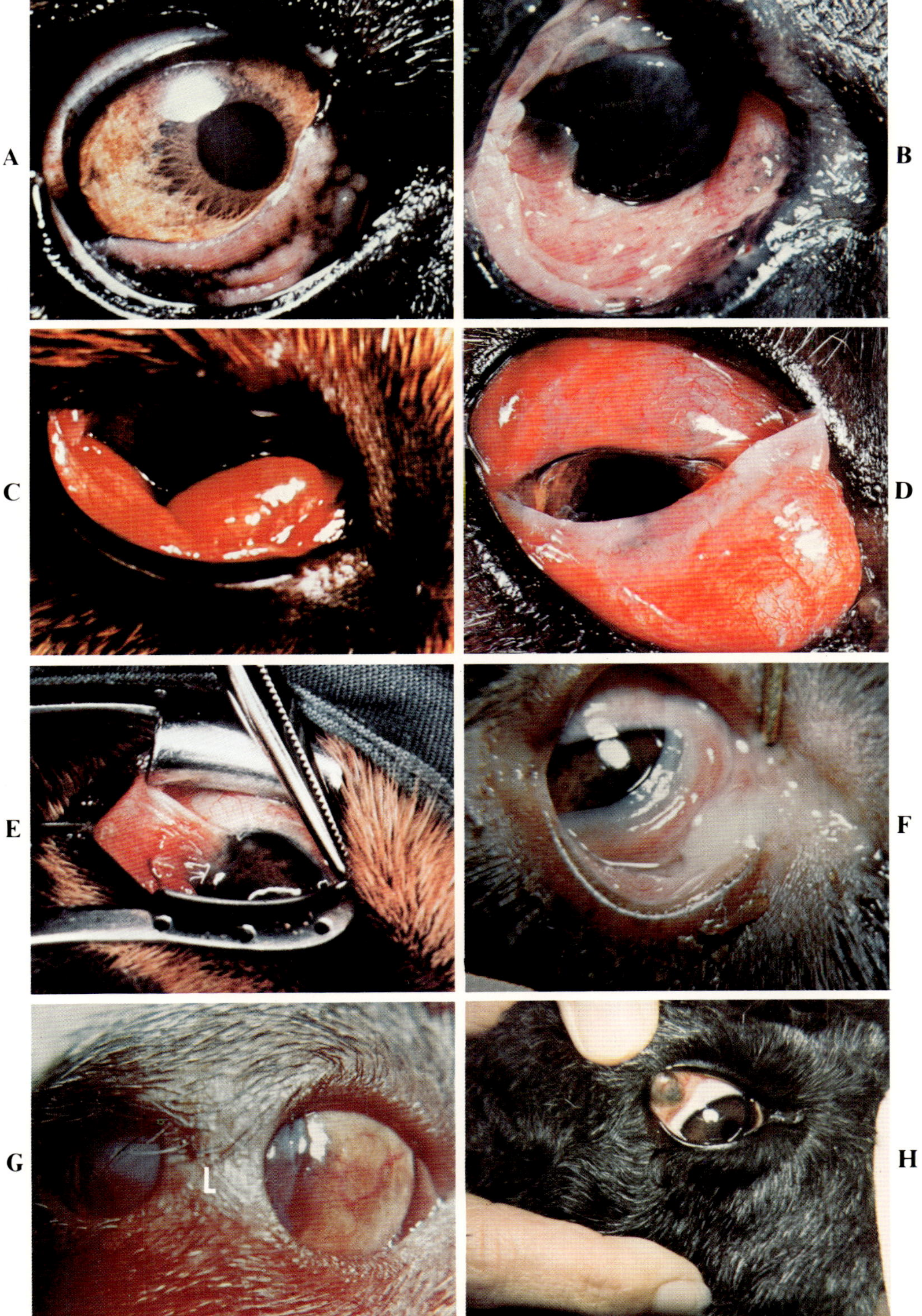

Plate 4

A. Chemosis.
B. Chronic purulent conjunctivitis.
C. Follicles on the external surface of the membrane nictitans.
D. Conjunctival hyperplasia encroaching onto the cornea.
E. Subconjunctival mast cell tumor
F. Meibomian gland adenocarcinoma involving the lid and conjunctiva.

Plate 4

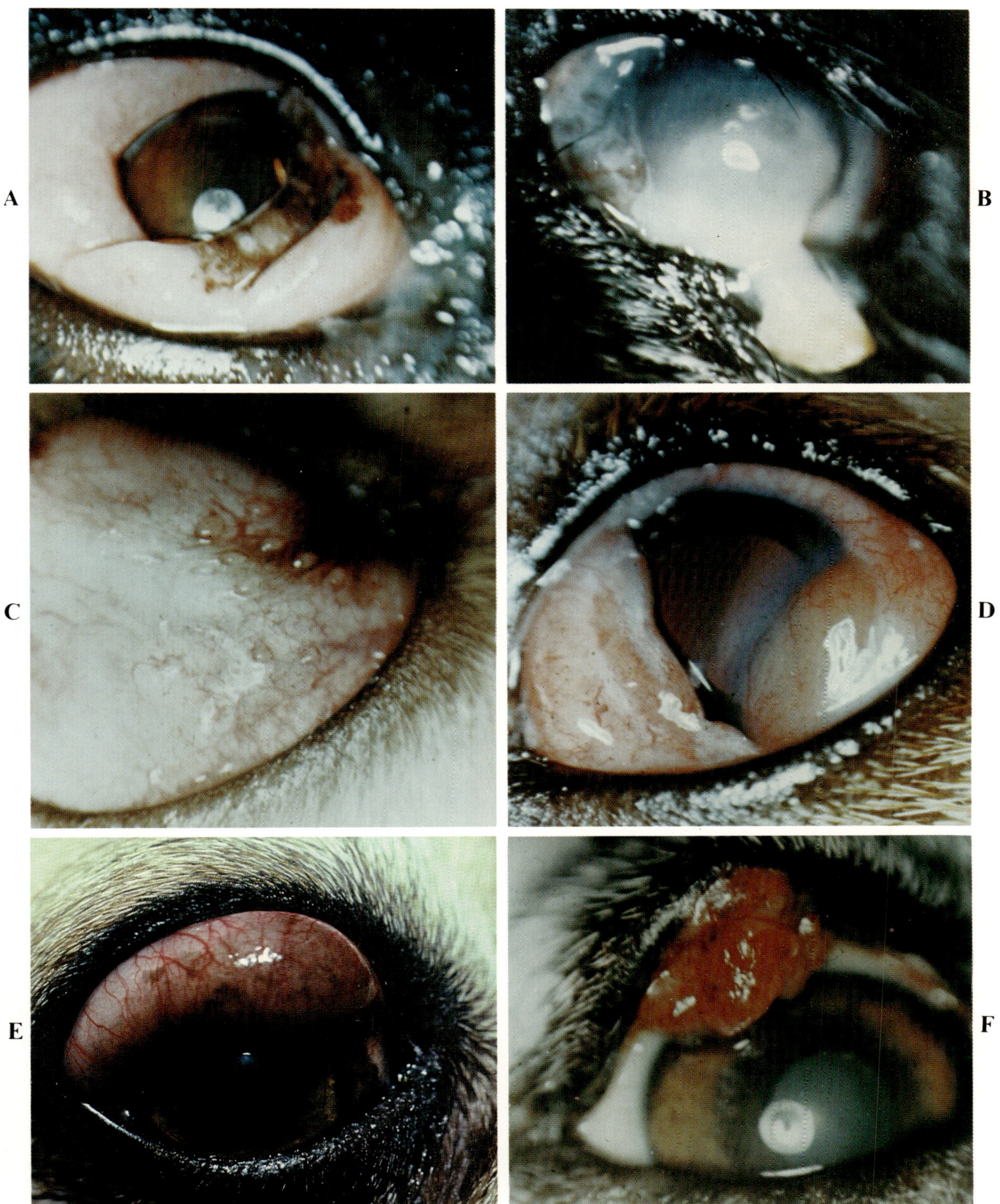

Plate 5

A. Entropion-ectropion anomaly. Note "rolling in" (temporal), "pagoda effect" (upper) and corneal damage.
B. Ecchymosis.
C. Erosion (excoriation) of the lids and skin at the medial canthus.
D. Imperforate punctum (lower).
E. Meibomitis-blepharitis. External view.
F. Meibomitis-blepharitis. Internal view.
G. Conjunctival dermoid.
H. Conjunctival hyperplasia.

Plate 5

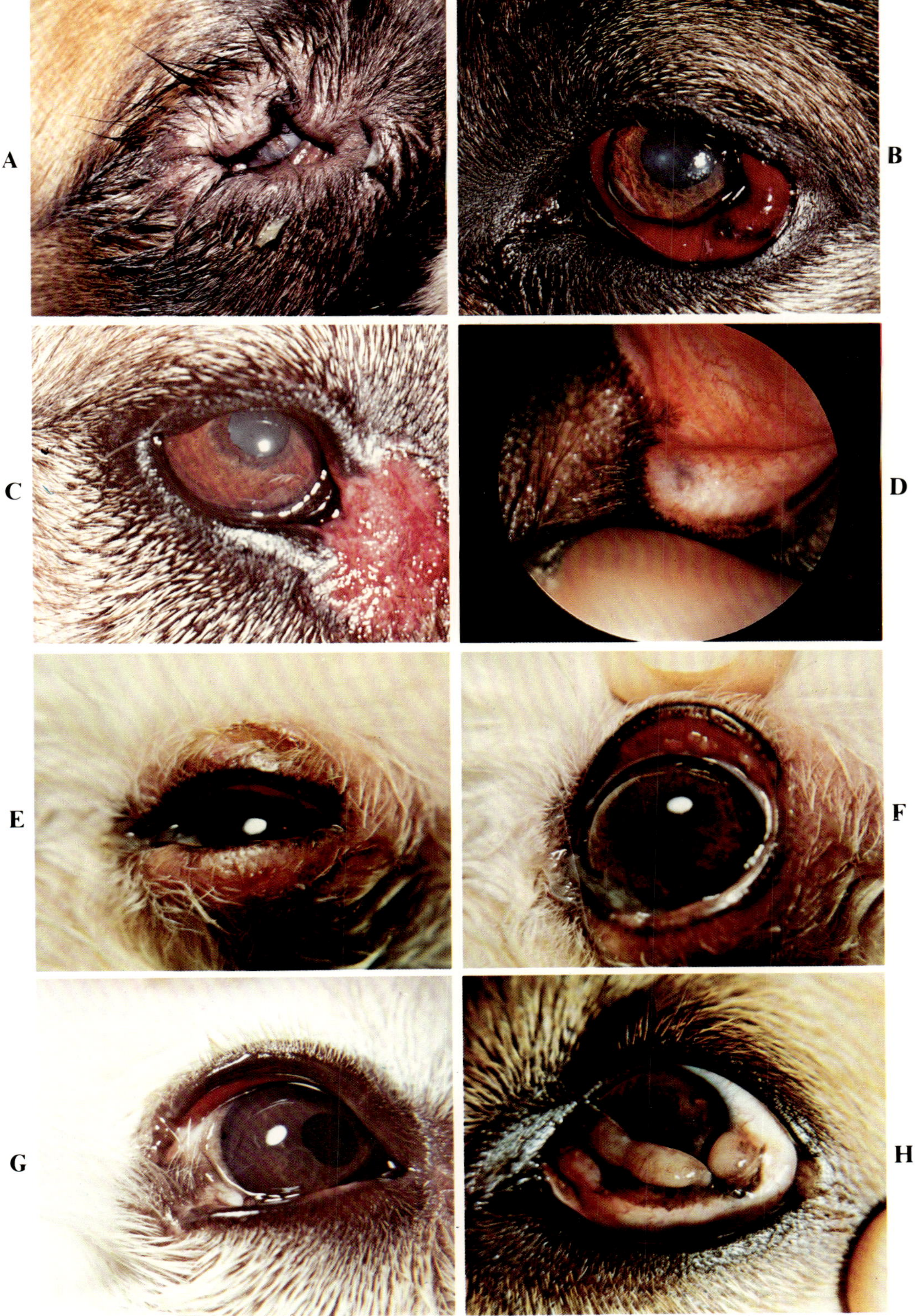

Plate 6

A. Dermoid cyst involving conjunctiva and cornea.
B. Corneal dystrophy.
C. Superficial vascularization of the cornea. Note extension from the bulbar conjunctiva.
D. Interstitial (deep) keratitis. Note "brush-like" invasion of the vessels and the opacity resulting from the severe corneal edema.
E. Pannus of the German shepherd. Right eye. Note invasion from the lateral limbal area.
F. Pannus and plasma cell infiltration of the third eyelid. Note "cobblestone" cornea and depigmented and swollen membrane nictitans.
G. Exuberant granulation tissue. Note large trunk vessels supplying the area.
H. Superficial corneal dystrophy in a 3-year-old German shepherd. It disappeared in a year.

Plate 6

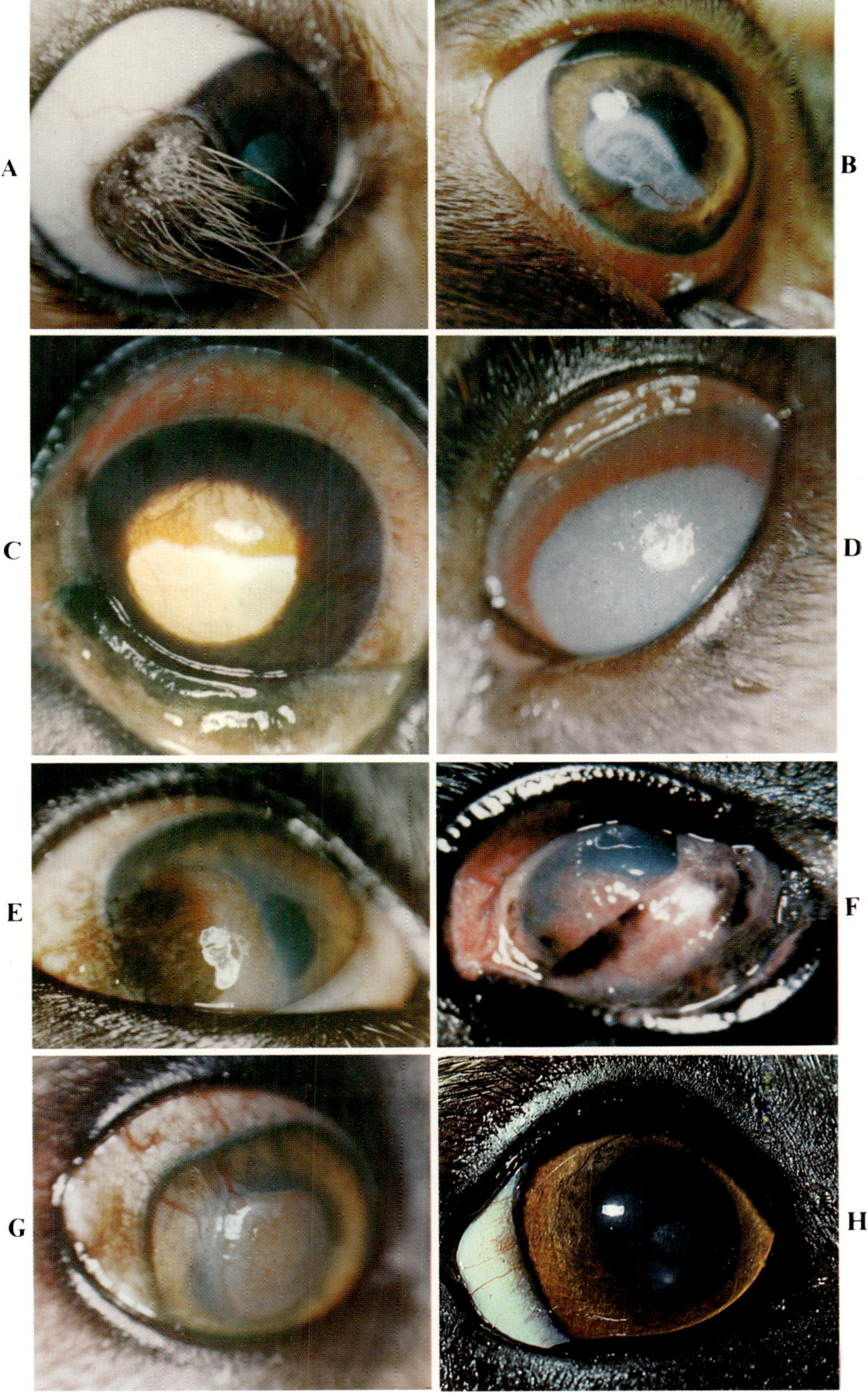

Plate 7

A. Bullous keratitis. Note clear area of cornea still remaining.
B. Deep ulcer (fluorescein stained), vascularization, and hypopyon.
C. Serpentine type of ulceration (fluorescein stained).
D. Keratomalacia. Note stained area and accompanying corneal edema.
E. Corneal erosion (fluorescein stained).
F. Detergent denudation of the cornea (fluorescein stained).
G. Chronic, non-healing ulcerative keratitis with granulation and pigmentation.
H. Leaking descemetocele (clear area center cornea) with ring of granulation.

Plate 7

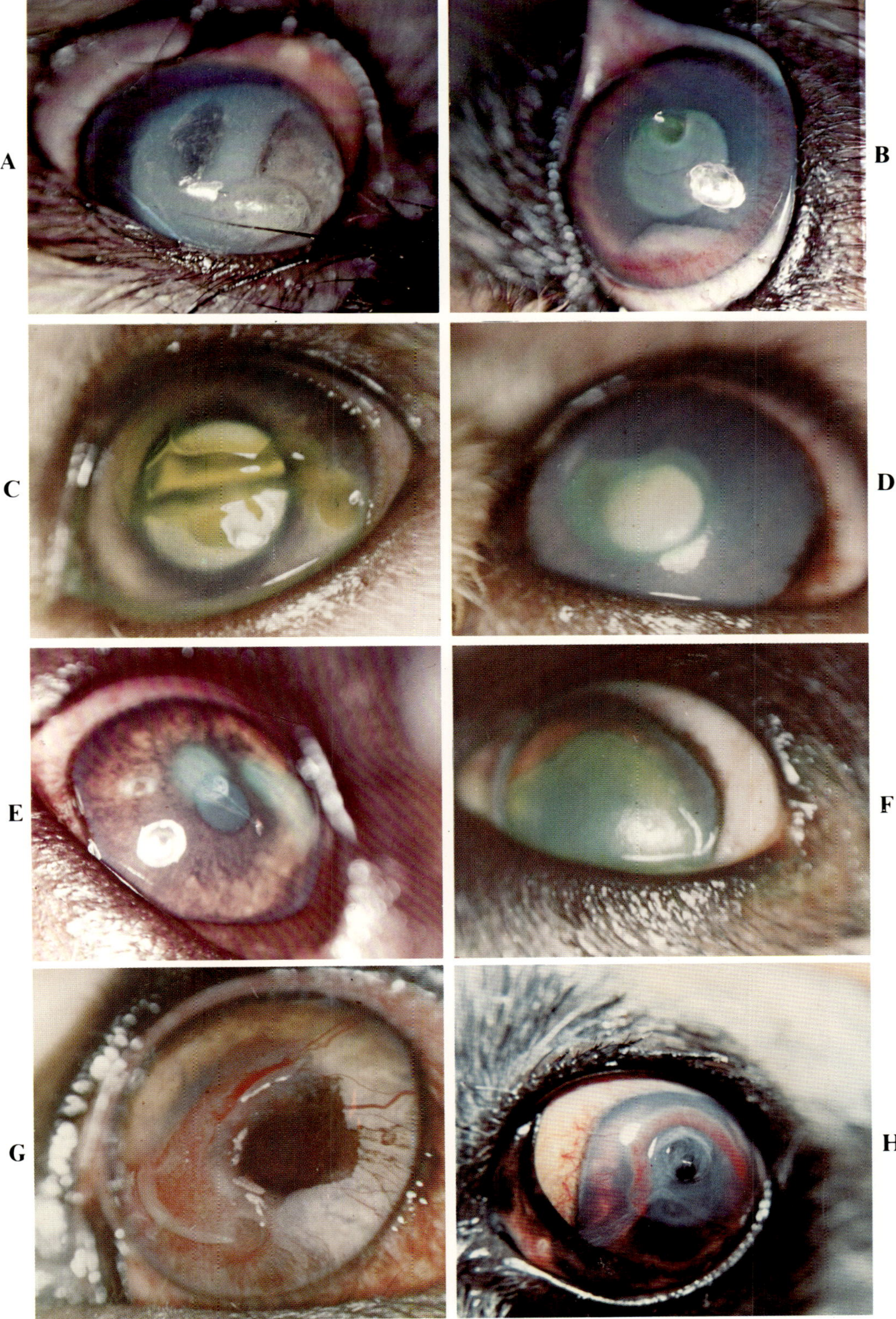

Plate 8

A. Iris prolapse.
B. Foreign body granuloma (result of embedded splinter).
C. Advanced pannus and blindness.
D. Nodular episcleritis (lower aspect of globe). Note accompanying corneal infiltration of vessels and pigment.
E. Right eye 5-year-old Scottie with bilateral keratoconjunctivitis sicca (KCS). Mucopurulent conjunctival discharge revealed neomycin-resistant Staph aureus on culture and sensitivity testing. Schirmer tear test value was 3 mm/min.
F. Left eye of *E.* Classic signs of KCS—a dry, lusterless cornea with adhering mucus. Moderate photophobia and blepharospasm were also present.
G. Intrascleral invasion of a malignant melanoma of the uveal tract.
H. Malignant lymphoma. Note intraocular growth and corneal-scleral involvement.

Plate 8

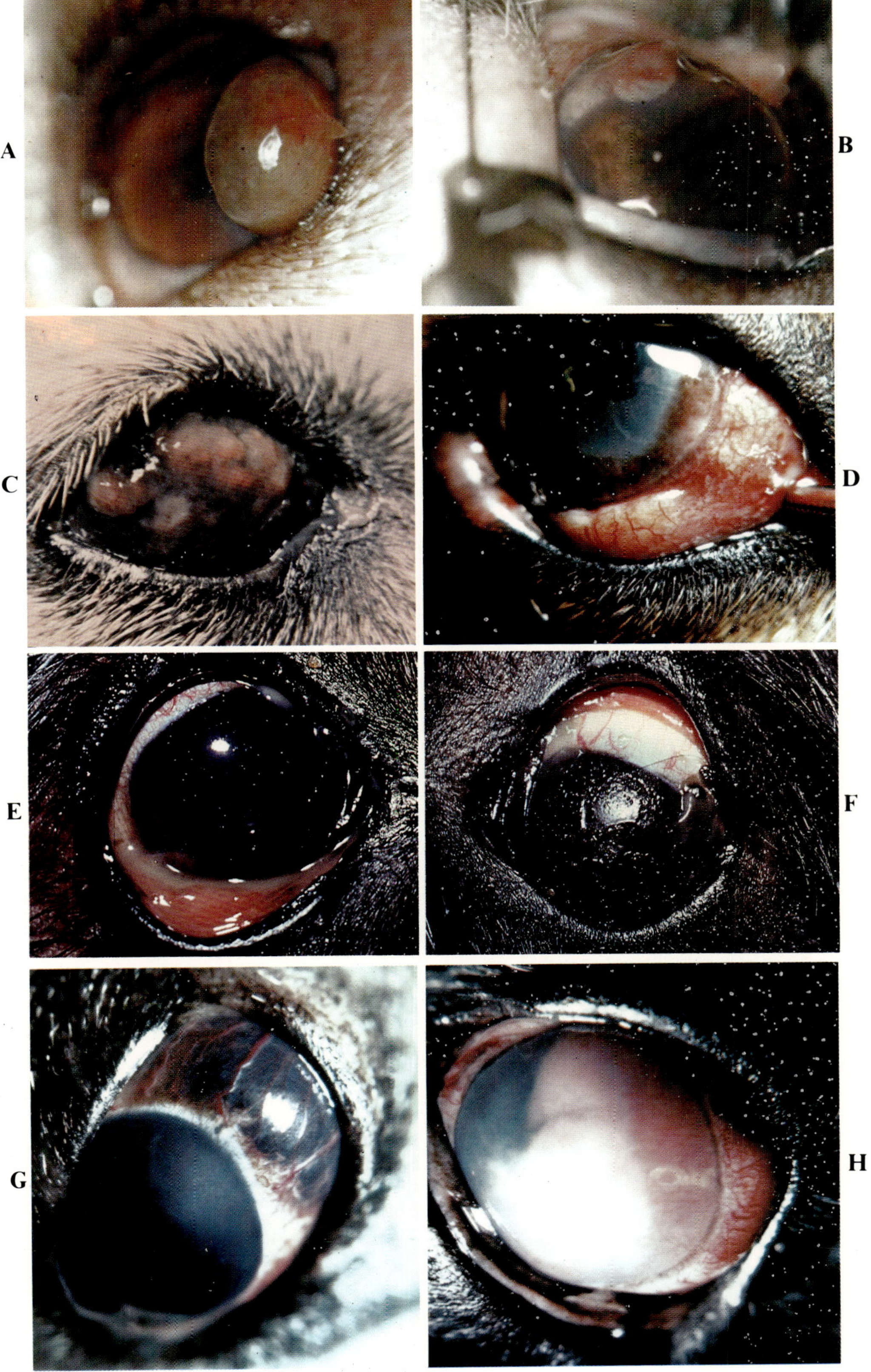

Plate 9

A. Superficial punctate keratitis (stained).
B. Superficial punctate keratitis. Stained areas are "doughnut-like" in appearance.
C. Localized endothelial (mesothelial) dystrophy (Boston terrier). The area of corneal edema is restricted to that portion of the cornea overlying the disturbed mesothelium.
D. Corneal edema due to endothelial dysfunction and hypopyon due to hepatitis vaccine reaction.
E. Leukoma caused by persistent pupillary membrane adherent to the endothelium.
F. Lateral view of *E* illustrating iris strands and attachment.
G. Neuroparalytic keratitis following luxation and replacement of the globe.
H. Boxer corneal erosion syndrome in late stage with corneal granulation.

Plate 9

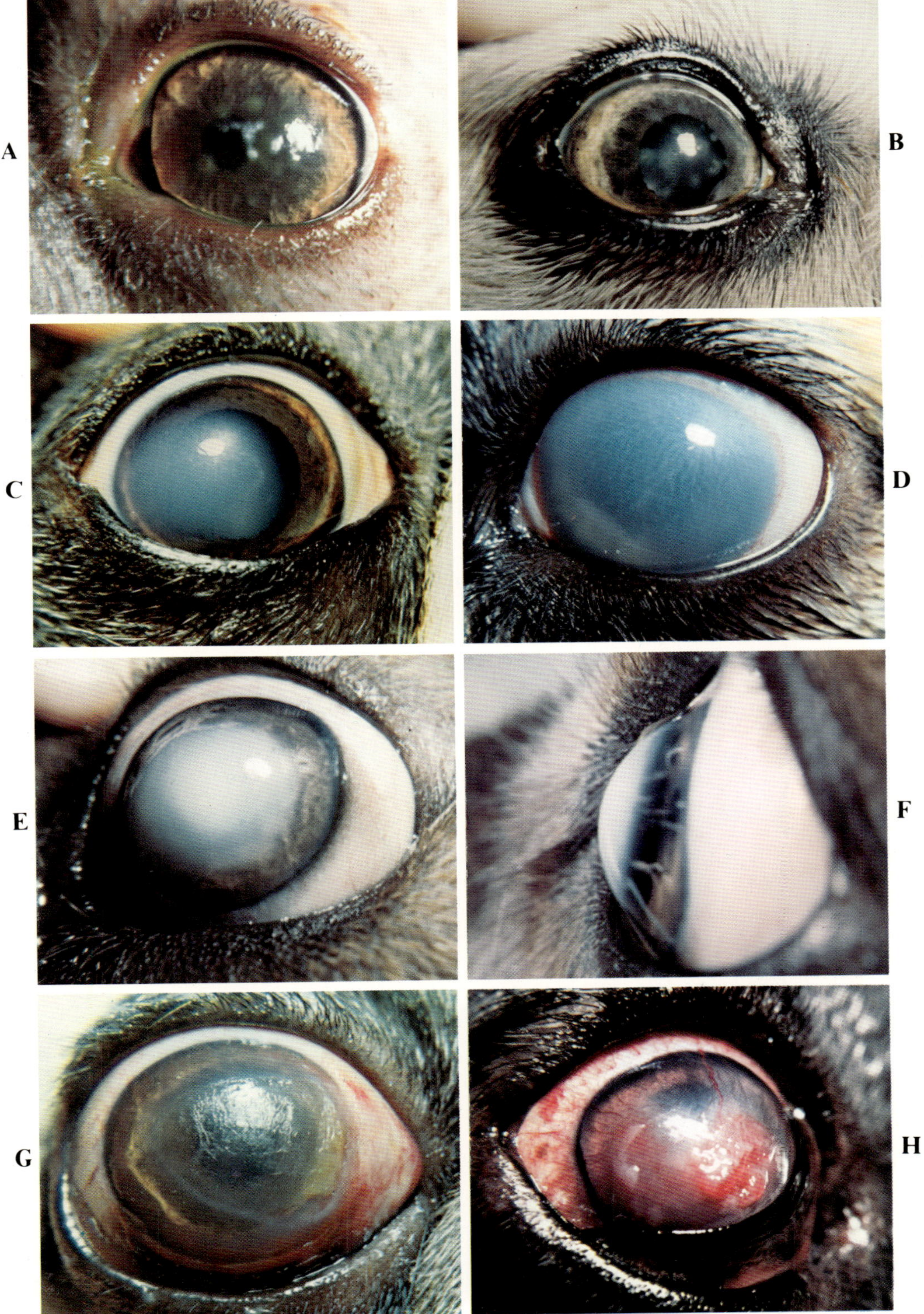

Plate 10

A. Epibulbar melanocytoma in a German shepherd.
B. Scleral melanosis syndrome in an aged Cairn terrier.
C. Persistent pupillary membrane adherent to the lens with an anterior capsular cataract.
D. Scleral staphyloma.
E. Corneal foreign body. Note associated inflammation.
F. Pigmentation associated with chronic keratoconjunctivitis sicca.
G. Corneal staphyloma, intraocular adhesions and cataract resulting from perforating injury.
H. Bullous keratopathy in chronic pannus (German shepherd). (Courtesy: Dr. J.J. Rosenthal, Vineland, N.J.)

Plate 10

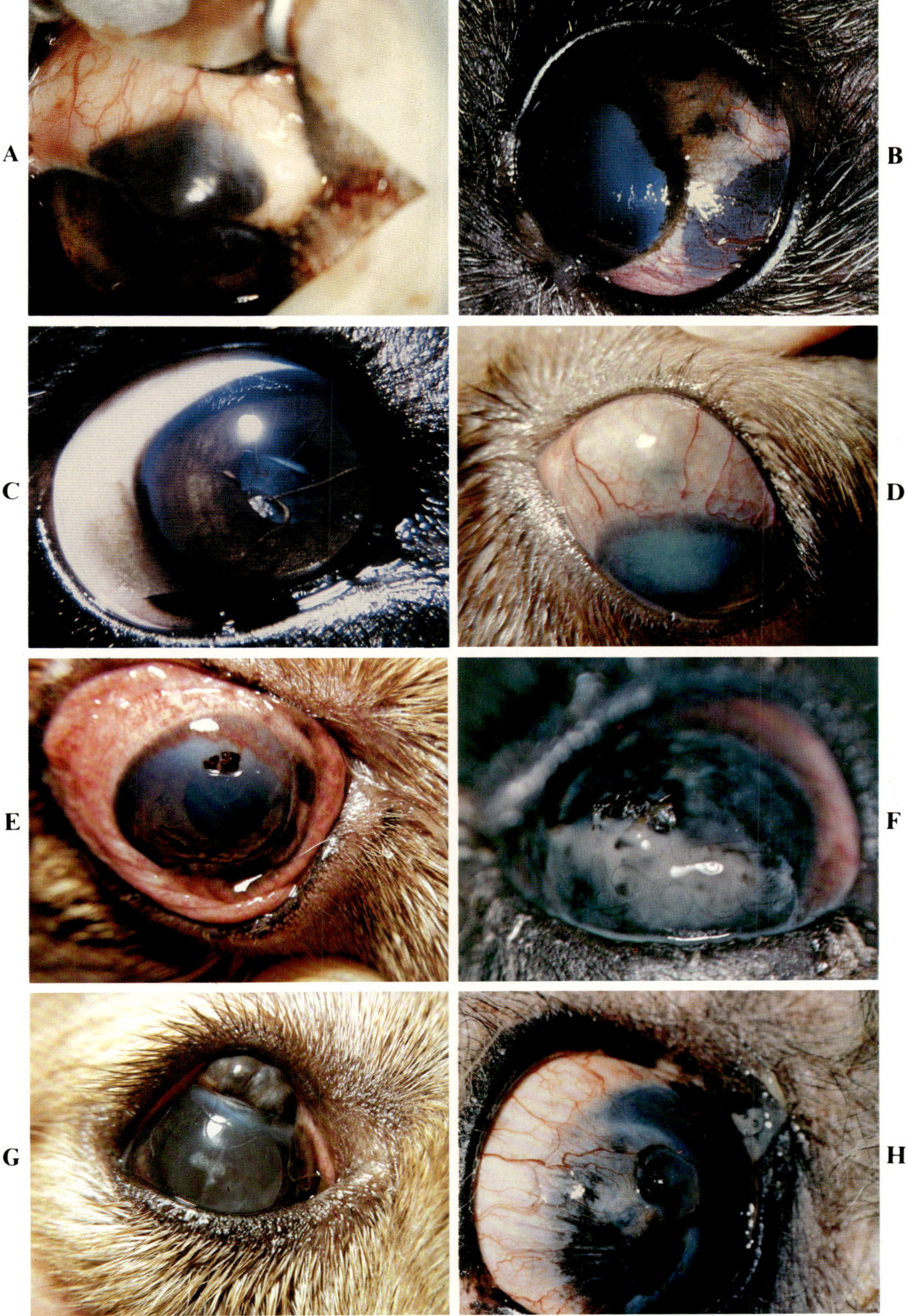

Plate 11

A. Heterochromia.
B. Iris cysts.
C. Iris atrophy in an aged poodle.
D. Acute iritis. Note exudate in anterior chamber opposite 1:00 o'clock; dull, lusterless iris; and miotic pupil.
E. Anterior uveitis. Note hemorrhage and exudate in area of the fixed pupil.
F. Iris bombé associated with anterior uveitis.
G. Panophthalmitis.
H. Staphyloma.

Plate 11

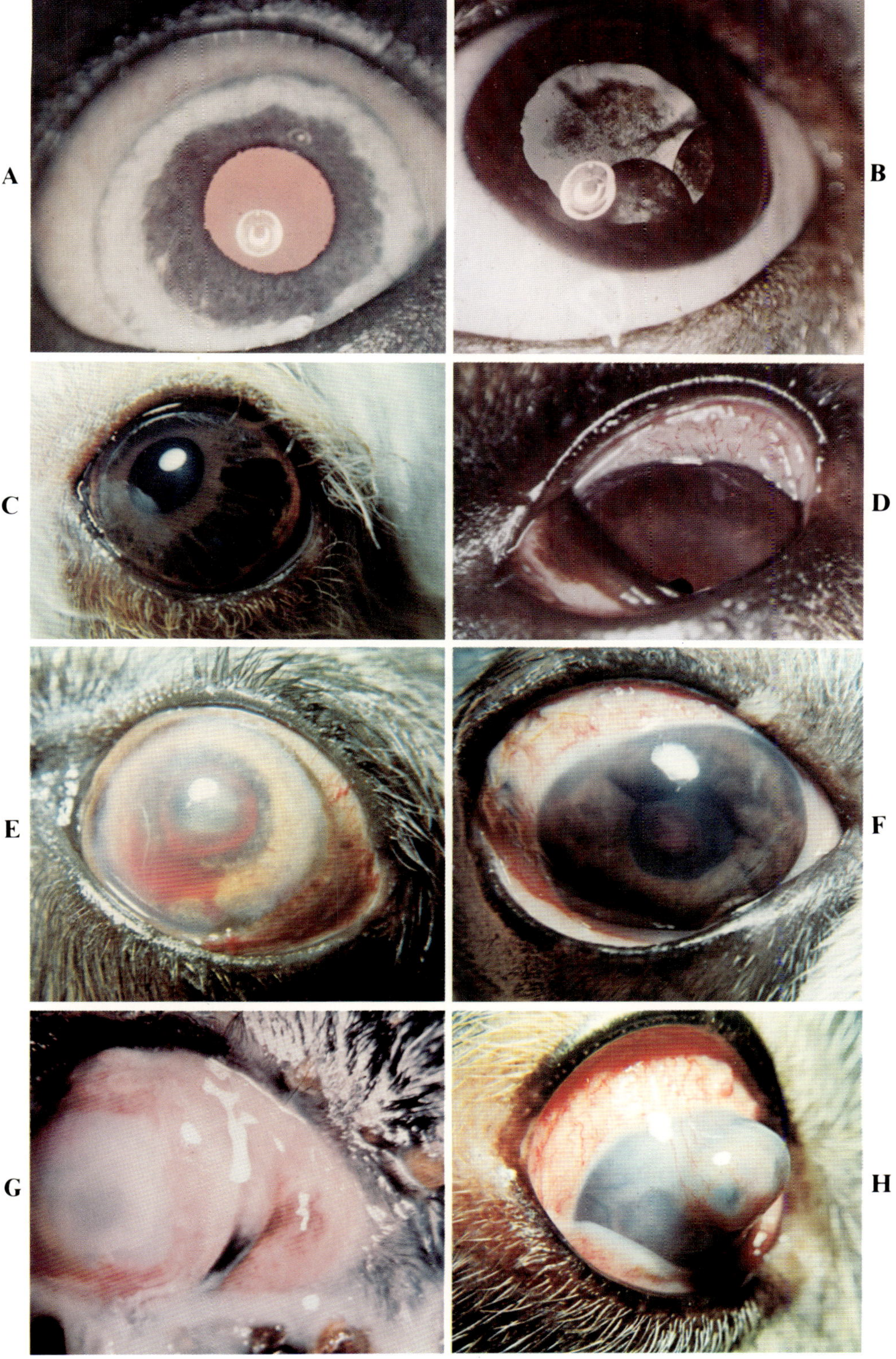

Plate 12

A. Iris atrophy and glaucoma.
B. Lens-induced uveitis with posterior synechia.
C. Cavernous hemangioma of the iris (entire upper half).
D. Pigmented nevi of the base of the iris with scleral and corneal invasion. There was no recurrence following surgical removal of the nevi from the involved structures.
E. Malignant melanoma of the iris and ciliary body. Extension from 11:00 to 2:00 o'clock.
F. Malignant melanoma of the uveal tract with secondary glaucoma.
G. Adenocarcinoma of the iris and ciliary body (below flash reflection).
H. Adenoma of the ciliary body (pupil artificially dilated).

Plate 12

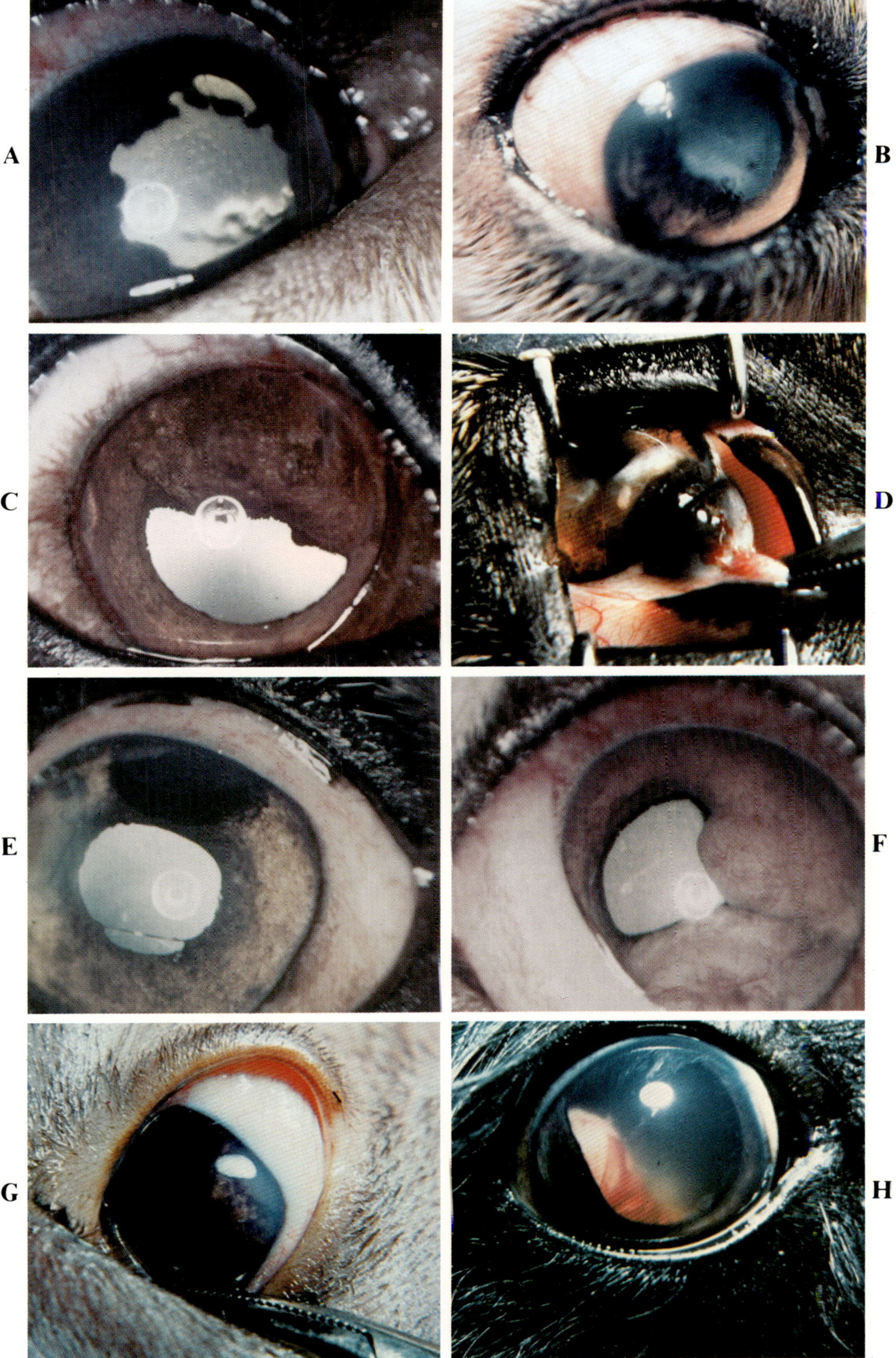

Plate 13

A. Strabismus (esotropia).
B. Luxation (prolapse) of the globe.
C. Retrobulbar abscess. Note conjunctival chemosis and exophthalmos.
D. Eosinophilic myositis. Note protrusion and drying of the membrane nictitans associated with the exophthalmos.
E. Retrobulbar malignant melanoma.
F. Retrobulbar embryonal rhabdomyosarcoma.
G. Retrobulbar rhabdomyosarcoma. (Courtesy: Dr. R. Sytek, Rockford, Ill.)
H. Enophthalmos. Note distance from medial canthus to the globe.

Plate 13

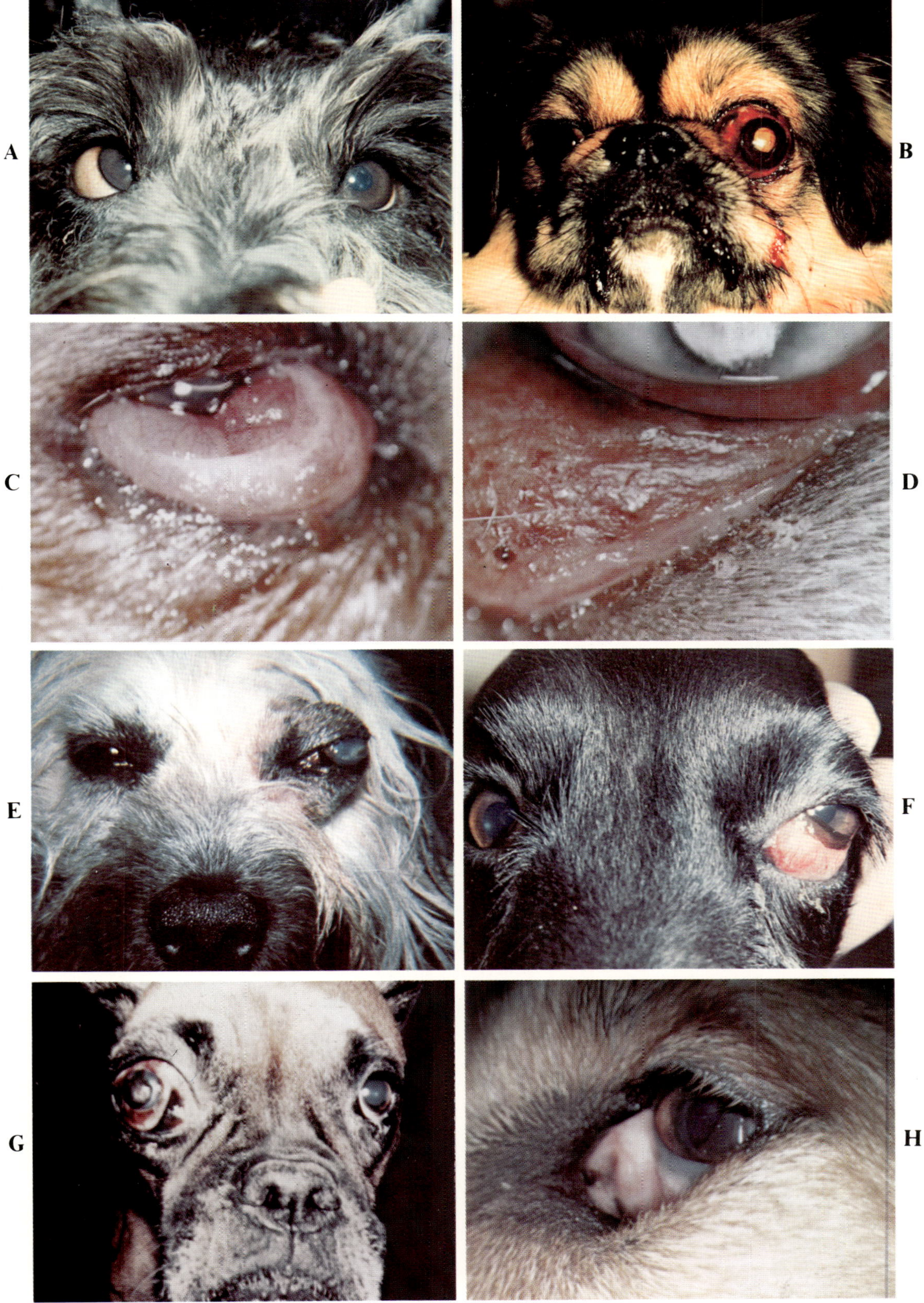

Plate 14

A. Hepatitis vaccine reaction resulting in glaucoma with buphthalmia (St. Bernard).
B. Lymphosarcoma of the eye and orbit. All superficial lymph nodes were enlarged.
C. Anophthalmos (right eye). Two-month-old mixed breed.
D. Microphthalmos (left eye) of *C.*
E. Phthisis bulbi as the sequel to uveitis.
F. Zygomatic gland enlargement (left). Pseudotumor (proliferative inflammation). Successfully removed.
G. Iris cysts (acquired senile).
H. Pseudotumor (tumorlike inflammation of iris). Successfully removed (iridectomy).

Plate 14

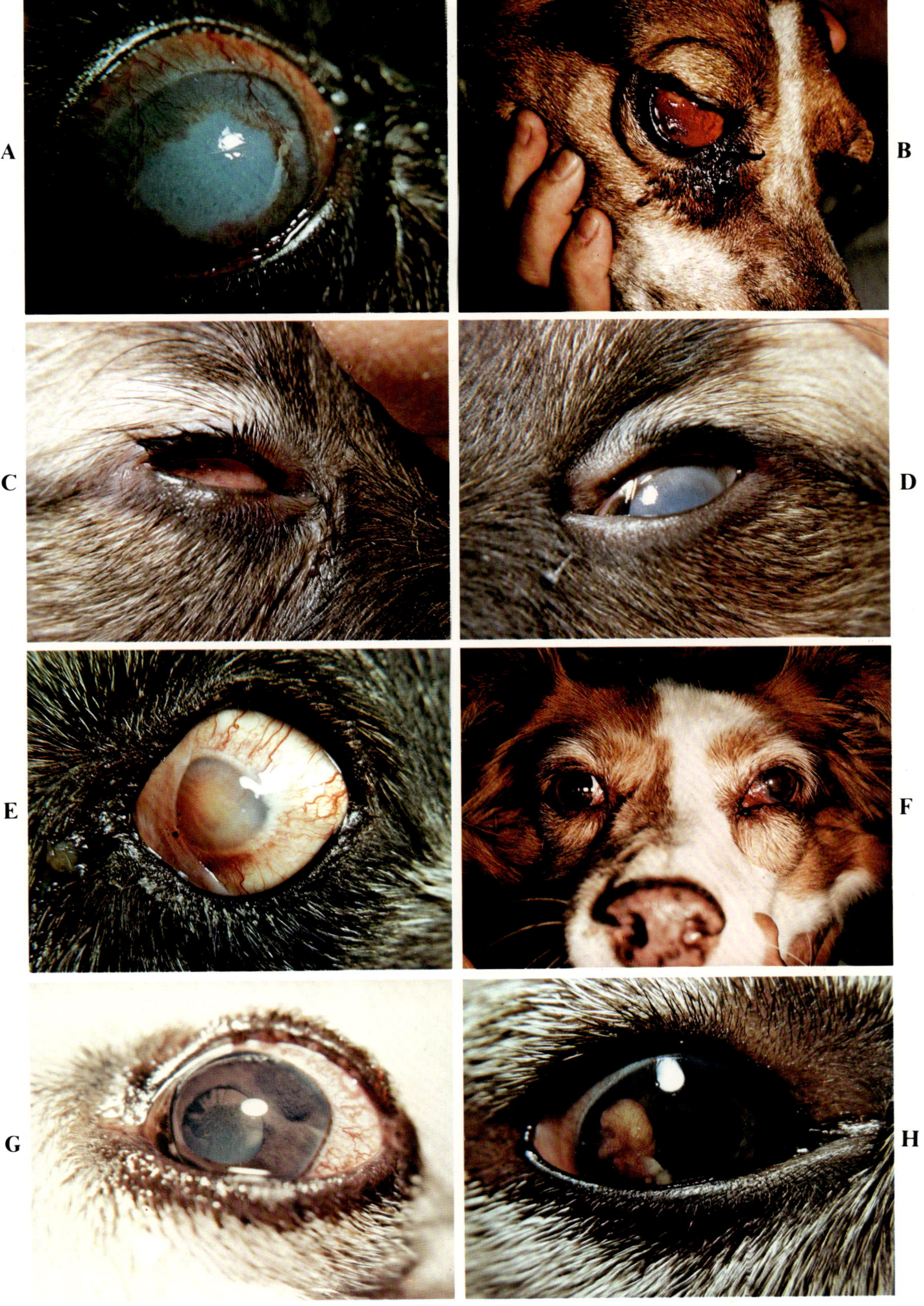

Plate 15

A. Acute congestive glaucoma. Note congestion and ejection of the conjunctival and episcleral vessels and dilatation of the pupil.

B. Subluxated lens and secondary glaucoma. Lens is displaced to the superior position with the lower border visible as an aphakic crescent.

C. Luxation of the lens into the anterior chamber. Note bluish "cast" to lens.

D. Absolute glaucoma with secondary iris atrophy.

E. Absolute glaucoma with secondary intraocular hemorrhage. Note congestion and ejection of the conjunctival and episcleral vessels, dilatation of the pupil (above the blood level), and bluish "cast" to the sclera (denotes thinning).

F. Iridencleisis bleb (3 months postoperatively). Note area of iridectomy and iris pillar under bulbar conjunctiva.

G. Basal, peripheral iridectomy opposite 10:00 o'clock.

H. Iridectomy (base to pupillary margin). Postoperative appearance following correction of secondary glaucoma resulting from an iris bombé.

Plate 15

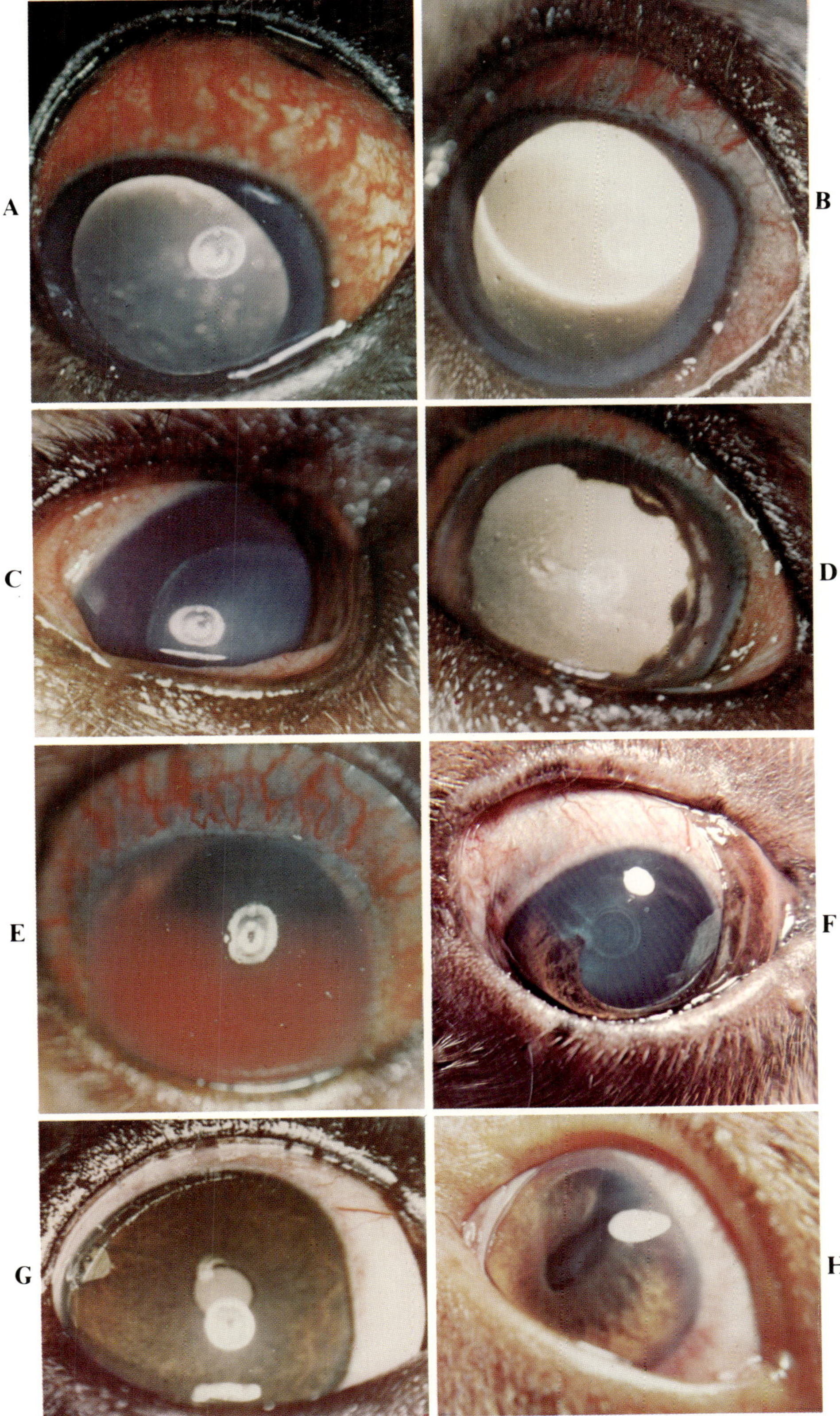

Plate 16

A. Morgagnian cataract. Pupil pathologically dilated due to a secondary glaucoma. Note tapetal reflection through the liquefied cortex, and the nucleus settled on the bottom. The upper corneal vascularization is indicative of this toxic stage.

B. Subluxated lens (inferior) with exposed ciliary processes. (Courtesy: Dr. M. Wyman, Ohio State University.)

C. Absolute glaucoma with striate pressure streaks of the cornea and intraocular hemorrhage.

D. Buphthalmos and exposure keratitis due to absolute glaucoma.

E. Absolute glaucoma and scleral staphyloma. (Courtesy: Dr. M. Wyman, Ohio State University.)

F. Gonioscopic view of drainage angle. *I,* iris; *PL,* pectinate ligament band; *IP,* inner pigmented band, *OP,* outer pigmented band.

Plate 16

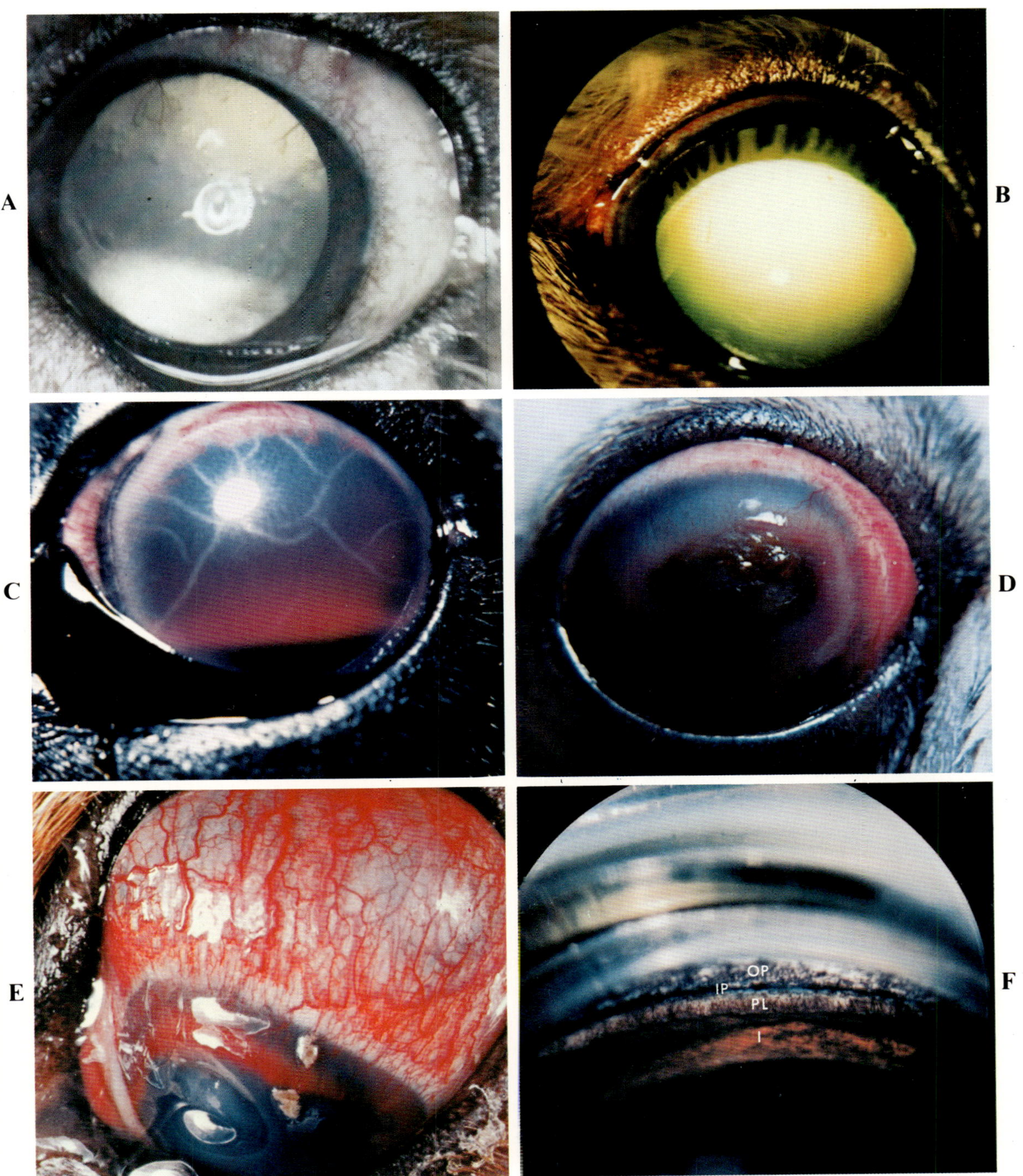

Plate 17

A. Juvenile cataract. Incipient stage. Pupil dilatation is artificial. Note tapetal reflection through unaffected portions of the lens.
B. Juvenile cataract. Immature stage. Pupil dilatation is artificial. Lens opacity diffuse but a "fundic reflex" is still discernible.
C. Senile cataract. Mature.
D. Hypermature cataract. Cortex liquefied.
E. Cataract secondary to progressive retinal atrophy in the poodle. Pupil dilatation is pathological. Note tapetal reflection still visible and accentuation of the "Y" suture. (Courtesy: D.K. Barnett, Cambridge University, England.)
F. Traumatic cataract. Note iris adhesion and lens opacity resulting from penetrating injury.
G. Congenital, stationary cataract (posterior cortical).
H. Nuclear sclerosis. Note "bluish" haze in pupillary area.

Plate 17

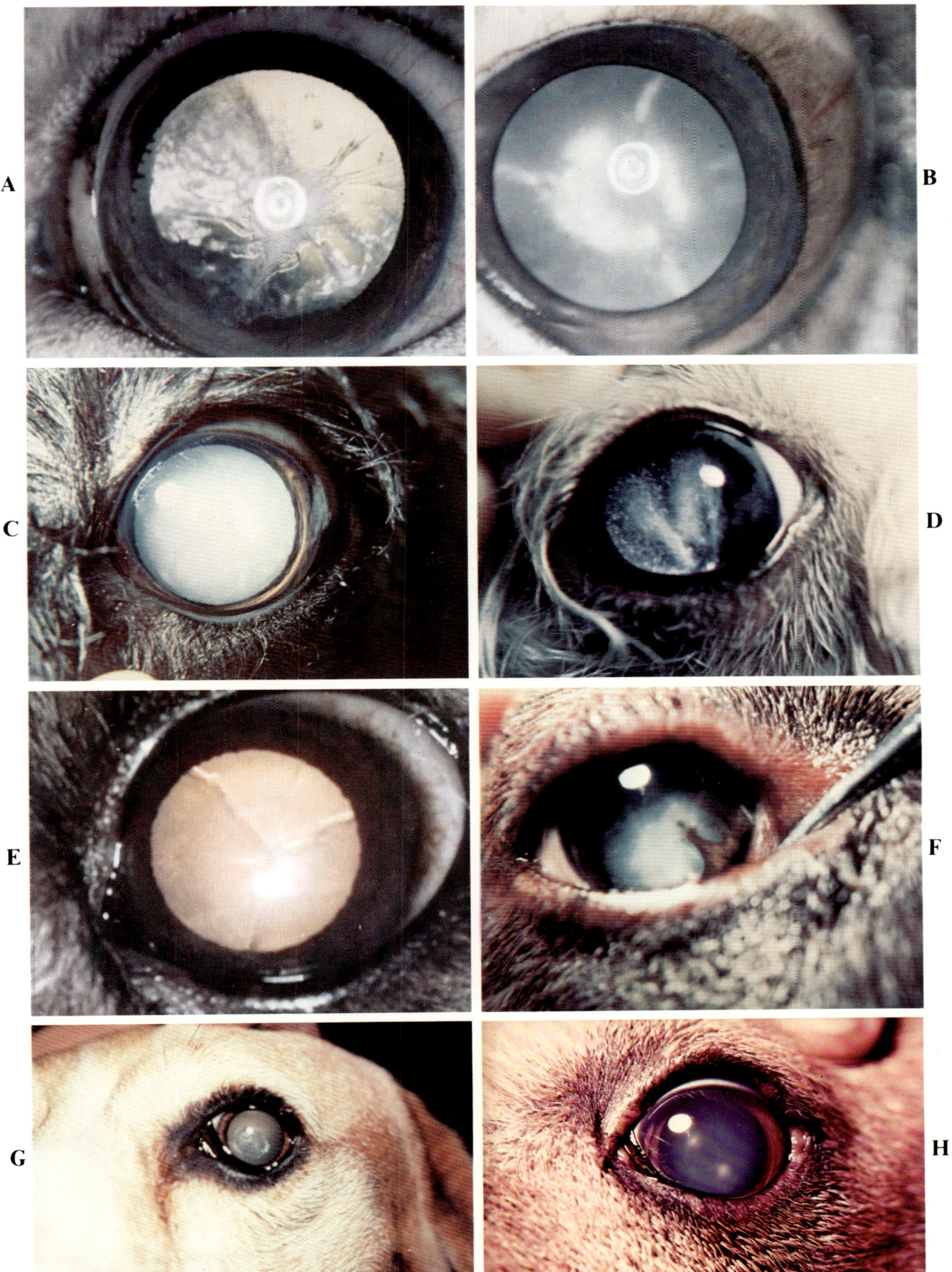

Plate 18

A. Detachment and disinsertion of the retina. The retina remains attached only at optic disc. (Courtesy: Dr. R. Trueman, Philadelphia, Pa.)

B. Complete serous retinal detachment (gross photograph). Note vessels within the retinal folds behind the dilated pupil. Retina lies near the posterior surface of the lens.

C. Generalized progressive retinal atrophy (poodle).

D. Central progressive retinal atrophy (Labrador retriever). (*C, D* from Barnett, K.C.: Primary Tapeto-Retinal Degeneration in Dogs *in* Graham-Jones, O. (Ed.): *Aspects of Comparative Ophthalmology.* London, Pergamon Press, Ltd., 1966.)

E. Retinal dysplasia in a Cocker spaniel.

F. Retinal dysplasia in a Springer spaniel.

G. Active focal retinochoroiditis. Note grey areas. (Courtesy: Dr. C. Fischer, Animal Medical Center, New York.)

H. Inactive retinochoroiditis. Note pigment clumping through eroded areas. (Courtesy: Dr. C. Fischer, Animal Medical Center, N.Y.)

Plate 18

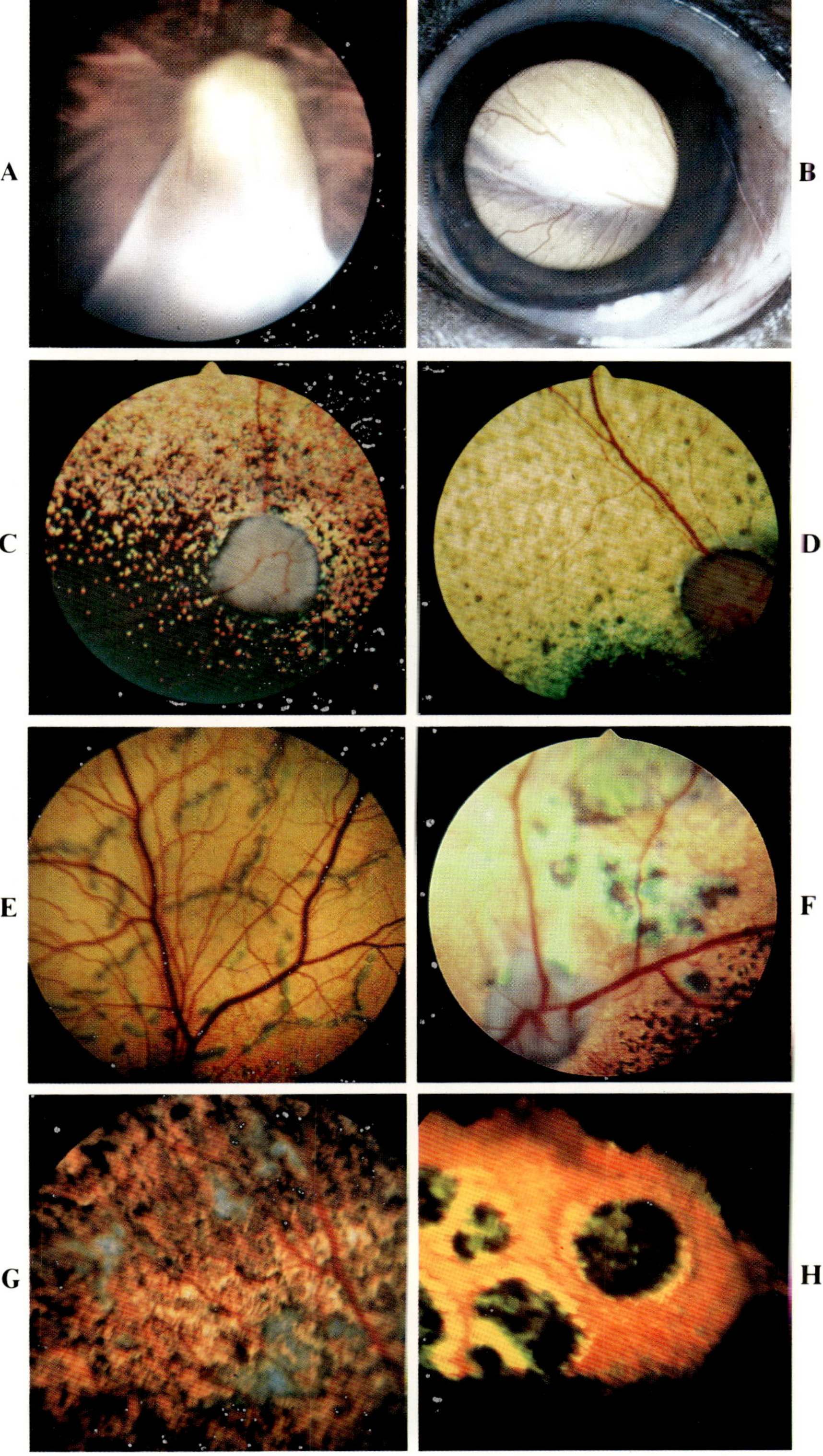

Plate 19

A. Active papillitis. *a,* indistinct disc borders which blend into peripapillary edema. *b,* peripapillary hemorrhage. (Courtesy: Dr. C. Fischer, Animal Medical Center, N.Y.)

B. Optic nerve hypoplasia. Note difference from normals (Plate 19C and D).

C. Normal fundus, 3-month-old collie pup. The blue color is typical of the immature fundus before the tapetum lucidum has developed. (Courtesy: Dr. S. Roberts, Stanford University.)

D. Moderate choroidal hypoplasia adjacent to a normal optic papilla. The choroidal vessels are visible against the white sclera. Courtesy: Dr. R. Donovan, Retina Foundation, Boston, Massachusetts.

E. Partial optic nerve coloboma.

F. Severe coloboma of the optic disc of a collie.

G. Intraocular hemorrhage associated with the collie eye anomaly.

H. Exposed choroidal circulation as a consequence of absence of choroidal pigment. Vision normal. Note retinal vessels overlying the choroidal circulation and blending of the optic disc into the surrounding area.

Plate 19

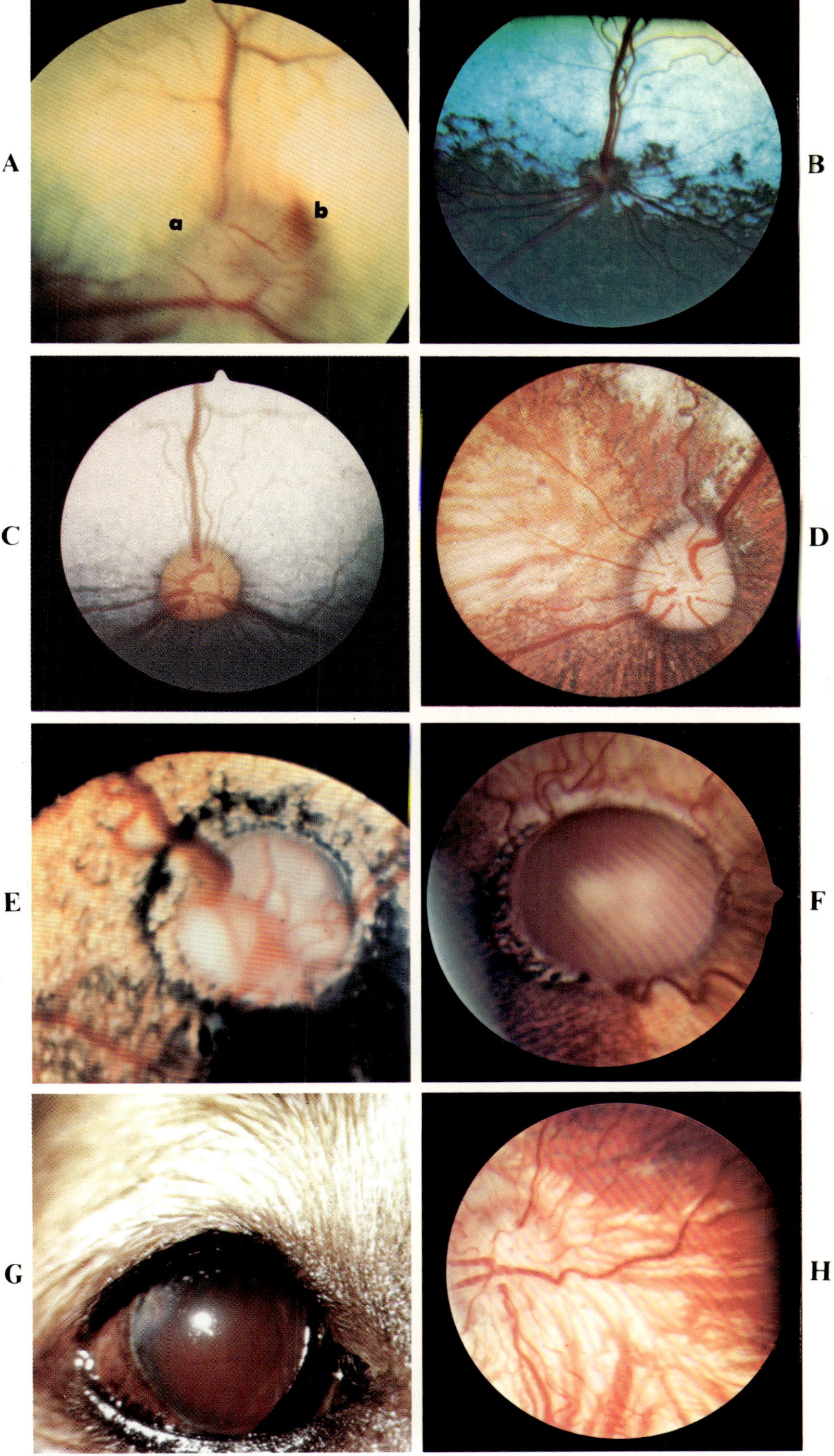

Plate 20

A. Clotted intravitreal hemorrhage.

B. Multiple asteroid bodies (asteroid hyalosis) in the vitreous obscuring easy visualization of the fundus.

C. Fundus of a 4-month-old beagle blinded by severe distemper retinopathy. There is extensive depigmentation of the non-tapetal fundus, hyperreflectivity of the tapetal fundus, constriction of the vascular tree, optic atrophy, and strands of glial tissue extending from the disc to the surrounding retina.

D. Retinochoroiditis. Fundus of a 3-year-old German shepherd. There is a wide hyperreflective area surrounding the optic disc, and some of the retinal vessels are narrowed. There were other hyperreflective zones in the fundus of both eyes, as well as some posterior cataract formation. The retinal lesions spread slowly.

E. Glaucomatous cupping. The retinal vessels are narrow, the tapetal fundus hyperreflective, and the depression of the disc is severe.

F. Thrombocytopenic purpura. The optic disc is swollen and multiple deep and superficial hemorrhages are present.

G. Cryptococcosis. Multiple black spots, representing cryptococcal chorioretinitis and some localized retinal detachments.

H. Large intravitreal hyaloid remnant attached at the optic disc (Bergmeister's papilla) and retinal atrophy. The grayish mass obscures complete visualization of the optic disc.

(A to H. Courtesy: Rubin, L., *Atlas of Veterinary Ophthalmoscopy.* Lea & Febiger, Philadelphia, 1974.)

Plate 20

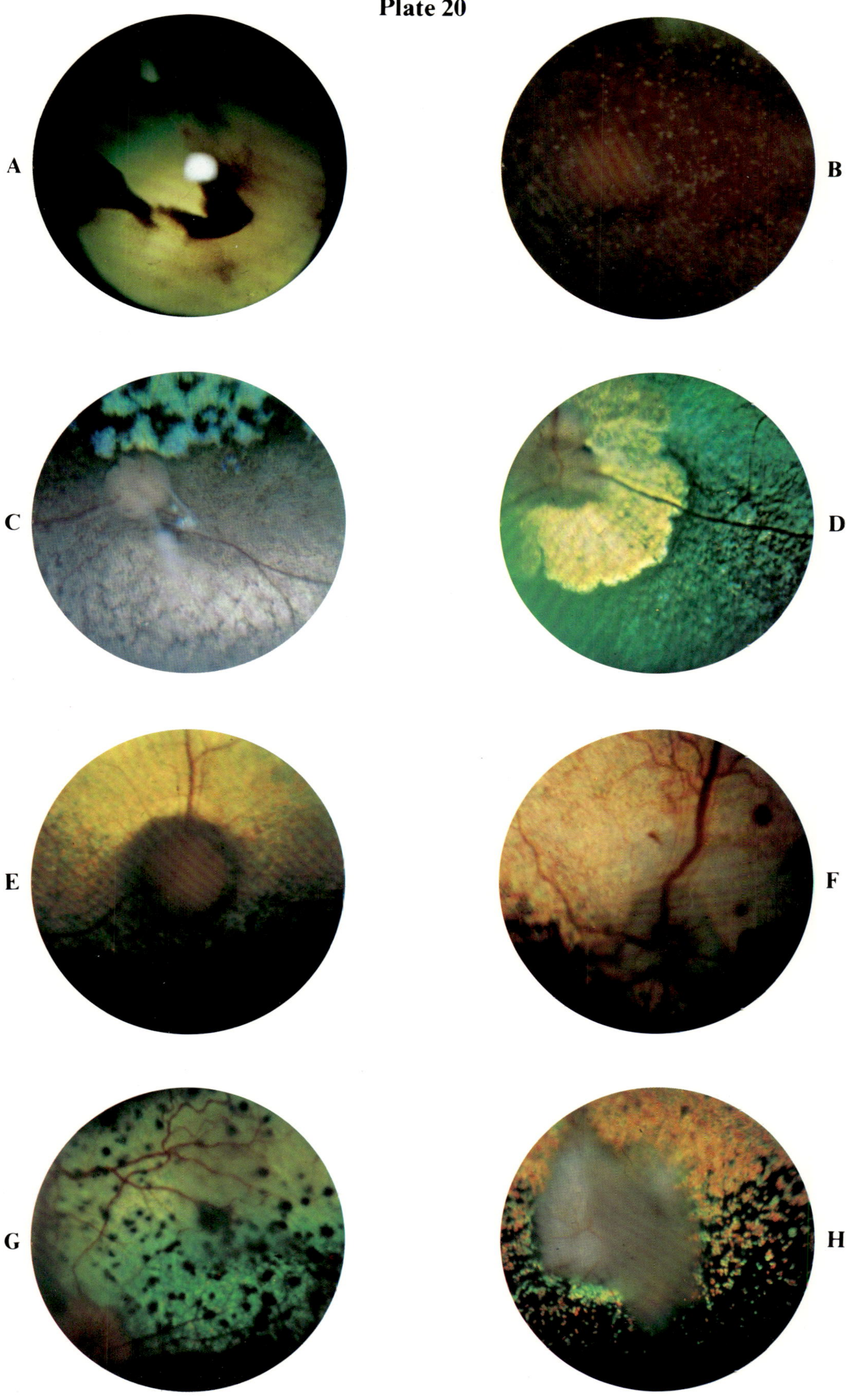

67. Roberts, S.R.: A Feasible Technic for Corneal Grafting, Mod. Vet. Pract., *44*:40–42, 1963.
68. Roberts, S.R.: Superficial Indolent Ulcer of the Cornea in Boxer Dogs, J.S.A.P., *6*:111, 1965.
69. Roberts, S.R.: The Nature of Corneal Pigmentation in the Dog, J.A.V.M.A., *124*:208, 1954.
70. Rubin, L. and Aguirre, G.: Clinical Use of Pilocarpine for Keratoconjunctivitis Sicca in Dogs and Cats, J.A.V.M.A., *151*:313, 1967.
71. Rubin, L. et al.: Clinical Estimation of Lacrimal Function in Dogs, J.A.V.M.A., *145*:947, 1965.
72. Runnquist, O. and Henricson, B.: Keratitis Superficialis Chronica hus Schäfer, Särtryck ur/Svensk Veterinärtidning, *15*:516–519, 1970.
73. Schmidt, G.: Corneal Inclusion Cyst Associated With Keratectomy in a Dog, J.A.V.M.A., *168*:144, 1976.
74. Schmidt, G.M., et al.: Intraocular Lead Foreign Bodies in Four Canine Eyes, J.S.A.P., *16*:33–39, 1975.
75. Schmidt, Gretchen, Magrane, W.G., and Helper, L.C.: Parotid Duct Transposition: A Follow-up Study of 60 Eyes, J.A.A.H.A., *6*:235–241, 1970.
76. Schramm, A.W.: How Scleral Contact Lenses Aid in Corneal Lesion Therapy, M.V.P., *48*:46, 1967.
77. Severin, G.A.: *Vet. Ophth. Notes,* Col. State U. Printing Service, 1975.
78. Slatter, D.H.: *Fundamentals of Veterinary Ophthalmology.* Philadelphia, W.B. Saunders Co., p. 375, 1981.
79. Slatter, D.N.: Keratoconjunctivitis Sicca in the Dog Produced by Oral Phenazopyridine Hydrochloride, J.S.A.P., *14*:749–771, 1973.
80. Slatter, D.H., Lavach, J.D., Severin, G.A., et al.: Uberreiter's Syndrome (Chronic Superficial Keratitis) in Dogs in the Rocky Mountain Area—a Study of 463 Cases, J. Sm. Anim. Pract. *18*:757, 1977.
81. Smelser, G.K. and Ozanies, V.: Effect of Local Anesthetics on Cell Division and Migration, Arch. Ophth., *34*:277, 1945.
82. Smythe, R.H.: *Veterinary Ophthalmology,* London, Baillière Tindall & Cox, p. 248, 1956.
83. Startup, F.G.: *Diseases of the Canine Eye,* London, Bailliere Tindall and Cassell, 1969.
84. Tripathi, R.C. and Bron, A.J.: Ultrastructural Study of Nontraumatic Recurrent Corneal Erosion, Brit. J. Ophth., *56*:73–85, 1972.
85. Überreiter, Von Otto: Ein besondere Keratitisform (Keratitis Superficialis Chronica) bein Hunde, Wien. Tierarztl. Mschr., *2*:65–78, 1961.
86. Überreiter, Von Otto: Examination of the Eye and Eye Operations in Animals, *Advances in Veterinary Science,* Vol. 5, New York, Academic Press, Inc., p. 52, 1959.
87. Überreiter, V.C., et al.: Zur Frage der Ätiologie der Keratitis Superficialis Chronica der Schäferhunde, Wien tierärztl Monatsschr, *58*:323–328, 1971.
88. Vestre, W.A., Brightman, A.H., Helper, L.Cl, et al.: Decreased Tear Production Associated with General Anesthesia in the Dogs, JAVMA, *174*:no. 9, 1006, 1979.
89. Vierheller, R.C.: Cataract Surgery in the Dog, Mod. Vet. Pract., *43*:45, 1962.
90. Weiner, M. and Scheie, H.: *Surgery of the Eye,* 3rd ed., New York, Grune & Stratton, 1952.
91. Wyman, M.: *Manual of Small Animal Ophthalmology,* New York, Churchill Livingstone, p. 160, 1986.
92 Yasuna, E.: Management of Traumatic Hyphema, Arch. Ophth., *91*:190, 1974.

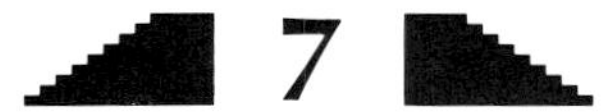

DISEASES AND SURGERY OF THE UVEAL TRACT

Anatomy and Physiology

7:1 The second or vascular coat of the eye (uvea or uveal tract) lies beneath the sclera (Fig. 7–1). It consists of three parts which are intimately associated. In the anterior portion the *iris* is clearly visible and assumes a perpendicular position in the globe. The second component part *(ciliary body)* and the third *(choroid)* are both attached to the internal surface of the sclera. There is no distinct line of separation between the iris and ciliary body, but there is a marked junction of the ciliary body with the choroid. This area is known as the *ora ciliaris retinae* (*ora serrata* in man).

7:2 The *iris* (Fig. 7–2) consists of spongy, connective tissue stroma, muscular fibers, and an abundance of vessels and nerves. It is covered anteriorly by endothelium and posteriorly by a pigmented epithelial layer that is continuous with the epithelium of the ciliary body and the retinal pigment epithelium. Iris color is dependent on the amount and location of the melanin pigment. In a brown iris, melanin is located throughout the thickness of the iris to the anterior surface. In a blue iris, the melanin is only on the posterior surface of the iris; light entering the eye passes through the iris stroma to the pigmented layer, and is reflected back toward the cornea. All of the wave lengths of light except blue, are absorbed by the iris stroma, and the observer sees a blue iris. Colors between brown and blue (e.g., green or yellow) are results of varying depth of the melanin in the iris.

7:3 The two muscles present in the iris are the *sphincter* which encircles the pupil near its edge and has parasympathetic innervation, and a *dilator* which extends from near the sphincter to near the iris root and has sympathetic innervation. The sphincter is the stronger of the two.

7:4 Purtsher[20] points out the significant differences between the iris of the dog and man. The canine iris possesses an immense arterial ring that is lacking in man. The peripheral part of the canine iris carries the important arteries and nerves that are intended for the ciliary body. Prince[19] states that the origin of this large vessel which forms a complete arcade around the iris is from the two long posterior ciliary arteries which reach it by passing right through the ciliary body. The dog appears to have a major but no minor arterial arcade in the iris.[19]

7:5 The iris regulates the amount of light admitted to the interior of the eye through the pupil. The size of the pupil may vary among breeds and at different ages. Normally the pupil is in a state of constant change, with many factors operating which influence the size. The behavior of the pupil during anesthesia has long been utilized to determine the depth of narcosis, a miotic pupil indicating stage 4 of surgical anesthesia. The iris lies in firm contact with the anterior capsule of the lens when the pupil is contracted or moderately dilated. When fully dilated, it is in less firm contact with the anterior chamber. The iris separates the *anterior* from the *posterior* chamber of the globe.

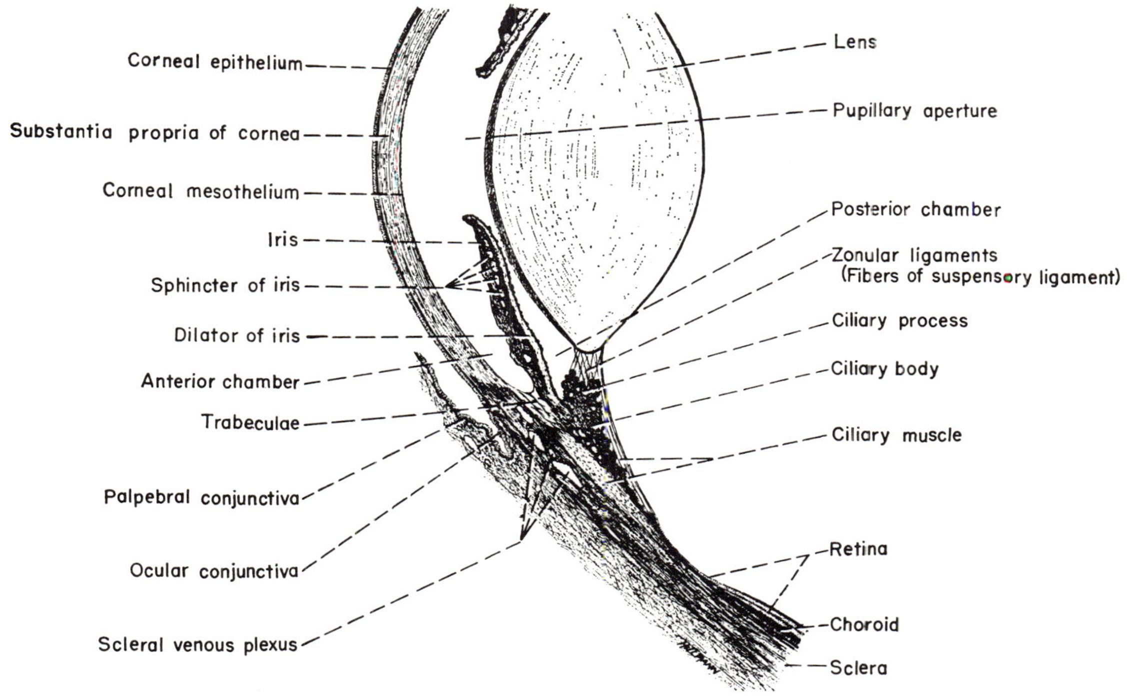

Fig. 7–1. Longitudinal section of anterior part of the eye showing relationship of uveal tract to cornea and lens. (Miller, *Anatomy of the Dog,* courtesy of W.B. Saunders Co.)

7:6 Most dogs' irides are brown or golden yellow with the pupillary border usually being more darkly pigmented. On its irregular posterior surface the iris is deeply pigmented with heavy radial striations. The color of the iris depends primarily on the amount and location of melanin in the iris, and the function of the iris stroma as a filter. An iris that appears blue has melanin only on the posterior surface. As light passes through the stroma and is reflected back by the pigment cells, all light frequencies except blue are absorbed and the iris appears blue. If melanin is present all the way to the anterior surface, the iris appears brown. Intermediate colors—green, yellow, etc.—indicate the presence of melanin at intermediate depths in the iris stroma. Human babies born with blue eyes may have a change in iris color as more pigment develops in the iris. In animals, it is not uncommon to have a blue or yellow iris change to a darker color as a result of pigment proliferation due to chronic uveitis. The depth of color of the iris plays a part in the reactions of the pupil to the various mydriatics. In dogs with lighter irides, the mydriatics are more prompt and longer lasting in their effect.

7:7 The *ciliary body* is that part of the vascular tunic which extends backward from the base of the iris to the anterior part of the choroid. It consists of the ciliary *muscle* and the ciliary *processes* covered by the ciliary epithelium. The ciliary muscle is poorly developed as compared to man and this is probably the greatest factor in the limitation of the dog's accommodation (Par. 1:3). The ciliary body is richly supplied with nerves.

7:8 The ciliary processes range in number from 70 to 80. The larger processes extend to as much as 2.4 mm in length, while the smaller ones situated between them may show in a section as little more than half of this. Their width will usually be 0.14 mm.[19] It is on these ciliary processes that the fine

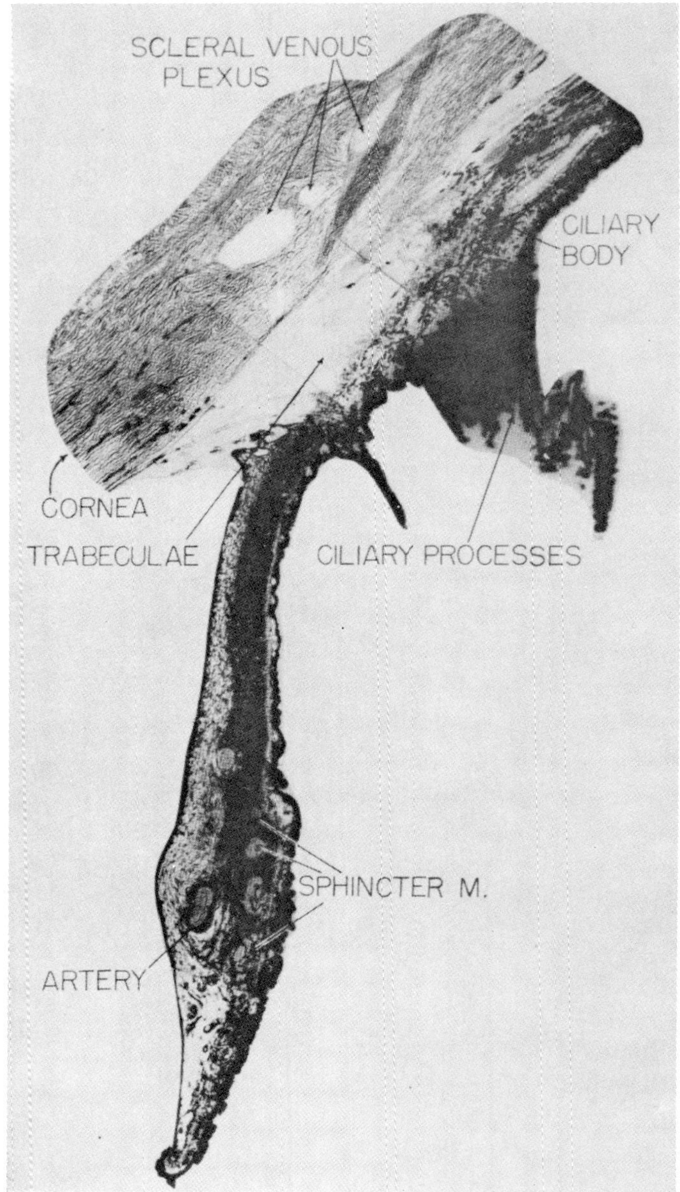

Fig. 7–2. Iris and relationship to the drainage angle. (Prince et al., *Anatomy and Histology of the Eye and Orbit in Domestic Animals,* courtesy of Charles C Thomas.)

suspensory or zonular ligaments *(zonules)*, which hold the lens, have their attachments. The ciliary processes are important in that the ciliary epithelium covering them secretes the nutrient fluid in the interior of the eye which, in turn, nourishes the cornea, lens and part of the vitreous. This fluid, the *aqueous* humor, under normal conditions, remains constant in amount and, by so doing, maintains a uniform intraocular pressure.

7:9 The aqueous is able to escape from the

eye by way of the trabecular meshwork into the intrascleral venous plexus (Fig. 7–2), thus carrying the waste products of lens and corneal metabolism with it. If, for some reason, this escape channel is blocked, the intraocular pressure rises, with glaucoma as the result, since the aqueous continues to be secreted by the ciliary processes. The aqueous humor is a much more dilute fluid than blood serum and contains considerably less protein and a low concentration of specific immune bodies. If, however, the anterior chamber is subjected to draining by paracentesis, the fluid which refills the anterior chamber contains a high percentage of protein and shows a high titer of antibodies (6:163). Secondary aqueous always contains a network of fibrin which, in all probability, results from disturbance of the blood-aqueous barrier. There also is a greater tendency for clot formation in the aqueous humor of the dog compared to man.

7:10 The *blood-aqueous barrier* is similar to the blood-brain barrier. The difference in composition of the aqueous and the plasma indicates its existence. In health it prevents entrance of substances of higher molecular weight into the anterior chamber. Its clinical importance lies in the fact that most antibiotics given systemically do not readily pass this barrier and blood levels of any particular substance are no indication of the aqueous level obtained (Par. 3:42).

7:11 The *choroid* constitutes the third and final component of the uveal tract. It is located between the sclera and the retina, extending from the ora ciliaris retinae to the opening for the optic nerve. The choroid is composed mainly of blood vessels and pigmented tissue and serves as a shield to absorb any light that passes through the retina or which is not reflected by the tapetum.

7:12 This vascular structure is bounded on either side by non-vascular membranes. Externally lies the suprachoroid, connected with the sclera by loose connective tissue. Underneath are several layers of large and medium sized anastomosing veins. Next comes a layer of capillaries *(choriocapillaris)* and, finally, *Bruch's* membrane lying between the choriocapillaris and the retinal pigment epithelium. The function then of the choroid is chiefly to serve as a nutrient organ for the retina, vitreous and lens.

7:13 The *tapetum* is a reflecting cellular layer of tissue situated in the choroid behind the retina. It serves to reflect light which has already passed through the retina, and to return it to the receptors so that they are doubly stimulated.[19] The tapetum (tapetum lucidum) varies in color and is responsible for the "eyeshine" so readily seen at night when the pupil is dilated and the dog stands facing a light. Some authors call the reflecting layer or tapetum the *tapetum lucidum,* and the non-reflecting part of the fundus, located inferior to the tapetum, the *tapetum nigrum.* This terminology does not seem to be correct, because there is no tapetum in this non-reflecting area. This lower area, below the tapetum, is better termed *non-tapetal.*

The Pupil

7:14 The normal pupil is circular and regular and is larger in the dog than in man (Par. 1:5). The size should equal that of its fellow and both should respond alike to light stimulation (Par. 2:26). The movements of the pupil are contraction and dilatation. Inequality of the diameter of the pupils is referred to as *anisocoria.*

7:15 The pupillary aperture serves to:

1. Adjust the intensity of retinal illumination. Constriction prevents dazzling of vision and possible retinal damage. Dilatation allows for sufficient light to reach the retina under conditions of subdued illumination.
2. Restrict the path of light rays to the central portion of the lens thus increasing the sharpness of the retinal image.
3. Influence the depth of focus of the lens system of the eye.

7:16 The contracting fibers of the iris (sphincter) are supplied by nerve fibers of the parasympathetic system that reach the eye via the *third* nerve. The dilating fibers (dilator) are supplied by the *sympathetic* system that reaches the eye via the cervical sympathetic trunk. Dilatation may be due to a decrease of third nerve tone or it may be due partially to stimulation of the dilator. Since the sphincter is the more powerful, the muscles are not equal antagonists. Contraction of the sphincter alone causes constriction of the pupil.

7:17 The rate of constriction varies, but the greatest part of the contraction occurs within the first few seconds and is completed within 5 or 6 seconds. When the light stimulus is removed, the pupil dilates quite slowly, the time for dilatation being at least twice that required for contraction. Failure of dilated pupils to contract upon being subjected to light stimuli indicates one of several pathologic conditions, provided mydriatics have not been used prior to the examination.

7:18 Pupil contraction from light stimulation may be direct or indirect. A *direct* light reflex is obtained by exposing an eye to increased illumination and observing the resulting contraction. The indirect reflex is obtained by observing the contraction in the fellow eye when the first is subjected to light stimuli. These reactions should be practically equal. The indirect contraction is explained by the fact that the light stimulus in one eye is carried by the optic nerve and passes to both optic tracts and in this way to the nucleus of the third nerve of each side. Blindness in one eye abolishes the direct reflex in this eye, but its indirect reflex from the contralateral eye is preserved.

7:19 A persistent dilatation may be a significant symptom of glaucoma in the dog (Par. 9:28). It is usually unilateral, however, and is accompanied by the other diagnostic signs of increased intraocular pressure. The dilatation of progressive retinal atrophy is, in contrast, bilateral, and no other gross lesions are evident, ophthalmoscopy necessarily being employed as a diagnostic adjunct.

7:20 McGrath[18] points out that dilatation is seen also in paralysis of the oculomotor nerve, irritation of the cervical sympathetics, and as a common symptom of canine encephalitis (bilateral constriction or anisocoria may occur).

7:21 Bilateral dilatation is seen in optic neuritis (Par. 11:111). In sphincter paralysis the pupil is widely dilated and does not react to light although it does contract after the instillation of a direct-acting miotic such as pilocarpine, but does not respond to a cholinesterase inhibitor such as humersol. Usually the mydriasis is associated with paralysis of other muscles that are innervated by the third cranial nerve but it also does occur without any other phenomenon.[12]

7:22 A miotic pupil may be seen in irritation of the oculomotor nerve, paralysis of the cervical sympathetics, and increased intracranial pressure (*e.g.* concussion, brain tumors). Miosis, usually unilateral, occurs in Horner's syndrome (Par. 12:24) and can also follow an injury to the area above the superior cervical ganglion.

7:23 A pupil that may be of normal size and yet fails either to dilate or contract suggests a posterior synechia (adhesion) of the iris to the anterior capsule of the lens (Par. 7:47). Iris atrophy, too, will result in an immobile pupil, the pupillary border of the iris, which possesses the sphincter fibers, being involved most conspicuously (Par. 9:40).

7:24 As a quick reference (Fig. 1–3):

1. *Disease between retina and optic chiasm.* No pupillary light response (PLR) in either eye when light is directed into eye on side of lesion. Light into contralateral eye—constriction in both. Eye on diseased side—pupil dilated a little more than normal in room light.

2. *Entire chiasm or both optic tracts destroyed.* Dilated pupils, no response of either and blind.

3. *Oculomotor nerve interrupted one side.* Pupil dilated on that side. Light response only in contralateral eye. Sight normal.

4. *Optic nerve and ciliary ganglion function destroyed (retrobulbar lesion).* Pupil on

affected side dilated and unresponsive to light directed into either affected or blind eye. PLR in unaffected eye only.

5. *Cortical lesion only.* PLR normal. Animal blind.

The Iris

7:25 *Congenital anomalies* of the iris include persistent pupillary membrane, heterochromia, polycoria, iris cysts, pigment spots or iris freckles and coloboma. These deviations from the normal are of interest but are only important from the standpoint of a differential diagnosis. No treatment is indicated or should be attempted.

7:26 *Persistent pupillary membrane* (Fig. 7–3). In the fetus the pupil is covered by a thin pupillary membrane, attaching to the anterior surface of the iris at the collarette, about midway between the base and free margin of the iris. This membrane and its vessels are gradually absorbed before birth. When this absorption is incomplete, shreds or strands remain. These strands, arising from the surface of the iris, may extend across the pupillary opening or, on occasion, can be found attached to an opaque spot on the anterior capsule of the lens (Par. 10:23) (Plate 10C) or to insert on the posterior cornea (Plate 9E,F). In most instances there is no significant change in iris mobility. A high incidence of the condition suggests a hereditary influence in the Basenji breed.[22]

7:27 *Heterochromia* (Plate 11A). Occasionally the two irides are of different color or

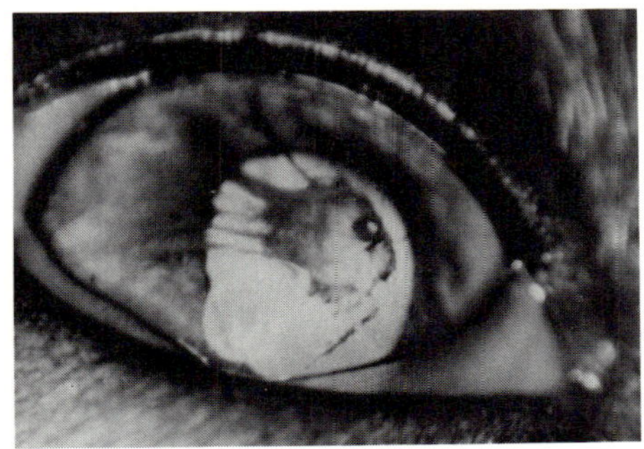

Fig. 7–3. Persistent pupillary membrane.

part of one iris may differ in color from the rest of that iris. There does not appear to be any associated lack of visual acuity. In several breeds of dogs, heterochromia has been shown to be associated with merle (or harlequin or dappled) coat color which is controlled by an autosomal dominant gene designated M. However, it appears that in beagles this pigmentary variation is independent of the dominant gene M.[25]

7:28 *Polycoria.* Rarely two or more pupils will be seen in one iris. To be a true polycoria each pupil must have its own sphincter fibers. Rarely iris coloboma, more often iris atrophy, is a more common reason for multiple holes in the iris (Par. 7:31).

7:29 *Iris cysts* (Plate 11B) Pigmented cysts, resembling varying sized "cannon balls," may be found loose in the anterior chamber or adhered to the iris. They can be congenital or acquired. They are seldom present in sufficient number to interfere with vision. It is important that iris cysts be differentiated from a melanotic tumor of the anterior segment. A misdiagnosis may result in an unwarranted surgical intervention. Iris cysts are hollow, and often can be transilluminated.

7:30 *Pigment spots or iris freckles* (iris nevi) appear as dark brown to black spots in and on the iris.

7:31 *Coloboma* of the iris is a notching which is usually present in the inferior half of the iris and is most often associated with coloboma of the choroid. It is very rare in the dog. Iris atrophy (Par. 7:86) is a much more common cause of holes or notching of the iris.

Anterior Uveitis (Iridocyclitis)
(Plate 11D,E)

7:32 Anterior uveitis refers to inflammations of the iris and ciliary body. Since inflammations of these structures are usually coexistent and cannot be differentiated on a clinical basis, those cases designated as iritis and cyclitis should be thought of as *iridocyclitis.*

7:33 Anterior uveitis has, in the past, been

classified or divided in various ways, depending on clinical signs. Such classification is arbitrary. The presenting signs are, in reality, a continuum from the slightest inflammation, characterized by a slightly reddened eye to a severely inflamed blind eye, and one not well correlated with etiology. Although blastomycosis, for example, is more likely than leptosporosis to result in severe exudative uveitis with blood and fibrin in the anterior chamber, there is no clear-cut relationship that allows etiologic diagnosis based on clinical signs. The clinical signs observed correlate to the degree of inflammatory response to the causative agent, rather than to the agent itself. It is important to note that much of the response is immune mediated, and that prostaglandins play an important role in the cascade of events that follow uveal tract insult or injury.[6,8,14,24]

7:34 *Etiology.* Acute uveitis usually follows or accompanies some systemic disorder. It is most important that considerable time be expended in careful history taking and in conducting a thorough physical examination, including laboratory tests, if a cause is to be determined. Even then, the cause of many cases presented will never be known. The source often depends upon a toxin or antigen derived from a septic focus in some part of the body. This includes, for example, infected tonsils, teeth, prostate, sinuses, and pyometra. Heartworm infestation is a fairly common cause in endemic areas. A classical chronic form of the disease has been seen as the result of toxoplasmosis and the systemic mycotic diseases. Blastomycosis, coccidioidomycosis, cryptococcosis and histoplasmosis are all capable of producing a subacute or chronic uveitis and blindness. But, as indicated above, although systemic disease may trigger a uveitis, the greater number of cases cannot be correlated to such disease. The present concept places the involvement of the anterior uvea as an immune-mediated reaction excited by pathogens elsewhere. The resultant tissue reaction within the uveal tract most likely follows the classical concept of the antigen-antibody reaction mechanism. The exact cause, or initiating antigen, is often obscure; therefore, the incrimination of a single specific agent is difficult. The fungus diseases, especially blastomycosis, coccidioidomycosis and cryptococcosis are exceptions to the generalization. In these diseases, uveitis is commonly accompanied by organisms in the affected eyes.

7:35 *Specific diseases* such as distemper, leptospirosis, and hepatitis may, in turn, initiate an iridocyclitis. The "blue eye" (corneal opacity) following a hepatitis attack stems from an iridocyclitis which, in turn, is caused by the hepatitis virus. Carmichael's[5] study showed that during the acute febrile stage of hepatitis there was a mild anterior uveitis without corneal involvement. The corneal opacity supervened during convalescence. Two fundamentally different modes of pathogenesis are postulated for the ocular lesions of the disease. During the acute phase of illness, prior to the onset of circulating antibodies, uveitis occurs that is related directly to effects of viral growth in vascular endothelium, and in reticuloendothelial elements of the anterior uvea. The severe iridocyclitis with corneal opacification that occurs in clinically recovered dogs possesses characteristics of the Arthus-type of antigen-antibody reaction.

7:36 *Vaccine-induced uveitis* and corneal edema ("blue eye") occurs occasionally, following the use of some modified live virus adenovirus hepatitis vaccines (CAV-1). The inflammatory process is similar to that produced by the virulent virus described above (Par. 7:35). One or both eyes may be slightly to severely affected. In the ordinary mild case affecting but one eye the opacity disappears within a few days. Some cases, however, persist for months or remain permanently. Severe involvement can predispose to a secondary glaucoma (Plate 14A).

7:37 The incidence of corneal edema recorded in one series[7] was 1 in 243 dogs vaccinated with live vaccine (approx. 0.4%). All ocular reactions occurred within one month of vaccination with a peak on days 12 and 13. At least half of these opacities persisted beyond one week, one third beyond 2 weeks, and one tenth beyond 2 months. The remainder were unresolved when examined at 6 months. In another study[1] pathogenicities of two adenoviruses (CAV) were compared. Results indicated that suitably attenuated CAV-2 should be used as a replacement for the vaccinal CAV-1 which are known to cause postvaccinal ocular lesions.

7:38 The use of Canine Adenovirus II (CAV-2) vaccines in the DHL combination is said to eliminate this complication. Other manufacturers,* using Canine Adenovirus-1 in the DHL vaccine, have modified the manufacturing process, so that the vaccine no longer causes the "blue eye" problem.

7:39 *Dirofilariasis* (heartworms) can produce an anterior uveitis ranging from mild to severe. In some cases, a severe "flare up" has occurred as the dog was being treated with the adulticide (Caparsolate sodium) or the microfilariacide (Dithiazanine iodide).

7:40 A *traumatic* iritis occurs as a result of accidental injury or following intraocular surgery. The seriousness and course depend on the degree of injury and whether infection takes place.

7:41 A *secondary* iritis, following inflammation of adjacent tissues, may be found in severe corneal ulceration (Par. 6:108), lymphosarcoma (Par. 12:47), (Plate 8H), and in neoplasia involving the uveal tract.

7:42 *Lens-induced uveitis* (phacoanaphylaxis) is caused by leaking of the lens protein into the aqueous and its subsequent contact with the anterior uvea. Since the lens protein is recognized as foreign to the eye, an antigen-antibody reaction results in a uveitis. Leaking can occur during the early stages of cataract formation, especially when the lens swells during rapid development (intumescence). It also may occur if liquified cortical material from a hypermature cataract leaks through the lens capsule. Lens-induced uveitis varies from a transient or mild inflammation, easily controlled by medical treatment, to severe, requiring vigorous treatment, even lens removal. Traumatic rupture of the lens capsule invariably results in a uveitis. If the tears in the capsule are small, the uveitis can often be controlled by medical treatment, as the lens material is absorbed by the aqueous over several weeks, especially in young dogs. In massive ruptures, reaction in some is severe, and surgical removal of the lens material is often required. Recurrent uveitis sometimes occurs in dogs that have undergone extracapsular cataract extractions months to years previously. It is associated with formation of new lens fibers ("Elschnig pearls") at the equator of the remaining lens capsule. Most cases can be controlled with medical treatment.

7:43 *Clinical Signs.* Anterior uveitis is characterized by pain, photophobia, blepharospasm, and increased tearing. The ciliary blood vessels are congested and can be differentiated from congested conjunctival vessels (Par. 5:05). In the examination, the examiner should decide whether there is congestion of ciliary vessels *in addition to* conjunctival vessel congestion, since ciliary vessel congestion is invariably accompanied by conjunctival vessel congestion. The cornea may have an overall haze. This is due to the possible presence of keratitic precipitates (leukocytes) clinging to the endothelium and, also, to the fact that damage has reduced effectiveness of the endothelial pump (Par. 6:12) with a resulting corneal edema. The contents of the anterior chamber show changes. There is frequently turbidity *(aqueous flare)* which, when viewed obliquely, can be likened to the dust particles seen in a room when the drapes are pulled and a ray of sunshine pours in (Tyndall effect). In some instances great numbers of leukocytes and exudate from the iris may pour into the anterior chamber producing hypopyon (Plate 7B).

7:44 The iris itself looks spongy, muddy, and lusterless. Its color is altered some as the

*Pitman-Moore & Co., Washington Crossing, New Jersey.

result of the congestion and exudation of cells and fibrin into the stroma. The pupil is contracted *(miosis)* as a result of the distention of the radial blood vessels and irritation of the sphincter muscle. If the pupil is both miotic and irregular, adhesions between the posterior surface of the iris and the anterior capsule of the lens *(posterior synechia)* should be suspected. Although the intraocular pressure in iritis is usually normal or below (hypotony), the presence of posterior synechia can result in iris bombé or peripheral anterior synechiae and a secondary glaucoma (Par. 9:75).

7:45 *Course.* When an attack of iridocyclitis is acute and is diagnosed and treated early, the response is most dramatic and a "quiet" eye can be expected within several days to a week. If, on the other hand, the history and objective symptoms indicate a chronic condition, response to the best therapy is slow, and serious complications can develop at any time, necessitating a change of medication or surgical intervention. Certain forms of iridocyclitis have a tendency to recur. Relapses are common because of the irritation effects of sequelae but probably more to the fact that the etiological factor has not been eliminated.

7:46 *Sequelae.* The usual complications following an attack of uveitis include: posterior synechiae, a cloudy film deposit upon the anterior lens capsule, complete seclusion of the pupil, occlusion of the pupil, iris atrophy, secondary glaucoma, vitreous opacities, lens opacities (cataract). Chorioretinitis of the same etiology as the anterior uveitis may also occur. An endophthalmitis (Par. 7:62) may develop with loss of the eye.

7:47 A partial posterior synechia is of little consequence to the dog, but if a complete synechia with seclusion of the pupil occurs *(iris bombé)* (Plate 11F), a secondary glaucoma may result. When the iris is bound down throughout its entire pupillary margin (Fig. 7–4), there is a loss of communication between the anterior and posterior chambers. Thus the aqueous secreted by the ciliary processes (Par. 7:8) is retained in the posterior chamber and causes the iris to billow forward,

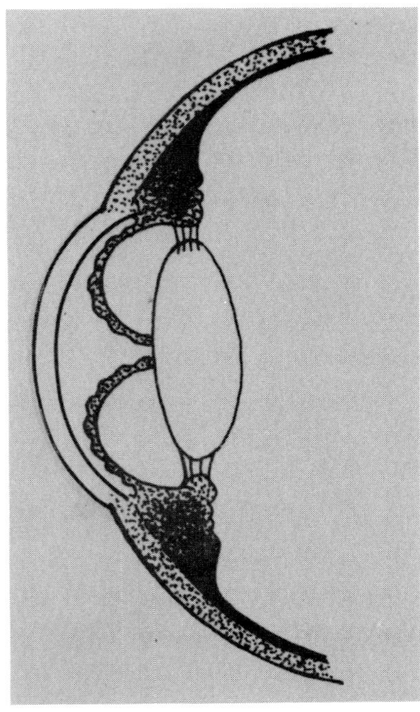

Fig. 7–4. Anterior section of the eyeball showing posterior synechia (iris bombé) and angle closure.

creating iris bombé (Fig. 7–4). The base of the iris closes the filtration angle and causes angle closure glaucoma.

7:48 Occlusion of the pupil is a filling in of the pupillary space with an opaque exudate or the entire iris may appear to obliterate the pupil area. Atrophy of the pupillary border and other sections of the iris stroma (Plate 12A) can, in turn, produce a secondary glaucoma because the sloughing pigment and iris debris clog the drainage angle. With atrophy of the iris, the base of the iris may also come forward causing angle closure glaucoma.

7:49 Strands of inflammatory exudate in the vitreous may persist for some time or permanently, and latent lens opacities can be expected in the chronic, recurrent forms of uveitis. Chorioretinitis is discussed in paragraph 11:31. The choroid and vitreous are often involved to some degree when anterior uveitis is severe. A vitreous tap (Par. 11:16) is often helpful in establishing a diagnosis. Fungal agents, especially Blastomyces sp., are commonly found in the vitreous when causing an anterior uveitis.

7:50 *Treatment.* Because of the serious complications and sequelae associated with this disease, appropriate therapeutic measures cannot be overemphasized.

7:51 The first consideration should be to alleviate the pain and get the inflammatory process under control. Determination of and elimination of the etiologic factor, whenever possible, are of importance, but no time must be lost in "putting out the fire," with the cause as the secondary consideration.

7:52 Atropine (2 to 4%) diminishes congestion of the iris, relieves pain by paralyzing the ciliary body, and prevents adhesions by its mydriatic action (Par. 3:23). In the initial stages atropine should be used every few hours, or until the pupil dilates well, and then twice a day. When the inflammation is severe, the pupil will not dilate readily. Use of a combination of 10% Phenylephrine HCL and .3% Scopolamine (Par. 3:30) every 20 minutes for 4 applications is indicated, if atropine is insufficient. If the pupil fails to budge, a synechia is probably present.

7:53 Steroids, like atropine, are specific for treatment. A subconjunctival injection of a repositol preparation (Par. 3:63) will afford the best control of the inflammation. If the etiology is obscure and fungus diseases are not ruled out, use of a short-acting steroid, such as Dexamethasone or Flumethasone* (Par. 3:65) subconjunctivally, daily, is preferred over a repositol preparation. If the response is favorable or when fungus disease is ruled out, a repositol steroid can be used. Topical corticosteroid-antibiotic combinations are helpful. In addition, systemic steroids, such as prednisolone, beginning at 1 mg/pound/day orally for 3 days, then at a gradual tapering of dosage over a several week period, should be begun if response to the mydriatic, subconjunctival and topical steroids is not satisfactory in 24 to 36 hours. *Note:* Blood samples should be collected for analysis before subconjunctival or systemic steroids are started, because the steroids will make interpretation of the WBC and differential blood counts difficult. In those instances where a systemic mycotic disease is responsible for the uveitis, corticosteroid use is contraindicated. In fact, the condition will worsen, a possible "tip off" as to the cause.

7:54 Since prostaglandins are important mediators of inflammation, prostaglandin inhibitors (Par. 3:66) are of value in treatment. Flunixin meglumine† at .25 mg/pound, IV, daily or aspirin, 10 mg/pound, orally, BID to QID are helpful. Banamine, although not approved for the dog, is used widely. It is more profound in action than aspirin, but should not be used for more than 3 days.

7:55 It is of utmost importance to treat the entire animal and not just the eye. Appropriate treatment of the underlying disease is imperative for long-term success in treating the eye disease and for the animal's well-being.

7:56 Some relief from the pain and photophobia can be attained by keeping the patient out of bright areas and by the administration of prostaglandin inhibitors (Par 7:54). Moist, hot compresses diminish the pain and inflammation (Par. 3:82). Hospitalization is to be recommended, at least for that period necessary to complete the diagnostic workup and bring the acute stage under control.

7:57 *Treatment of sequelae.* To repeat an old cliché, the best treatment is prevention. If, however, a posterior synechia results in a secondary glaucoma, an iridectomy (Par. 7:98) will ordinarily re-establish communication between the posterior and anterior chambers, and allows reopening of the filtration angle by getting the iris back in normal position. Secondary glaucoma will probably necessitate the performance of cyclocryosurgery (Par. 9:129) or other surgical procedures for glaucoma. Lens opacities may be disregarded if vision is satisfactory in either of the two

*Flucort, Syntex, Palo Alto, California.

†Banamine, Shering Corporation, Kenilworth, New Jersey.

eyes. The damage resulting from chorioretinitis commonly results in retinal scars, but does not usually cause blindness. Enucleation may be necessary in an endophthalmitis, but other appropriate therapy should be tried first.

Choroid

7:58 There is a wide variation of normal in the appearance of the non-tapetal choroid as viewed through the retina with the ophthalmoscope. The pigmentation of the choroid is, as one would expect, more aligned with iris color than hair coat color. The choroidal color along with pigment in the retinal pigment epithelium may appear dark brown or gray (Plate 1B,C), or have such sparse pigmentation that the choroidal vessels are visible over all of the non-tapetal fundus (Subalbinotic fundus) (Plate 19H). Considerable variation also occurs in the vascular pattern. Large choroidal vessels are visible on the white scleral background in some dogs (Plate 19H), while others have a fine, velvety, red appearing fundus. The tapetum itself varies in size and, in general, is larger in large breeds, extending to below the optic disc, and smaller in small breeds. Absence of the tapetum is probably familial, but is considered a normal variation and not an anomaly. The only significant anomaly of the choroid is the choroid hypoplasia that occurs in Collie eye anomaly. It is characterized by absence of pigment and even choroidal vasculature temporal to the optic disc (Par. 11:86). Since coloboma of the optic disc and retinal detachment are the serious aspects of the disease, it is discussed in Chapter 11.

Choroiditis (Plates 18G,H; 20C,D)

7:59 When posterior uveitis occurs independently in conjunction with or as an aftermath to an involvement of the iris and ciliary body, it is not recognizable without the use of the ophthalmoscope. If the ocular media is not clear, and it usually is not in uveitis, then it remains for clearing to occur before ophthalmoscopy can be employed to assess the choroidal damage. In animals that have an anterior uveitis in one eye, examination of the fundus of the fellow eye for choroidal retinitis can be helpful in diagnosis, as some diseases produce rather characteristic chorioretinal lesions. Since choroiditis essentially always involves the retina (chorioretinitis), see further discussion beginning Par. 11:29.

7:60 *Etiology.* Any cause listed for anterior uveitis (Par. 7:35) must be considered.

7:61 *Treatment* of choroiditis in the active stage is as recommended for uveitis in general (Par. 7:50). Steroids and other therapy must be given systemically because topical and subconjunctival therapy does not provide adequate drug levels in tissues posterior to the ciliary body.

Endophthalmitis

7:62 This disease is also known as purulent uveitis and is an infection of the interior of the eye by pyogenic organisms. The infection may be of either internal or external origin.

7:63 *Internal Origin: Clinical Signs.* In the initial stages the purulent exudate fills the vitreous, often with little or no external evidences of inflammation. If bilateral, blindness may be the presenting sign. A dirty yellowish reflex is obtained from the interior of the eye. Within a short time the purulent exudate fills the whole interior, with pus in the anterior chamber, and all the symptoms of an acute uveitis most apparent. The patient exhibits considerable pain, may be generally ill, and shows conjunctival congestion, chemosis, lid swelling, and a cloudy, vascularized cornea. When all structures of the eye are involved, the condition is referred to as a *panophthalmitis* (Plate 11G).

7:64 If treatment fails or an enucleation is not performed, the purulent mass degenerates, the eyeball softens and the process ends with atrophy of the eyeball *(phthisis bulbi)* (Plate 14E).

7:65 *Treatment.* Regardless of the stage or severity it is usually impossible to save any vision. If diagnosed early, and before the whole eye is involved, an occasional eye might be preserved for cosmetic purposes. Vitreous tap (Par. 11:16) for direct examination, culture and sensitivity should be followed by systemic and subconjunctival chloramphenicol until sensitivity results are available. Then subconjunctival and systemic treatment with the appropriate antibiotic should be started, and even intravitreal injection might be considered.

7:66 *External Origin: Clinical Signs.* Endophthalmitis of external origin is the result of infection introduced through a penetrating wound, either accidental or surgical. The introduction of infection is usually into the anterior chamber, and the initial sign is an anterior uveitis with pus in the anterior chamber. Paracentesis and/or culture of the wound are helpful to select a proper antibiotic. Chloromycetin should be administered topically, QID, subconjunctivally (25 to 37 mg) and orally at 25 mg/pound, TID pending sensitivity results.

7:67 If medical treatment fails to alleviate the symptoms described, with noticeable improvement within a week, an enucleation should be performed.

7:68 Treatment of any accidental penetrating wound of the cornea or sclera as a potential endophthalmitis (Par. 6:143) is important in preventing this serious complication. Some veterinary ophthalmologists include systemic antibiotics in their regimen following intraocular surgery. We do not, and have had only 2 cases of post-surgical intraocular infection in 20 years.

Sympathetic Ophthalmia

7:69 Involvement of a normal eye with an inflammation of the uveal tract, often resulting in blindness due to the effects of an inflammation in the first eye, is referred to as sympathetic ophthalmia. It occurs most often after trauma to the anterior uveal tract and is an immune mediated disease. It occurs in man and other primates, but has not been reported in other animals.

7:70 Sympathetic ophthalmia, as it occurs in man, should not be confused with sympathetic irritation in which the unaffected eye of the dog waters more than usual and may exhibit some photophobia.

Injuries

7:71 Injuries to the iris and uveal tract may be of the perforating or nonperforating type. In perforating wounds of the globe, in which there is an iris prolapse, the prolapse should be excised (Par. 6:133). Lacerations of the cornea or sclera with prolapse of a part of the uveal tract may need to be sutured following excision (Par. 6:145).

7:72 Non-perforating injuries (concussion) may cause a transient or permanent mydriasis from paresis or paralysis of the motor nerve fibers supplying the sphincter and the ciliary muscle. Concussion can cause an *iridodialysis,* a separation of the iris from its attachment to the sclera. In these instances a black crescentic area will be noted at the site of detachment and there will be some displacement of the corresponding pupillary border. This type of injury usually produces an accompanying hyphema.

Hyphema

7:73 Hyphema is defined as blood in the anterior chamber. The most common cause is trauma. Other causes include clotting disorders, including dicoumarin (Warfarin) poisoning; disorders such as thrombocytopenia that increase bleeding time; detached retina with bleeding from retinal vessels; and intraocular tumors. Severe anterior uveitis may be accompanied by blood-tinged exudate in the anterior chamber, but that is covered elsewhere (Par. 7:50).

7:74 Frank hemorrhage into the anterior chamber following trauma usually comes from the anterior uvea and forms a clot in the anterior chamber. Slow continual hemorrhage, such as from a detached retina or tumor, and hemorrhage associated with bleeding and clotting disorders, commonly does not clot.

7:75 *Diagnosis.* The owner's concern is that the eye looks "all red." Examination reveals a clear cornea (unless there is concurrent corneal disease or elevated intraocular pressure) and blood in the eye. The amount of blood may appear uniform throughout the anterior chamber or there may be some red blood cells inferiorly, where they have settled out. (If the dog is turned on its side this unclotted blood will shift as the dog is turned.) Clotted blood often appears darker red or even black.

7:76 Determination of etiology is based on history of injury, breed predisposition to retinal detachment, previous lens extraction, evidence of bleeding elsewhere, and laboratory findings concerning bleeding and clotting disorders. Ultrasonography may be helpful in detecting an intraocular tumor. Cage rest with or without sedation may allow unclotted blood to settle enough to allow visualization of the iris, pupil and deeper structures in the eye.

7:77 *Treatment.* If due to bleeding or clotting disorders, treat these appropriately. There is no satisfactory treatment to stop the slow bleeding from retinal detachment. Surgical removal of blood or clots by paracentesis is not helpful and may predispose to further bleeding. If due to trauma, measure the intraocular pressure, and, if elevated, treat for glaucoma (Par. 9:91). If the pressure cannot be controlled medically, then and only then should surgical intervention for clot removal be considered. Treat for traumatic uveitis with topical antibiotic and steroids and, if the pressure is normal or subnormal, with topical atropine (Par. 7:50). Use of systemic enzymes to speed clot resolution is not especially helpful. However, the dog should be kept quiet and a collar or restraint around the neck should be avoided to prevent further bleeding. Intraocular prosthesis could be considered in a blind eye in which bleeding from a detached retina or other intraocular disorder persists for several months and the owner considers the continual blood-filled eye objectionable. The removed uveal tract can also be examined for neoplasia. Enucleation is indicated if an intraocular tumor is present.

7:78 *Sequelae.* The clot following traumatic hypema will usually resolve in 14 to 21 days. The first favorable sign is retraction of the clot, with clear aqueous visible around the periphery of the anterior chamber. The presence of an indirect light refex from the affected to the normal eye is a favorable sign. If damage to the ciliary body is severe, phthisis bulbi may occur.

LIPEMIC AQUEOUS

7:79 The aqueous may become cloudy due to lipid material entering the aqueous in dogs with marked lipemia. It may be unilateral with an associated uveitis in the affected eye or may be bilateral without evidence of uveitis, although there must be some alteration in the blood aqueous barrier in these cases as well. The history may be of impaired vision after a heavy intake of fat or just cloudy aqueous.

7:80 *Treatment.* Dietary control and evaluation of thyroid function with correction of hypothyroidism, when present, are indicated, as well as treatment of any underlying uveitis.

Tumors

7:81 Primary tumors of the iris and uveal tract include benign melanomas, melanocytomas, cysts, hemangiomas, epitheliomas (adenomas), adenocarcinomas, malignant melanomas and lymphosarcomas.

7:82 Although of uncommon occurrence, uveal tumors in the dog cannot be considered rare even though comparatively few intraocular tumors have been documented in the veterinary literature of the world. Individual case reports appear,[3,11,26,27] but the files of the Armed Forces Institute of Pathology allowed a study[2,23] of pigmented and nonpigmented tumors in greater depth.

7:83 Malignant melanoma of the uveal tract is by far the most common malignant intraocular tumor found in man, and occurs mostly in advanced middle age.[13,21] Those involving the iris alone comprise only approximately 5 to 8% of all uveal melanomas. Iris melanomas rarely metastasize and mortality is much less than in similar tumors of the ciliary body or choroid. Being easily seen they are ordinarily removed at an early stage. Whereas melanomas in the human eye most often arise from the choroid, in the dog, they most often arise from the iris or ciliary body.

7:84 In a necropsy study of over 2000 eyes (man) with malignant melanomas of the uveal tract, it was found that in 21% of the affected eyes the media were opaque at the time of enucleation. Thus the tumor could not be visualized clinically. In 11% of those eyes proved to contain malignant melanomas of the choroid or ciliary body, there was not even the clinical suspicion of the presence of an intraocular neoplasm. In more than 90% of such unsuspected melanomas, the eye was glaucomatous.[15]

Cases

7:85 Magrane's series includes over 30 assorted intraocular neoplasms. These cases were received mostly by referral and were certainly not to be considered common in occurrence. However, it became evident in the study that neither should they be considered rare because: 1. in most instances either no diagnosis or an erroneous diagnosis had been made, 2. similar cases are known to have been euthanized because of blindness or discomfort without a diagnosis being established, and 3. of the incidence of intraocular new growths reported in man. There was no particular breed incidence and, although the usual age represented was from 8 to 12 years, one individual was but 2 years of age.

1. Benign Non-pigmented

7:86 One case of iris hemangioma (cavernous)[16] and four of epithelioma of the ciliary body were treated surgically with preservation of the globe and vision.

7:87 The hemangioma involved the entire upper half of the iris and filled the upper anterior chamber (Plate 12C). Because the hemangioma is progressive in nature, vision was about to be lost because of filling of the pupillary space.

7:88 The epitheliomas (Plate 12H) were visible on pupil dilatation. They occupied the posterior chamber area and in each instance were crowding against the lens and were pushing the iris forward.

7:89 Hemangiomas of the iris must be considered rare in occurrence. Ferry[9] is of the opinion that "the only convincing case of iridic hemangioma occurred in an animal."[16] Epitheliomas, which arise from the nonpigmented epithelium of the ciliary processes, are more common, but are usually found accidentally in the microscopic examination of eyes removed for other causes in the human. Among 10,000 pathologic specimens the tumor was found 48 times in man.[27] The author felt that epithelioma occurs frequently, is always benign, and probably represents a secretory adenoma of the ciliary epithelium.

7:90 Verwer[26] points out that tumors of the ciliary epithelium can be diagnosed clinically because they are circumscribed and have a characteristic pink color. In any event, there is a similarity in the gross clinical findings between some benign and malignant intraocular growths. This, then, necessitates exploratory surgical intervention.

2. Malignant Pigmented

7:91 Of this group the majority were confirmed malignant melanomas. In each instance only one eye was involved and the growth observable in the iris was usually an extension from the remainder of the uveal tract (Plate 12E,F). A secondary glaucoma resulting from drainage angle occlusion by the tumor was either present at the time of the initial examination or followed with continued progression of the growth. It became necessary to eventually enucleate the eyes with malignant tumors. In one instance, however, it appeared on gross clinical examination that only the iris was involved. An iridectomy, including the lesion, was performed with no extension or recurrence discernible eighteen months following surgery.

7:92 A complete follow-up until death was not possible in each instance, but the malignant nature of the primary intraocular growth was demonstrated in the case of a male, 8-year-old cocker spaniel. Two-thirds of the iris was involved and the growth extended anteriorly to the cornea (Plate 12F). A secondary glaucoma was present. The fundus was normal. The eye was enucleated and histologically the growth was found to involve the iris and ciliary body and was classified as a highly malignant melanoma of the epithelioid type. Eight months later euthanasia was performed because of a progressive respiratory involvement and rapid tumorous enlargement of the upper gum. Generalized metastasis to the nasal sinuses, turbinates, lungs, stomach and adrenal gland was noted.

7:93 In each of the eyes examined the cornea was clear and recognition of the new growth was not difficult. Aids to recognition included one or more of the following:

1. an irregular pupil or loss of pupillary space;
2. filling in of a part of the anterior chamber and drainage angle;
3. increased pigmentation of the part;
4. iris thickened and/or thrown into irregular undulating folds;
5. episcleral congestion and increase in pressure;
6. scleral ectasia opposite the ciliary lesion.

7:94 Each case of intraocular new growth must be evaluated individually. In the very old dog it may be best to reserve enucleation for those cases in which a secondary glaucoma and discomfort to the animal make it necessary. Melanomas of the uveal tract are known to metastasize slowly in most instances. Thus, early enucleation would only be imperative in the young to middle aged dogs. If only the iris appears to be involved, an iridectomy may well save vision and a globe. If, on the other hand, at the time of surgical procedure or sometime following, it is learned that there is further invasion of the uveal tract, there still remains the alternative of enucleation.

7:95 New techniques for removal of iris tumors include iridocyclectomy and corneosclero-iridocyclectomy. In the latter procedure a corneoscleral button, together with the iris and ciliary body tumor, is removed. A donor graft of cornea and sclera replaces the host structure.

Iris Atrophy

7:96 *Essential iris atrophy.* A progressive atrophy of the iris, characterized initially by thinning and finally by holes through the iris (Plate 11C) is not an uncommon incidental finding in middle age and older dogs. The cause is unknown. An irregular pupillary border and loss of round-shape of the pupil during constriction are the other features. Secondary glaucoma can be, but rarely is, a complication of iris atrophy. It is caused by the relaxed base of the iris coming forward, causing angle closure or by blocking of this angle with iris debris. A differential diagnosis between essential iris atrophy with a secondary glaucoma and an iris atrophy secondary to glaucoma (Par. 9:40) may be difficult in long-standing cases.

SURGERY OF THE IRIS

7:97 Surgical excision of iris prolapse is the most commonly performed procedure. This has been described (Par. 6:133).

7:98 *Iridectomy*, excision of a portion of the iris, is often performed in both cataract and glaucoma surgery. Because of the nature of the iris in the dog, a profuse hemorrhage usually follows the cutting or removal of a portion of the iris (Par. 7:4). For this reason the electroscalpel is routinely used (Par. 3:87) to perform an iridectomy.

7:99 An iridectomy will be pupillary or peripheral depending upon the type condition being operated on. For example, a complete pupillary iridectomy, with removal of a seg-

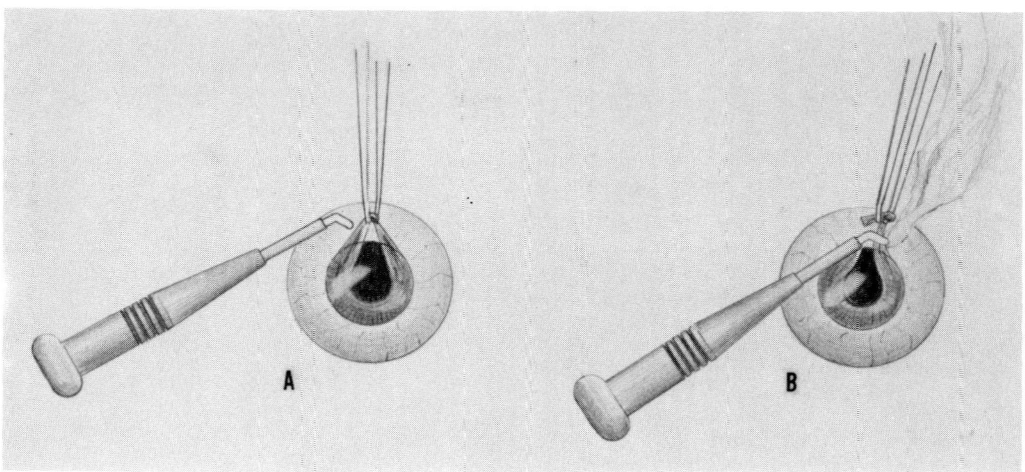

Fig. 7–5. Iridectomy with electroscalpel. *A.* First cut from base to pupillary border. *B.* Completing excision of iris wedge.

ment from the pupillary border to the base of the iris, would be the surgical procedure of choice in an iris-lens adhesion (iris bombé) (Plate 15H). A peripheral iridectomy (Plate 15G) may be performed in an acute congestive glaucoma (Par. 9:105). This type of iridectomy is more appropriately referred to as a basal iridectomy since it involves the iris base. A pupillary iridectomy is occasionally used to afford more working space in cataract extractions (Par. 10:104).

7:100 In nearly every instance a limbal based conjunctival flap is prepared prior to the section into the anterior chamber and performance of a complete iridectomy. One or more preplaced sutures (Par. 9:140) are usually used. Following the section into the anterior chamber, the iris is withdrawn with a dull iris hook, eye tissue forceps, or iris forceps. With the assistant holding the conjunctival flap out of the way, the electroscalpel is used to complete the iridectomy (Fig. 7–5).

7:101 If a peripheral iridectomy is to be performed, a small curved iris forceps or Calibri forceps is barely introduced into the anterior chamber, the surface of the iris is grasped just beyond its base and pulled just far enough into the wound so that the bottom of the forceps escapes the wound margin. The electroscalpel can then be used to excise a portion of the base, although extra caution must be exercised to avoid burning the surrounding structures. If either the electroscalpel or small curved iris scissors are used for the cutting, the excision should be as close as possible to the iris forceps so as to include in the cut only that part of the iris close to its base, avoiding the cutting of the iris sphincter and the major arterial arcade.

7:102 As with any and all specialized intraocular procedures mentioned in this book, the reader is urged to pursue the technique further in one or more of the splendid, well-illustrated ophthalmic surgery texts and to enlist the aid of an ophthalmic surgeon in his initial attempts.

REFERENCES

1. Appel, M., et al.: Pathogenicity of Low-Virulence Strains of Two Canine Adenovirus Types, Am. J. Vet. Res., *34*:543, 1973.
2. Barron, C.N. and Saunders, L.Z.: Primary Nonpigmented Intraocular Tumors, Cancer Research, *19*:1171–1174, 1959.
3. Bellhorn, R.W.: Ciliary Body Adenocarcinoma in the Dog, J.A.V.M.A., 9:1124–1128, 1971.
4. Borley, W.E. and Miller, W.W.: Iridocyclectomy, A.J.O., *60*:829, 1965.
5. Carmichael, L.E.: The Pathogenesis of Ocular Lesions of Infectious Canine Hepatitis, Path. Vet., *1*:73–95, 1964.

6. Cole, D.F., and Unger, W.G.: Prostaglandins as Mediators for the Response of the Eye to Trauma, Exp. Eye Res., *17*:357, 1973.
7. Curtis, R., and Barnett, K.C.: The Ocular Lesions of Infectious Canine Hepatitis, J.S.A.P., *14*:737–745, 1973.
8. Eakins, K.R., and Whitlock, R.H.: Prostaglandin-like Activity in Ocular Inflammation, Br. Med. J., *3*:452, 1972.
9. Ferry, A.P.: *Hemangiomas of the Iris and Ciliary Body, International Ophthalmology Clinics,* Boston, Little, Brown and Co., 1972.
10. Fischer, C.A.: Lens-induced Uveitis in Dogs, J.A.A.H.A., *8*:39–49, 1972.
11. Gelatt, K.N., et al.: Excision of an Adenocarcinoma of the Iris and Ciliary Body in a Dog., J.A.A.H.A., *6*:59–70, 1970.
12. Haessler, F.H.: *Eye Signs in General Disease,* Springfield, Charles C Thomas, 1960.
13. Hogan, M.J. and Zimmerman, L.E.: *Ophthalmic Pathology,* 2nd Ed., Philadelphia, W.B. Saunders Co., 1962.
14. Jampol, B., Neufeld, A.H., and Lears, M.L.: Pathways for the Response of the Eye to Injury, Invest. Ophthalmol. Visual Sci., *14*:183, 1975.
15. Makley, T.A. and Teed, R.W.: Unsuspected Intraocular Malignant Melanomas, Arch. Ophth., *60*:475–478, 1958.
16. Magrane, W.G.: Cavernous Hemangioma of the Iris, No. Am. Vet., *35*:516, 1954.
17. Magrane, W.G.: Tumors of the Eye and Orbit in the Dog, J.S.A.P., *6*:165–169, 1965.
18. McGrath, J.T.: The Neurologic Examination of the Dog with Some Clinico-Pathologic Observations, University of Pennsylvania Vet. Ext. Quart., *54*:5–47, 1953.
19. Prince, J.H., Diesem, C.D., Eglitis, I. and Ruskell, G.L.: *Anatomy and Histology of the Eye and Orbit in Domestic Animals,* Springfield, Charles C Thomas, 1960.
20. Purtscher, C.: The Large Arteries of the Canine Iris, Berl. U. Munch. Tierärzt. W. Schr., *74*:(22) 436–438, 1961.
21. Reese, A.B.: *Tumors of the Eye and Adnexa,* A.F.I.P., Washington, D.C., 1956.
22. Roberts, S.R., and Bistner, B.S.: Persistent Pupillary Membrane in Basenji Dogs, J.A.V.M.A., *153*:533, 1968.
23. Saunders, L.Z. and Barron, C.N.: Primary Pigmented Intraocular Tumors in Animals, Cancer Research, *18*:234–245, 1958.
24. Schlaegel, T.F., Jr.: *Current Aspects of Uveitis.* Boston, Little, Brown & Co., 1977.
25. Shively, J.N. and Phemister, R.D.: Fine Structure of the Iris of Dogs Manifesting Heterochromia Iridis, A.J.O., *66*:1152, 1968.
26. Verwer, M.A.J. and Ten Thije, P.A.: Tumors of the Epithelium of the Ciliary Body in the Dog, J.S.A.P., *8*:627, 1967.
27. Wallnoefer, A.: Benign Adenoma of the Ciliary Body, Klin. Mbl. Augenh., *150*:851, 1967.

8

DISEASES AND SURGERY OF THE ORBIT

Anatomy

8:1 Prince[23] describes the canine orbit in somewhat the following manner. The shape of the head has some influence on the proportions and shape of the orbit, and the bones that constitute it. In the brachycephalic group for instance, the lacrimal bone does not reach the orbital margin, but leaves an edge of the maxilla in the position it would otherwise occupy.

8:2 Ordinarily six bones form the dog's orbit: the frontal, lacrimal, sphenoid, palatine, zygomatic and maxillary (Fig. 8–1). But the last bone only encroaches into the orbital region to a small extent in the extreme anteroventral region, and even then it is well external to the periorbita and true orbit.

8:3 On the frontal bone, there is a rudimentary process called the zygomatic process, and on the zygomatic bone below it, there is another prominence called the frontal process. These two are joined by a bridge of fibrous tissue containing a few bands of smooth muscle, called the *orbital ligament*. This ligament alone completes the lateral closure of the orbit, which otherwise merges into the temporal fossa.

8:4 The size of the dog or of the dog's head has little relationship to the size of its orbit, an important detail to know when planning surgery of the extraocular muscles or an enucleation. A large headed dog may have a larger eye than a smaller breed, but the orbit may not necessarily increase in diameter to an equal extent.

8:5 The contents of the orbit consist of the eyeball and optic nerve, the extraocular muscles, the lacrimal gland, blood vessels and nerves; the spaces between these are filled with fat and fasciae. The contents are wholly enclosed within a conical fibrous *periorbital* membrane.

8:6 The various orbital foramina through which the orbital nerves and blood vessels pass differ considerably in size and shape. The *optic foramen* is the pathway for the second or optic nerve and the internal ophthalmic artery.

8:7 The *orbital fissure*, separated from the optic foramen by a bridge of bone about 1 mm wide, is the largest of three adjacent foramina. It carries the third, fourth, and sixth nerves, the ophthalmic division of the fifth nerve, and the orbital vein.

8:8 Because the dog does not possess a complete bony orbit, there are several nerve trunks, which although they do not serve the orbit in any way, are only separated from its contents by the thin periorbita. This close apposition means they are in a surgically vulnerable position. The sphenopalatine nerve, the sphenopalatine ganglion, infraorbital nerve, sphenopalatine artery, infraorbital artery, deep facial nerve, and zygomatic gland (Par. 8:9) are those structures which have to be carefully considered in this respect.

8:9 In addition to the lacrimal and nictitans glands which are common to all of the animals, the dog has a *zygomatic gland* situated in the orbital region. In most animals the dor-

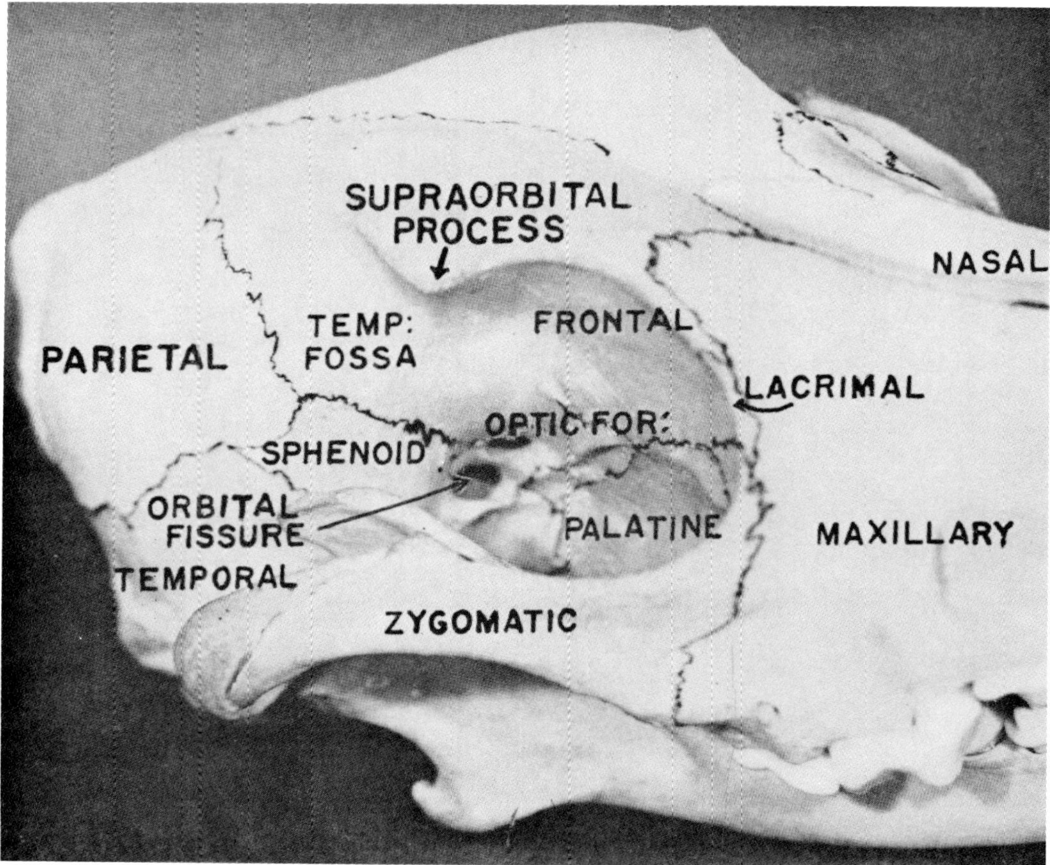

Fig. 8–1. The orbital bones. (Prince, et al. *Anatomy and Histology of the Eye and Orbit in Domestic Animals*, courtesy of Charles C Thomas.)

sal and ventral buccal glands extend along the cheek. In the dog the dorsal buccal gland lies inferior and lateral to the orbit, against the internal surface of the anterior portion of the zygomatic arch. For this reason it is referred to as the zygomatic gland although its salivary secretions pass through the ducts to empty into the mouth near the last upper molar.

8:10 The *lacrimal gland* lies within the periorbita (Fig. 1–10), is well demarcated, and is shaped like the tip of a spatula. Its long axis is directly against the orbital ligament and almost symmetrically situated anteriorly and posteriorly from it. The dorsal end is just below the tip of the zygomatic process of the frontal bone and further down it has a tendinous anchorage to the frontal process of the zygomatic bone. It has an appearance very similar to muscle. From fifteen to twenty small ducts open from it into the conjunctival sac at the superior fornix where they are not easily seen. The lacrimal gland usually has a maximum width of 12.5 mm, a depth (dorsoventral) of 15 mm, and is fairly flat.

Diseases

8:11 Affections of the orbit and globe-orbit relationship include: (1) congenital anomalies, (2) displacement of the eyeball (*i.e.* proptosis, exophthalmos, enophthalmos), (3) cellulitis and periostitis, (4) tumors, and (5) injuries.

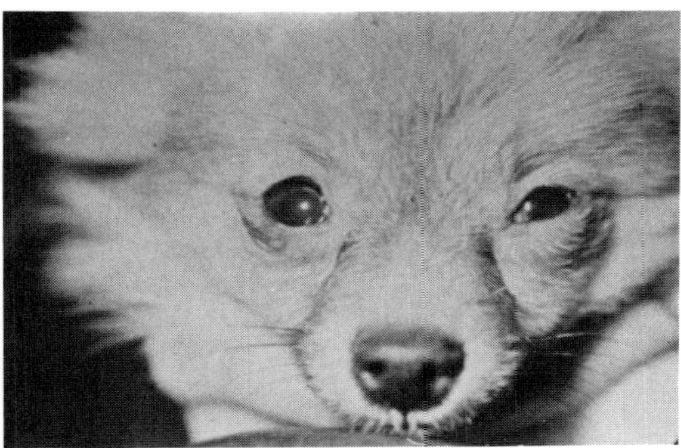

Fig. 8–2. Congenital microphthalmos (left eye).

8:12 *Congenital anomalies* of the eyeball include: (1) anophthalmos, (2) microphthalmos, and (3) congenital glaucoma. *Anophthalmos* (Plate 14C) is rare. The globe is replaced by a small solid or cystic mass. In *microphthalmos* (Fig. 8–2) (Plate 14D) the eyeball is diminished in size in all diameters. This condition cannot be considered rare, may occur in any breed, but is seen more frequently in the Pekingese, poodle, miniature schnauzer, collie, Australian shepherd, and Chihuahua breeds. On occasion there is a concurrent congenital keratitis sicca (Par. 6:67). Two conditions frequently accompany microphthalmia in collies. One is unilateral or bilateral strabismus, almost always convergent, and the other is a horizontal nystagmus of fine amplitude and great frequency.[26] Microphthalmia and multiple colobomas were detected in 45 Australian shepherd dogs.[7] In addition, many of these eyes had heterochromia irides, cataracts and retinal detachments. *Congenital glaucoma* (Par. 9:88) is uncommon. It results in an enlarged eyeball (buphthalmos, hydrophthalmos) and is due to an interference with the filtration from the eye as a consequence of a congenital defect in the angle of the anterior chamber.

8:13 *Strabismus* (squint) is a deviation of one or both globes from the normal visual axis (Plate 13A). It may be either congenital or acquired. The congenital form is most often seen in the Pekingese, pug, Boston terrier, and Chihuahua breeds. There does not appear to be any visual impairment. Acquired strabismus may result from orbital injury, luxation of the globe, cellulitis, sinusitis, or retrobulbar neoplasia.

8:14 *Treatment* of strabismus depends upon the cause. In the congenital form, involving both eyes, the owner seldom requests correction. If, however, one eye is straight and the other deviated, the appearance may be improved by repositioning the extraocular muscles. In my hands this procedure has resulted in permanent straightening in some instances but in a return to the strabismus in others. Undoubtedly the poorly developed and comparatively weak extraocular muscle structure of the dog is chiefly responsible for failures. Strabismus resulting from trauma to the extraocular muscles often corrects itself in time. On the other hand, serious muscle(s) rupture, most often of the medial rectus muscle, may leave a globe permanently deviated. An attempt should be made to effect correction as soon as possible (Par. 8:81).

8:15 *Displacement of the eyeball.* The most important signs of diseases of the orbit are *exophthalmos* (proptosis or protrusion of the eyeball from the orbit) and *enophthalmos* (recession of the eyeball into the orbit). As compared to the human there are, of course, many variations of the normal in the dog. Some eyes are naturally recessed, *e.g.* the collie breed, while others naturally protrude, *e.g.* Pekingese, pugs, Boston terriers. It is, therefore, important to compare one eye with the other in the same animal, observing the eyes from every aspect (Par. 2:16).

Exophthalmos

8:16 Exophthalmos is a common sign in affections of the orbit. The globe often appears to be larger or glaucomatous but it is the widening of the palpebral fissure that produces this illusion. There is not an increase in intraocular pressure. Exophthalmos is usually unilateral, except in orbital edema in which it is bilateral. Differentiating between exophthalmos and buphthalmos (enlargement of the globe) is important when an eye or eyes appear enlarged.

8:17 There are a number of conditions of the orbit and periorbital structures in which varying degrees of exophthalmos are exhibited. It is quite possible to confuse these and arrive at a hasty and incorrect diagnosis. Since the treatment for each differs greatly and the dog's life may well depend upon the correct diagnosis and proper treatment, it becomes imperative that exophthalmos not be considered lightly. A differential diagnosis is often difficult to make. An accurate history is important. Palpation of the orbital and oral cavities may be helpful. Comparing the differences in which the affected eye and fellow eye can be retropulsed (pushed into the orbit) helps delineate the size of space-occupying lesions in the orbit. Roentgenographic studies are often needed to disclose osteolysis, changes in soft tissue densities, or the presence of foreign bodies. Ultrasonography, especially B-scan, may be helpful in identifying soft tissue orbital masses. Orbital angiography has been used in diagnosis and localization of orbital neoplasms, localized inflammations and vascular anomalies.[6]

8:18 1. *Lid Abscesses* (Fig. 4–30A). Infection of the lid (Par. 4:89) causes but a moderate degree of exophthalmos but the swelling is fluctuating and painful. This condition must be distinguished from a true orbital cellulitis (retrobulbar abscess). Treatment of lid abscesses consists of surgical drainage, curettage, and the instillation of an antibiotic (Par. 4:89).

8:19 2. *Orbital Cellulitis* (retrobulbar abscess) (Plate 13C). Exophthalmos is a prominent symptom when an abscess develops in the retrobulbar area. In addition, there is swelling of the lids, inflammation and protrusion of the membrane nictitans, chemosis, impairment of mobility of the eyeball, subjective pain when pressure is applied, and often the dog will exhibit extreme pain when an attempt is made to open its mouth. A conjunctival discharge ranging from simple epiphora to a blood-stained mucopurulent exudate can be expected. General depression, a temperature rise and anorexia accompany the severe forms.

8:20 The cause of orbital cellulitis is often obscure but a number of possibilities must be considered. Awns have a way of working up through the mouth into the retrobulbar area. Extension of disease of the nasal accessory sinuses may be a factor. Infection of the maxillary sinus from dental disease is a probable cause. The mites of the genus *Pneumonyssus* found in the nasal and paranasal sinuses were believed to have precipitated a chronic orbital cellulitis with associated exophthalmia and periorbital edema in one instance.[24] Involvement of the zygomatic gland of the dog (Par. 8:9) cannot be discounted.

8:21 *Treatment* of retrobulbar abscesses consists of surgical drainage behind the last upper molar on the affected side, local instillation and systemic administration of penicillin.

Technique

(1) Administer general anesthesia and insert mouth speculum.
(2) Palpate soft area posterior to the last upper molar. There is often a red, raised area evident.
(3) Incise with No. 11 Bard Parker blade.
(4) Insert smooth probe to retrobulbar area

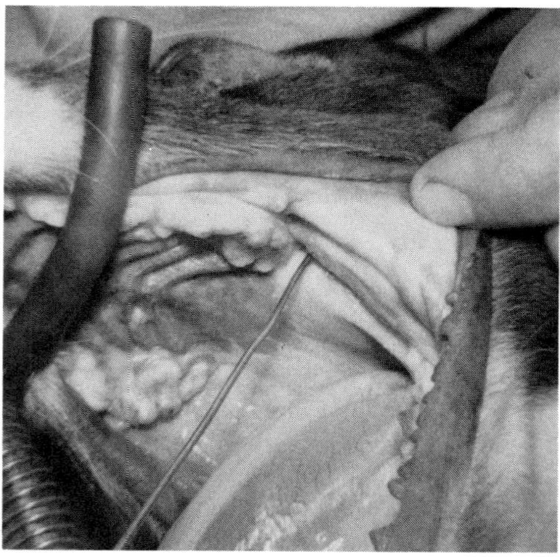

Fig. 8–3. Direction of probe to left retrobulbar area.

(Fig. 8–3). Pus may follow its withdrawal. Enlarge opening by spreading tips of long hemostatic forceps.

(5) Collect material for cytologic examination and culture.

(6) Instill 500,000 units of penicillin G (crystalline-potassium) into incision site and toward retrobulbar area with 2-inch, 22-gauge needle.

(7) Intramuscular injection of long acting penicillin.

8:22 Sometimes the abscess has not organized and little or no pus will follow the incision and probing. In either event there is noticeable improvement within 24 hours and complete recovery within several days to a week. The exophthalmos, membrane nictitans protrusion, and lid and conjunctival swellings subside quickly. An antibiotic ointment without steroids should be applied B.I.D. to protect the cornea. Hot packs to the orbit, twice a day, are helpful to speed resolution. It may be necessary to administer systemic penicillin more than once or to even re-establish drainage of the surgical site in the severely involved cases.

8:23 3. *Eosinophilic Myositis* (Plate 13D). This is a less common, but strikingly similar disease to orbital cellulitis. Whereas the symptoms are quite alike, this disease causes death in many instances. The blood picture may reveal a substantial increase in the eosinophil count and the disease presents a characteristic clinical picture. There is symmetrical swelling of the masseter, temporalis, and pterygoid muscles. As in orbital cellulitis, there is a variable degree of exophthalmos, edema of the lids, hypertrophy and protrusion of the membrane nictitans, and the mouth may be held open slightly. According to Winter and Stephenson,[31] the enlarged pterygoid and temporalis muscles press on the retrobulbar tissue and cause the exophthalmos.

8:24 From our observations and those of others, there are clearly differences in the manifestations of eosinophilic myositis. Great importance has been placed by some on eosinophil levels, with an increase of between 12 and 20% thought to be significant. Yet, Harding and Owen[9] examined the blood of 50 German shepherd dogs which had never suffered from eosinophilic myositis and found 11 with eosinophil levels between 10 and 28%. They believe a blood examination might prove deceptive. Their cases include six German shepherds and one Bedlington terrier. During attacks it was possible to open the jaws to their full extent, although it appeared to cause pain.

8:25 We have encountered the disease primarily in the German shepherd and weimaraner breeds. Aside from the increase in eosinophil count, present in some cases, we have noted that in the acute, severe cases it became *impossible* to open the jaws to their fullest extent, even when the animal was placed under deep general anesthesia. This, of course, would not be true in a case of orbital cellulitis. Moderate leukocytosis (primarily a neutrophilia and elevation of serum muscle enzymes) may be present. Finding muscle degeneration and neutrophil and eosinophil infiltration in a biopsy of the temporalis or other affected muscles is diagnostic.

8:26 Attacks of eosinophilic myositis last from 10 to 21 days. Spontaneous recovery may occur or the animal may well succumb without proper treatment. One or both eyes may be involved, regardless of whether the attack is mild or severe.

8:27 *Treatment.* Thus far, no factors which might have initiated attacks of eosinophilic myositis have been discovered. It would appear unlikely that an infectious agent is directly responsible, but that the disease falls into the category of immune-mediated. The systemic use of the steroids has proved to be specific. An initial administration of an intravenous steroid is suggested. This is followed by the oral preparation in gradually diminishing dosage until all symptoms have disappeared. In recurrent cases, continued low doses of steroid may be required. In recovered cases, one can expect wasting of the temporalis and masseter muscles. Atrophy can, in turn, create an enophthalmos (Plate 13H) (Par. 4:55).

8:28 4. *Retrobulbar Tumors.* Neoplasms of the orbit in man, although not considered rare, are still not so common that single institutions can collect a large series. The same can be said for cases occurring in the dog. Smythe[29] mentions osteosarcoma of the orbit causing exophthalmos and eventual blindness. Williams et al.[30] reported that a retrobulbar glioma of the optic nerve developed along the course of the left optic nerve to the optic nerve to the optic chiasm and then along the course of the right optic nerve. Micheletto[21] has encountered myxoma and sarcoma in the orbit. A retrobulbar and chiasmal meningioma produced exophthalmia, protrusion of the optic disc into the vitreous, and blindness in a middle aged poodle.[1] A meningioma originated from the meninges of the suprasellar area in a sixteen-month old German shorthair pointer, extended from the cranium along the optic nerves into the orbit, and resulted in blindness and retinal degeneration.[5] Exophthalmos and blindness were associated with a benign meningotheliomatous meningioma originating from the meninges of the optic nerve just behind the eye.[15] An asymptomatic nasal adenocarcinoma with direct extension into both the orbit and the eye produced a strabismus and exophthalmos.[8]

8:29 In a previously reported series[18] each of the retrobulbar tumor cases exhibited one or all of the following, depending on the stage of development:

1. exophthalmos, globe deviation, diminished movement;
2. swellings around the globe;
3. prominent, hypertrophied membrane nictitans;
4. pupil dilated and/or eccentric;
5. exposure keratitis;
6. blindness.

8:30 Age range was from 4 to 11 and six breeds were represented. Tumors included neurogenic sarcoma, chondrosarcoma, squamous cell carcinoma, meningioma, adenocarcinoma of salivary gland origin, and a rhabdomyosarcoma. The seventh did not come to necropsy. All were unilateral except one (squamous cell carcinoma) (Fig. 8–4). A boxer with the rhabdomyosarcoma (Plate 13G) presented a very prominent papilledema (Par. 11:105) along with the early exophthalmos. This type tumor is considered rare in man.

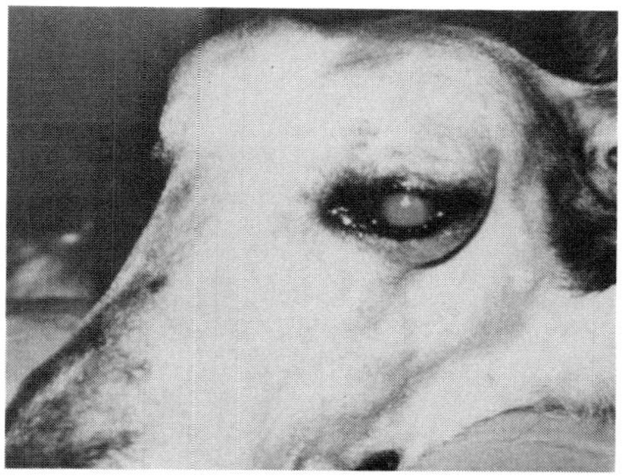

Fig. 8–4. Bilateral, retrobulbar squamous cell carcinoma. Note swellings above and around the eyes.

8:31 A later series included cases of malignant melanoma, neurogenic sarcoma, embryonal rhabdomyosarcoma and several lymphosarcomas involving the retrobulbar area. The malignant melanoma (Plate 13E) occurred in a young mixed breed dog that was presented early, underwent an immediate exenteration and still died 1 month later of generalized metastasis.

8:32 Most of the cases had a prior diagnosis of glaucoma when first seen, yet the intraocular tension was normal or below in each instance. Exophthalmos was confused with buphthalmos. A diagnosis of retrobulbar tumor is relatively easy to arrive at and is based on the history and *gradual* onset of the exophthalmos.

8:33 In recent years, orbital tumors removed at the University of Illinois have included undifferentiated adenocarcinoma; lymphoma; fibrosarcoma; undifferentiated sarcoma; adenocarcinomas, one arising from the lacrimal gland and one from the gland of the third eyelid; and periosteal osteosarcoma of the ramus of the mandible, with a concurrent orbital cyst filled with mucinous material.

8:34 *Treatment.* Whereas surgery for removal of a postorbital tumor with preservation of the globe is possible, most often exenteration of the orbit (Par. 8:52) will be necessary to insure patient comfort or prevent metastasis when a primary involvement is suspected. Exploratory surgery can certainly be planned and if the situation appears hopeless the surgeon can proceed to the exenteration. The majority of those tumors reported in the human and veterinary literature are of the malignant type and offer a poor prognosis.

8:35 The occasional exception is dramatized by the case of the embryonal rhabdomyosarcoma in a 1-year-old English cocker (Plate 13F) in which the globe and vision were preserved. In this case a circular skin incision was made anterior to the orbital ligament. The ligament was cut and the inferior retrobulbar area was exposed. The tumor tissue was removed by excision and curettage. Within 2 weeks following surgery the periorbital swelling was completely gone and the globe had resumed its normal position in the orbit. No regrowth of the tumor was evident 18 months postoperatively. Aside from a slight enophthalmos, there was no alteration in appearance and the eye was completely functional.

8:36 Non-neoplastic lesions of the orbit, *e.g.* cysts, may also manifest an exophthalmos and are amenable to surgery.[10] Knecht[12] describes both a dorsal and lateral approach to the retrobulbar area. The incision for the dorsal approach approximates the frontal bone margin of the periorbita. In the lateral approach a curved incision is made over the dorsal rim of the zygomatic arch, the orbital ligament is incised and the arch is excised with bone rongeurs. Slatter described a radical approach that allowed good visualization of the orbit and its contents.[28] The Krönlein procedure (temporary loosening and displacement of the external orbital wall) is the usual approach to the retrobulbar region in man.

8:37 *Diseases of the Zygomatic Gland.* As mentioned (Par. 8:20) sialoadenitis with bacterial infection can be a cause of retrobulbar abscess. In addition, neoplasia and cysts of the gland will produce exophthalmos and deviation of the globe.[3] The gland and tumor tissue may be excised by either the dorsal or lateral approach[12] (Plate 14F).

8:38 Other less common causes for exophthalmos include frontal sinus tumor,[13] retrobulbar foreign bodies, and vascular abnormalities.[14,25] I as well as others[22] have noted bilateral exophthalmos caused by orbital edema in dogs with heartworms. Treatment with Lasix and Prednisolone caused resolution within 3 days in two cases so treated.

Enophthalmos (Plate 13H)

8:39 Enophthalmos is an uncommon sign in affections of the orbit. The eye appears smaller but is not necessarily. It is the narrowing of the palpebral fissure, recession of the globe and subsequent elevation of the third eyelid that effects this appearance.

8:40 *Causes.* While not as common as exophthalmos, there are a number of possible causes for enophthalmos. Following trauma or surgery of the orbit, the orbital fat (Fig. 1–10) may absorb, thus allowing the eye to sink back. A hematoma of the orbit may encapsulate, slowly absorb and then result in an enophthalmos. Whereas absorption of the postorbital fat is given as the cause of enophthalmos in man, the cause in the dog is more obscure. In addition to the fat and other orbital tissue, the globe is held in position by the tone of the retractor and rectus muscles, which pull the eye into the orbit. These muscles are counteracted by a less well-defined cone of muscle or muscles, surrounding the rectus muscles, the contraction of which tends to push the eye forward. Trauma or orbital surgery may damage the nerves or muscles, upsetting the balance of muscle tone and cause enophthalmos. The ability to retropulse the dog's eye deeply into the orbit, and the immediate dramatic enophthalmos that occurs after injury, imply that it is more than retrobulbar fat that maintains the position of the dog's eye. Cicatricial contraction following orbital injuries and cellulitis may cause a recession of the eyeball. While not common to the dog, blunt external force to the orbital contents may cause a "blowout" of the thin orbital floor (periorbital membrane Par. 8:5) by transmission of sudden pressure. This results in a recession and inferior deviation of the globe. In one case, we rebuilt the inferior supportive structure of the orbit of a dog injured by a car but the eye remained enophthalmic. Enophthalmos is also one of the signs associated with Horner's syndrome (Par. 12:24).

8:41 Enophthalmos is a distinct possibility in the dog recovered from eosinophilic myositis (Par. 8:28) due to the atrophy of the surrounding muscles and postorbital fat. An atrophy of the head muscles seen in older dogs, especially German Shepherds and Weimaraners, in the absence of clinical evidence of eosinophilic myositis, has resulted in enophthalmos and elevation of the third eyelid, requiring surgical correction (Par. 4:55) (Fig. 4:22).

8:42 Reduction in size of the eyeball due to congenital microphthalmos (Par. 8:12) (Plate 14D) or phthisis bulbi (Plate 14E) causes apparent enophthalmos.

8:43 The possible effects of enophthalmos include (1) epiphora (excess tearing) because the puncti are no longer in the proper position to drain the tears; (2) mucous accumulation in the lower conjunctival cul-de-sac; (3) some alteration in overall vision because of the position of the eyeball and the elevated third eyelid (Par. 4:55); and (4) corneal drying because the lids are not in approximation with, and thus able to distribute, the precorneal film. This does not usually occur, unless the third eyelid has been removed.

Operations and Procedures Involving the Eye and the Orbit

Enucleation

8:44 *Indications* for enucleation include (1) the presence of suppurative panophthalmitis following foreign body penetration or disease process; (2) irreplaceable and/or gangrenous luxated eyeball with nerve and vessel rupture; (3) severe irreparable injuries in which the form of the eyeball cannot be preserved; (4) pain in a blind eye which cannot be relieved by less radical means; an intraocular prosthesis (Par. 8:61) rather than enucleation is the preferred treatment for an enlarged and painful glaucomatous eye; (5) massive anterior staphyloma, if the eye is blind, troublesome, and disfiguring (for cosmetic improvement); (6) the occurrence of chronic conjunctivitis, corneal, or eyelid disease due to an acquired phthisis bulbi or congenital microphthalmia; and (7) the presence of an intraocular or retrobulbar malignant neoplasm not amenable to surgery or radiation therapy.

8:45 In the practice of veterinary medicine, many enucleations have been and are being performed unnecessarily. Enucleation is selected as the procedure of choice in several conditions which will respond beautifully to the proper medical or surgical procedure. In addition, enucleation is often the consequence of a poorly conceived and executed line of treatment. The one-eyed dog is often a long living example of some veterinarian's apathy or inability to cope with an often simple ocular problem. In most instances, prolapse of the iris as the result of injury or ulcer, badly ulcerated eyes, scarred and pigmented corneas, luxated globes, and glaucoma are *not* indications for enucleation.

8:46 *Technique.* A true enucleation is performed by removing the eyeball from Tenon's capsule and the bulbar conjunctiva, leaving the extraocular muscles and soft parts of the orbit intact. This procedure (subconjunctival ablation) is preferable to the commonly practiced near exenteration (Par. 8:52) in which conjunctiva, muscles and adjacent structures are removed. By preserving these tissues a better cosmetic result is achieved since there is far less depression following final healing. In addition, this technique offers the advantage of preparing the socket for the insertion of an implant within the conjunctiva and Tenon's capsule, with still less depression resulting, or, for the use of an implant and prosthesis or artificial eye (Par 8:70).

8:47 *Steps:*

1. The eye is proptosed (Par. 6:157), if this is possible. A canthotomy (Par. 4:12) (Fig. 4–4) will facilitate the performance of this step. An incision is made near the limbus through the conjunctiva and Tenon's capsule down to the sclera. The released structures are either *(a)* grasped in the four quadrants with small Allis forceps, or *(b)* held away from the globe by eye tissue forceps or retention sutures.
2. The conjunctiva and Tenon's capsule are undermined with tenotomy scissors, severing the extraocular muscle attachments as the undermining proceeds to the posterior part of the globe (Fig. 8–5A).
3. With the globe exposed and the conjunctiva reflected, a regular tonsil snare, or, preferably one operated from an electrosurgical unit, is used to encircle the globe and to sever the optic nerve and accompanying vessels (Fig. 8–5B).
4. The eyeball is removed and the extraocular muscles, conjunctiva and Tenon's capsule are left to help fill the resultant cavity. Suturing of the conjunctiva or Tenon's capsule is not necessary. If, however, an implant is to be used, it is placed within the confines of the conjunctiva and Tenon's capsule. These structures, then, must be sutured over the implant.
5. If no implant is used, the third eyelid and its gland are then severed and removed at its base with the electrotonsil snare, electroscalpel or scissors (Fig. 8–5C).
6. Approximately ¼ inch of the margins of the lids are removed and the wound edges apposed with the suture material of choice. Particular care should be exercised to include the medial canthus (caruncle) area (Fig. 8–5D) else a permanent opening remains. If a prosthesis is to be used (Par. 8:54), the third eyelid is left intact and the lid margins, of course, are not cut or sutured.
7. A pressure pack of gauze or wound cotton is placed so as to depress the skin and suture line well into the orbit. This is held in place by bandaging in the conventional manner (Fig. 3–6). The bandage is left intact for 2 or 3 days. After removal of the bandage no further care is required until the sutures are removed.

8:48 Ordinarily there is little hemorrhage or serum accumulation attending the procedure as described, especially when the electrosurgical tonsil snare and pressure bandaging are used. This technique eliminates the need for packing the cavity prior to suturing of the lids and/or the draining of serum accumulation in the postoperative period.

8:49 Complications of enucleation are infrequent. They include: postoperative hemorrhage; infection; and a chronic discharge due to retention of glandular material. Orbital emphysema has been reported[20] and noted by me on one occasion. The orbit filled with air, ballooning the skin. Simple air aspiration by needle is insufficient. Surgical exploration to determine and seal off the source, usually a patent nasolacrimal duct, is necessary.

Evisceration

8:50 This operation differs from enucleation in that in evisceration entire contents of the eyeball are removed, but the cornea and sclera are left intact. The indication for this procedure is when an intrascleral implant is to be used as an artificial eye (Par. 8:56), or to provide a stump to lend mobility to an externally placed prosthesis (Par. 8:70).

8:51 The operation is contraindicated in malignant tumors of either the eye or retrobulbar area, in shrunken eyeballs, or when a generalized panophthalmitis is present.

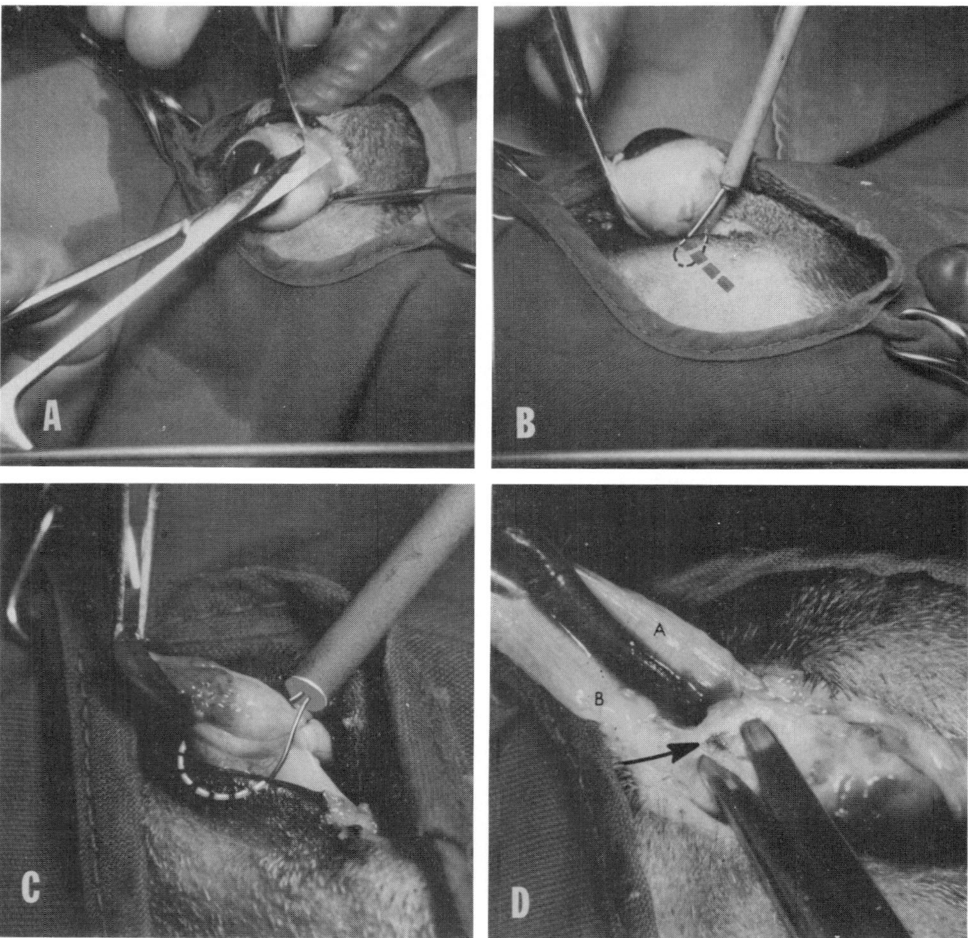

Fig. 8–5. Enucleation. *A*. Undermining the bulbar conjunctiva of the proptosed globe. *B*. Electrotonsil snare severance of globe. *C*. Removal of third eyelid and gland with electrotonsil snare. *D*. Upper *(A)* and lower *(B)* lids have been cut. Removal of the caruncle (arrow) and medial lid juncture completes the excision.

Exenteration

8:52 Exenteration of the orbit includes removal of the globe, conjunctiva, extraocular muscles, and surrounding structures within the orbit. The only indication for this radical procedure is in certain cases of malignancy, *e.g.* retrobulbar neoplasia or extension of a uveal tract tumor into the orbit itself. Loppnaw and Link[16] describe a case in which a malignant melanoma of the iris and ciliary body necessitated enucleation. Several months later the orbital cavity was found to be involved. On a subsequent necropsy, metastasis to the lungs, heart muscle, and kidneys was disclosed. A simlar case of mine has been alluded to (Par. 8:31).

8:53 Following exenteration of the orbit the closed lids and skin retract into the orbit with disfigurement, but the patient's life may well be saved by virtue of this procedure (Par. 8:34). Cosmetic improvement may be attained by burying various silicone and inert plastic preparations manufactured for that purpose.

Artificial Eyes

8:54 When confronted with the clinician's decision that a severely injured or diseased eye should be enucleated, the average pet owner almost invariably inquires as to whether an artificial eye can be used to replace the original. Eye prostheses have seldom been used in the dog despite the fact that prosthetic devices to simulate the enucleated eye were developed and used as long ago as the latter part of the nineteenth century. The operation has never become standard procedure in the dog because of economic factors, the nuisance of maintaining the devices, and a high percentage of failures.

8:55 Two types of artificial eyes may be used: (1) The permanent intrascleral implant; and (2) the external shell-shaped prosthesis in common use by human subjects following enucleation. This type is removed for cleansing purposes and reinserted.

8:56 1. *The Intrascleral Implant.* From the practical standpoint, a permanent, reasonably priced, extrusion free and maintenance free type artificial eye is to be desired. To achieve natural mobility, appear cosmetically attractive, and eliminate the need for continual care, only an intrascleral prosthetic device can be considered.

8:57 This fact has been previously acknowledged. Attempts have been made to replace the cornea and intraocular contents by several means. Simpson's[27] method involved the use of a plain black prosthesis with a tantalum mesh backing. The prosthesis was united with the sclera by sutures.

8:58 Keil[11] describes the use of a plastic intrascleral implant consisting of two parts. An iris and pupil can be painted on to the back of the anterior portion to "match" the other eye. When joined by a peg to the rim-like posterior part, the implant is held in place by a stainless steel purse string suture.

8:59 Magrane and Helper[19] constructed a prosthesis of ¾ of a silicone rubber ball covered by Dacron felt and a front piece composed of lucite, secured to the ball with silicone cement.

8:60 All of the above attempts included removal of the cornea. All failed in weeks to months, because of poor attachment[11,27] or gradual separation at the junction of the sclera and the prosthesis, probably brought on by low-grade infection.[19]

8:61 An inexpensive, easily inserted cosmetic intraocular prosthesis has recently been devised that is installed after eviscerating the globe.[2] Since it is entirely inside the globe, there is no scleral-tissue junction, and rejection has not been encountered. Dr. Richard Huff is credited with pioneering the original investigation. Installation is shown in Figure 8–6.

Procedure[2]

8:62 The horizontal diameter of the cornea of the normal eye is measured with a metric caliper or ruler and a sterile black silicone ball prosthesis* of this diameter or 1 mm larger is selected (Fig. 8–6A). After the patient has been placed in lateral recumbency and draped, a canthotomy is done. A lid speculum can be used to provide maximum exposure, or the globe may be proptosed to facilitate exposure and to render it taut for the incision. The conjunctiva and Tenon's capsule are incised with a knife and/or tenotomy scissors in an anterior to posterior direction, starting 2 to 3 mm from the limbus (Fig. 8–6B). The dorsolateral aspect of the globe is considered to be the best site for the incision. An alternate procedure is to make the incision 2 to 3 mm back of the limbus and parallel to it.

8:63 The incised conjunctiva and Tenon's capsule are spread and two stay sutures of 4–0 nylon are placed parallel to the proposed incision site (Fig. 8–6B). A stab incision is made 2 to 3 mm from the limbus with a No. 65 Beaver blade and enlarged in a posterior direction with the tenotomy scissors (Fig. 8–6C). The incision should be 1 or 2 mm longer than the previously measured corneal diameter.

8:64 Evisceration of the globe is accom-

*Jardon Plastics Research Corp., 17100 W. 12 Mile Road, Southfield, MI.

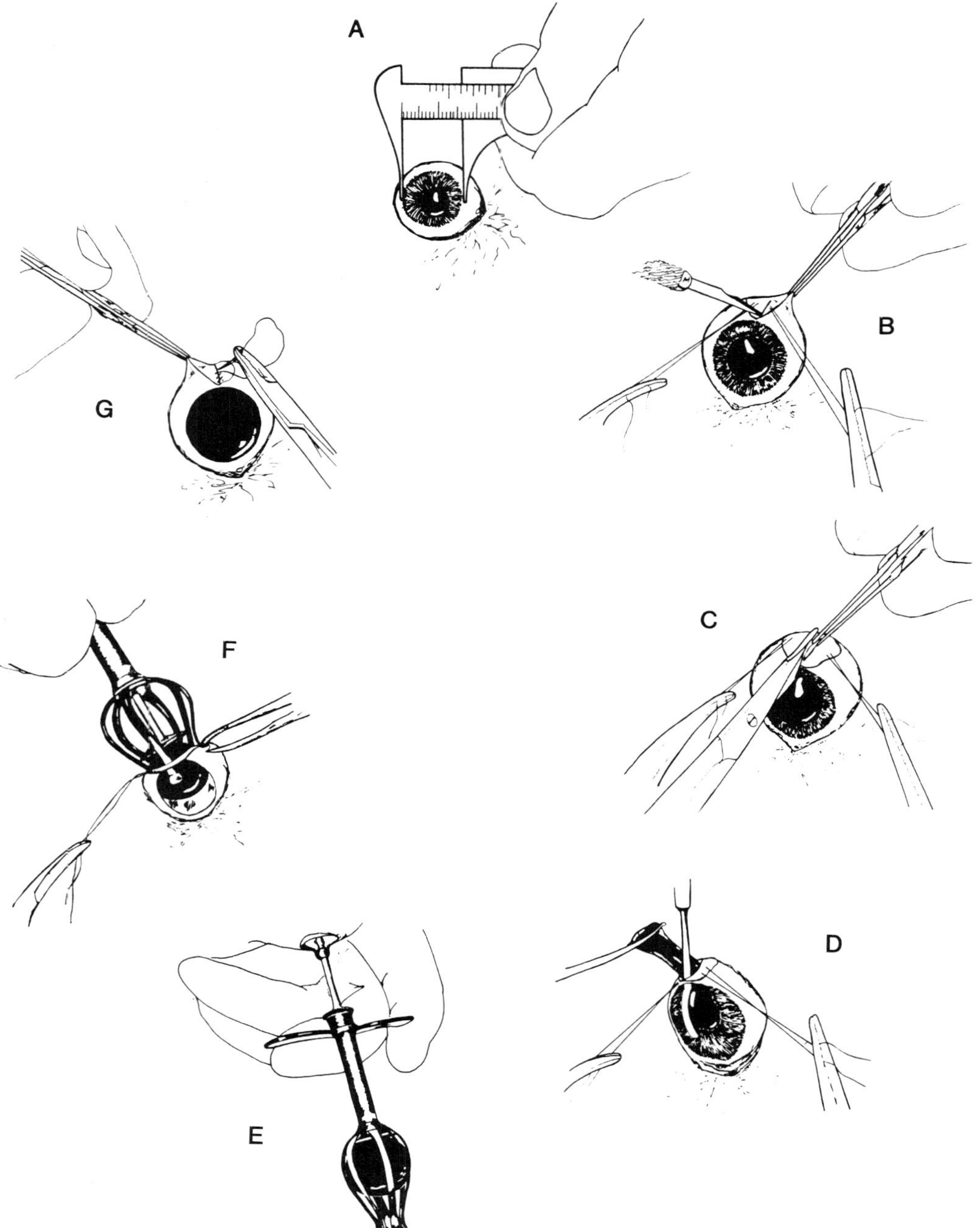

Fig. 8–6 *A,* Metric calipers measuring the corneal diameter. *B,* The conjunctiva and tenons have been incised. Stay sutures have been placed and a stab incision of the sclera is made. *C,* The scleral incision is enlarged with tenotomy scissors. *D,* The uveal tract is removed with forceps and a cyclodialysis spatula. *E,* Sphere holder and introducer. *F,* The silicone prosthesis is introduced into the globe. *G,* The scleral wound is closed with a continuous pattern after removal of the stay sutures.

plished by grasping the exposed iris and ciliary body, applying traction and sweeping them from the globe with a cyclodialysis spatula (Fig. 8–6D). Ordinarily the lens and most of the vitreous are expelled in the manipulation of the uveal tract. No attempt is made at hemostasis but occasional sponging may be needed to visualize the interior of the globe. Vitreous, blood clots and debris are now sponged or flushed from the globe. Low vacuum suction can be used to remove these materials. Any remaining uvea and retina are removed with forceps.

8:65 The prosthetic ball, equal to or a millimeter greater than the diameter of the cornea of the normal eye, is placed in a sphere holder and introducer* (Figs. 3–15X and 8–6E).

8:66 The sphere introducer is carefully placed through the incision site and the prosthesis is injected slowly into the globe (Fig. 8–6F). The stay sutures are removed and the sclera is closed with 6–0 dexon in a continuous pattern (Fig. 8–6G). The conjunctiva and Tenon's capsule are closed with a single continuous suture. To close the canthotomy, 4–0 nylon in a simple interrupted pattern is used. A temporary tarsorrhaphy (Fig. 9–15) is applied after surgery to protect the cornea, and an antibiotic ointment is applied topically.

8:67 *Aftercare.* The eye is usually bandaged (Fig. 3–6) for the first 24 hours to further protect the eye and to minimize swelling. The tarsorrhaphy suture may be left in place for 5 to 7 days if the eye was buphthalmic; otherwise it is removed prior to discharge of the dog from the hospital on the first or second day after surgery. An antibiotic or antibiotic-steroid ointment is dispensed for twice a day application for 7 to 10 days following surgery.

8:68 A buphthalmic globe will shrink down to the size of the prosthesis within several weeks to a month. The final appearance of the cornea is dependent on its appearance before surgery. It is seldom clearer than before surgery, and is often somewhat more cloudy, but quite cosmetically acceptable.

8:69 *Contraindications.* The major contraindication is a sighted eye. A prosthesis should be considered only in an *irreversibly blinded* eye. Other contraindications are active intraocular infection or intraocular tumor. The removed uveal tract should be submitted for histopathologic examination if the tumor is considered a possible cause of glaucoma, hyphema or other indication for prosthesis.

8:70 *The External Prosthesis.* The externally placed, shell-shaped prosthesis used in the human subject can be used successfully in the dog as well (Fig. 8–7). It is less desirable than the intraocular prosthesis, but could be considered in cases requiring enucleation in which the owner insists on an eye. Following enucleation (Par. 8:46) a ball of either glass, plastic or silicone intended for this purpose is inserted in the cavity and the edges of the conjunctiva and Tenon's capsule are drawn together over the implant. The membrane nictitans and lid margins are left intact.

8:71 A "conformer" is then placed underneath the lids and the membrane nictitans and the area bandaged in the conventional

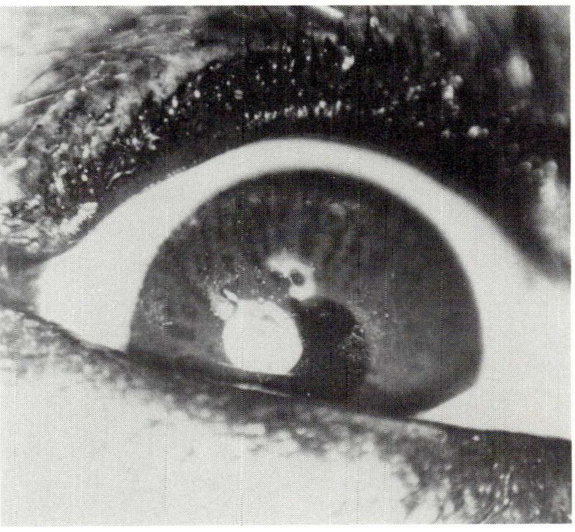

Fig. 8–7. The shell-shaped human prosthesis adapted for use in the dog.

*Carter Sphere Introducer and Holder, Storz Instrument Co., St. Louis, MO.

manner (Par. 3:90) (Fig. 3–6). Dressings are changed at 2- to 3-day intervals with removal, cleansing, and replacing of the conformer at each dressing. After approximately 3 weeks the cavity has healed sufficiently to allow fitting of the "glass eye." A regular "stock" prosthesis may be used, but to insure a good fit and matching eye a custom-made shell is preferable.

8:72 When this type of prosthesis is placed underneath the lids, with the membrane nictitans serving as an additional aid to its retention, the average dog tolerates it quite well. However, as is the case in the human, the "eye" should be removed at least once a day for the purpose of cleansing the cavity and the prosthesis. Needless to say, the average owner is reluctant to assume the expense and bother associated with this type of surgical procedure.

8:73 Success with this depends upon the observance of (1) complete asepsis in the operative procedure; (2) incising the conjunctiva and Tenon's capsule close to the limbus; (3) control of bleeding before the implant is inserted; and (4) placing the implant within Tenon's capsule as well as the conjunctiva, with the closure of these membranes over the implant made without undue tension.

Luxation of the Globe (Plate 13B)

8:74 Luxation or proptosing of the eyeball occurs most frequently in the brachycephalic breeds as a result of automobile injuries or encounters with larger dogs. Shortly after luxation the eyeball becomes inflamed and congested and the chemotic conjunctiva protrudes beyond the lid margins. Since the lids cannot close properly over the proptosed globe, corneal desiccation occurs. A subconjunctival hemorrhage may be present as the result of a tooth puncture. In severe cases a retrobulbar hemorrhage is usually present.

8:75 *Treatment.* The treatment and prognosis are largely dependent upon the degree of damage to the extraocular muscles and to the blood and nerve supply to the eye. It is usually difficult to ascertain the extent of vessel and nerve injury at the time of the accident. The first consideration should always be to replace the globe as quickly as possible. Permanent damage, requiring enucleation, will be evident within several days.

8:76 An evaluation based on pupil size is helpful. A pinpoint pupil indicates a normal response to pain and is a good sign. A dilated pupil occurs when sympathetic innervation is undisturbed and there is severe damage to the oculomotor nerve or to the ciliary ganglion. This offers a guarded to poor prognosis for vision. A direct response to light stimuli is not usually present, but a consensual response to the fellow eye is an encouraging sign. In any event, saving of the globe for cosmetic purposes is paramount. An evaluation of visual function may not be possible until several weeks following the luxation.

8:77 In simple and recent cases of luxation, replacement of the globe is easily accomplished following simple cleansing and lubrication with an antibiotic ointment. Under short-acting anesthesia, the lids are elevated with forceps or lid retractors, a pad of wet cotton is applied to the globe, and moderate pressure is applied with the fingers as the lids are pulled out over the eyeball. If the eyeball "snaps back" into the orbit with no tendency to protrude, no further treatment is needed. If the eye still appears somewhat exophthalmic, one or two temporary tarsorrhaphy sutures (Fig. 9–15) should be applied while the dog is still under anesthesia.

8:78 In the more complicated cases, and in those instances in which the globe has been luxated for several hours or a day, the following routine has been used with considerable success.

8:79 *Technique:*

(1) *Canthotomy* (Par. 4:11) (Fig. 4–4). Elongation of the palpebral fissure not only facilitates replacement of the globe, but failure to perform this initial step may make it impossible to do so.

(2) *Lid suture placement.* Three temporary

tarsorrhaphy sutures (Fig. 9–15) are placed through the skin opposite the lid margins at the medial (nasal), lateral (temporal) and center positions. These are left untied until the globe is replaced.

(3) *Replacement of the globe.* The eyeball is returned to the orbit in the manner described (Par. 8:77). If this becomes impossible because of the retrobulbar swelling, the lids and lid margins are carefully worked into position over the proptosed globe and the sutures are brought into place and tied. The canthotomy incision is closed with one or more interrupted sutures. By completely covering the eye in this manner, it remains protected until the postorbital swelling is reduced and it can assume its normal position in the orbit. A drop of atropine and an antibiotic preparation are instilled prior to the final closure.

8:80 *Aftercare.* Usually in 48 hours the swelling has reduced to the degree that either a lateral or medial suture can be removed. This enables the clinician to "take a peek" at the cornea, ascertain globe viability, and as to whether the eye is "saved" or must now be enucleated. As the swelling recedes a second peripheral suture may be removed. Finally, when it appears that the globe will be protected by the natural opening and closing of the lids, the center suture is removed.

8:81 In some instances the globe is deviated because of tearing of the extraocular muscle attachments. This deviation is usually to the temporal side and, unless it is severe, the eyeball most often straightens itself in time. When considerable muscle damage and deviation are noted at the time of the luxation, it is best to attempt correction along with replacement. This entails undermining the bulbar conjunctiva on the nasal side, finding the torn muscle ends and bringing them together. When this becomes impossible to do, an inverted mattress suture of stainless steel or monofilament nylon is placed in the deep episcleral tissue near the limbus on the nasal side, is brought through the membrane nictitans, and is tied over a button or pad in the nasal fold. This suture is allowed to remain for a week or more.

8:82 A transient paresis with incomplete closure of the lids *(lagophthalmos)* is frequently a sequel to luxation of the globe. This results in exposure and consequent injury to the cornea. To protect the cornea until healing and lid function return, a tarsorrhaphy (Par. 4:103, Fig. 4–35) (Plate 3G) is indicated. When the attachment is severed after several months a smooth cornea and functional globe can be expected.

REFERENCES

1. Barnett, K.C., et al.: Retrobulbar and Chiasmal Meningioma in a Dog, J.S.A.P., *8*:391, 1967.
2. Brightman, A.H., Magrane, W.G., Huff, R.W., et al.: Intraocular Prosthesis in the Dog, JAAHA, *13*:481–485, 1977.
3. Buyukmihci, N., Rubin, L.F. and Harvey, C.E.: Exophthalmos Secondary to Zygomatic Adenocarcinoma in a Dog, J.A.V.M.A., *167*:162–165, 1975.
4. *Canine Medicine*, 2nd ed., Santa Barbara, American Veterinary Publications, Inc., pp. 528–530, 1959.
5. Firth, C.H.: Meningioma in a Young Dog Resulting in Blindness and Retinal Degeneration, VM/SAC, *70*:307–310, 1975.
6. Gelatt, K.N.: *Veterinary Ophthalmology*, Philadelphia, Lea & Febiger, p. 246, 1981.
7. Gelatt, K.N. and McGill, L.D.: Clinical Characteristics of Microphthalmia with Colobomas of the Australian Shepherd Dog, J.A.V.M.A., *162*:393–396, 1973.
8. Gelatt, K.N., et al.: Nasal Adenocarcinoma with Orbital Extension and Ocular Metastasis in a Dog, J.A.A.H.A., *6*:132–142, 1970.
9. Harding, H.P., and Owen, L.N.: Eosinophilic Myositis in the Dog, Jour. Comp. Path. & Therap., *66*:109, 1956.
10. Harvey, C.E., et al.: Orbital Cyst with Conjunctival Fistula in a Dog, J.A.V.M.A., *153*:1432, 1968.
11. Keil, J.H., Jr.: Mobile Ocular Prosthesis, Jen-Sal Small Animal Topics, *13*:21–24, 1959.
12. Knecht, C.D.: Treatment of Diseases of the Zygomatic Salivary Gland, J.A.A.H.A., *6*:13, 1970.
13. Koch, S.A.: The Differential Diagnosis of Exophthalmos in the Dog, J.A.A.H.A., *5*:229, 1969.
14. Komar, G. and Schuster, A.: Exophthalmos Pulsans in a Dog, Berl. Münch. Tierärztl. Wschr., *80*:359, 1967.
15. Langham, R.F., et al.: Primary Retrobulbar Meningioma of the Optic Nerve of a Dog, J.A.V.M.A., *159*:175–176, 1971.
16. Loppnaw, H. and Link, E.: Berl. U. Münch. Tierärzt. Wschr., *174*(16):317–321, 1961.
17. Magrane, W.G.: Diseases of the Orbit, Vet. Med., 449–451, 1957.
18. Magrane, W.G.: Tumors of the Eye and Orbit in the Dog, J. Sm. A. Pract., *6*:165–169, 1965.

19. Magrane, W.G. and Helper, L.C.: *Evaluation of Intrascleral Prosthesis in the Dog*, Proceedings Am. Coll. Vet. Ophth., 1972.
20. Martin, C.L.: Orbital Emphysema, VM/SAC, *66*:986–987, 1971.
21. Micheletto, B.: Clinical and Histopathological Contribution to the Tumors of the Orbit of Dog and Cat, Atti della Soc. Italiana della Scienze Vet., *18*:296, 1964.
22. Noyes, Jack: Personal Communication, 1977.
23. Prince, J.H., Diesem, C.D., Eglitis, I. and Ruskell, G.L.: *Anatomy and Histology of the Eye and Orbit in Domestic Animals*, Springfield, Charles C Thomas, pp. 65–71, 1960.
24. Roberts, S.R. and Thompson, T.J.: Pneumonyssus caninum and Orbital Cellulitis in the Dog, J.A.V.M.A., *155*:731, 1969.
25. Rubin, L.F., and Patterson, D.F.: Arteriovenous Fistula of the Orbit in a Dog, Cor. Vet., *55*:471, 1965.
26. Saunders, L.Z.: Pathology of the Eye, Joest's Hanbuch der speziellen pathologischen Anatomie der Haustiere, Paul Parey, Berlin, 1968.
27. Simpson, H.D.: Reconstructive Surgery of the Canine Eye, No. Am. Vet., *37*:1060–1065, 1956.
28. Slatter, D.H.: Lateral Orbitotomy by Zygomatic Arch Resection, Proc. Am. Coll. Vet. Ophthalmol., Dallas, TX, 1977.
29. Smythe, R.H.: *Veterinary Ophthalmology*, London, Bailliere Tindall & Cox, p. 163, 1956.
30. Williams, J.O., Garlick, E.C. and Beard, D.C.: Glioma of the Optic Nerve of a Dog, J.A.V.M.A., *138*:377–378, 1961.
31. Winter, H. and Stephenson, H.C.: A Case of Eosinophilic Myositis in a Dog, Cornell Vet., *42*:531, 1952.

9 GLAUCOMA

9:1 Glaucoma is not a disease. It is a series of diseases with different etiologies but one common sign—elevation of intraocular pressure. Glaucoma should, perhaps, be referred to as *the glaucomas.* It is a leading cause of blindness in the middle aged dog. Since glaucoma is an emergency type disease, with irreversible blindness ensuing within hours to several days, it becomes extremely important that the veterinary clinician understand this condition. Accuracy in diagnosis, classification, and knowledge of the proper medical or surgical procedures to fit the classification will save or prevent loss of vision. For this reason, the importance of a disease cannot be overemphasized.

Anatomy and Physiology

9:2 Certain parts of the eye are particularly important in any consideration of the physiologic mechanisms, the pathology, and the medical and surgical treatment of the glaucomas. These structures are in the anterior segment of the globe (Fig. 7–1) and include the iris and ciliary body, the anterior and posterior chambers, the filtration angle, and the intrascleral drainage plexus (Fig. 7–2).

9:3 The iris divides the aqueous cavity into an *anterior* and *posterior* chamber. The ciliary body, via its ciliary processes, secretes the *aqueous humor* (Par. 7:8). The aqueous humor fills the anterior and posterior chambers and drains through the filtration angle into the intrascleral venous plexus (Fig. 9–1).

9:4 The filtration angle (angle of the iris) (iridocorneal angle) is a circular recess where cornea, sclera, the ciliary border of the iris and the ciliary body meet. In the angle a peculiar framework of *trabeculae* with irregular spaces (spaces of Fontana) are found. The trabeculae are also called the *pectinate ligaments* of the iris. Troncoso describes the trabeculum of the dog as being in contact with a well-developed venous plexus known as the intrascleral vascular plexus *(plexus venosus sclerae).* This plexus is formed by a thick network of large interlacing veins lodged in large canals inside the scleral wall. Its superficial branches spread over the inner scleral surface and are in contact with or run between the trabeculum fibers. They are called trabecular veins and it is through them that the aqueous filling the sinus is absorbed by the blood. These vessels function in a manner similar to the canal of Schlemm in man.

9:5 Considerable research has been conducted in aqueous drainage in the dog. The existence of the continual current of aqueous from the anterior chamber into the episcleral vessels was postulated by Leber,[19] mainly by experimental work in animals. Friedenwald and Pierce,[7] working with a modified Leber manometer, have shown by experiments that in dogs there is a constant current of liquid from the chamber into the episcleral veins. They also showed experimentally that other ocular tissues, especially the iris, take part in the elimination of the aqueous. Intraocular tension tends to lower when the iris is under vasodilatation as in acute iritis (Par. 7:44), and when the cornea is irritated.

Methods of Diagnosis

9:6 Normal intraocular pressure is that which is compatible with the continued health and function of the eye. In the dog, however, we must give more emphasis to sta-

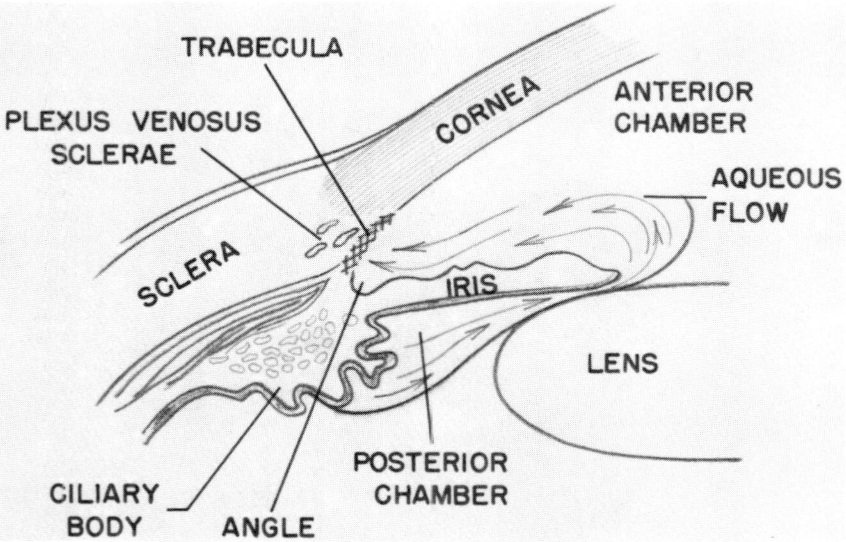

Fig. 9–1. Mode of aqueous production and flow from the posterior to the anterior chamber and then to the drainage angle.

tistical averages in our computation of normal pressures because of our inability to perform perimetry and other exact visual function tests.

9:7 A distinction has been made between the use of the terms "pressure" and "tension" in relation to the eye. The term "intraocular pressure" refers to the pressure of the intraocular fluid within the eye which can only be measured by means of a manometer. The "tension" of the eye is a measure of the state of tension of its tunics, being estimated either digitally or by means of a tonometer. In addition to intraocular pressure, tension depends upon the thickness and rigidity of the tunics, the surface area, and probably other factors.

9:8 Manometry is not practical for use in clinical ophthalmology, whereas digital palpation and tonometry are.

9:9 The term *intraocular pressure (IOP)* has, in use, become synonymous with ocular tension, and is the term used, regardless of the method of measurement.

Tonometry

9:10 Tonometry is the measurement of the impressibility of the tunics of the eye by deforming forces applied to these tunics. The impressibility depends on the resistance of the eyeball to stretching at a given intraocular pressure. Thus, tonometry gives a measure, however approximate, of the intraocular pressure.

9:11 In digital tonometry (Par. 2:29) (Fig. 2–16), the two index fingers are placed upon the dog's upper lid. By alternating pressure on the globe from one finger tip to the other, pressing more downward than backward, one can get some idea of the degree of tension by comparison with the other eye, if normal, or with a healthy eye of another dog. By way of comparison, a glaucomatous eye will feel like a hard apple, while an eye with normal tension will feel soft like a grape. Digital tonometry is especially useful in detecting very high or very low IOP, but is not adequate for detecting the minor or moderate elevations so important in the diagnosis and treatment of glaucoma.

9:12 Instrumental tonometry is by far the

more accurate means of measuring intraocular pressure and should be used routinely (Par 2:32) (Fig. 2–18).

9:13 In almost all dogs, readings can be made following instillation of topical anesthetics.

9:14 The dog should be placed on a table in a sitting position. An assistant, or the owner, restrains the animal's head in such manner that the eyes are directed upward, the lids are separated and the tonometer is allowed to rest by its own weight upon the center of the upturned cornea. In the separation of the lids, undue pressure must not be exerted on the eyeball itself, thus influencing the reading. The nictitating membrane often proves a deterrent to the accurate placement of the footplate of the tonometer and many readings will, of necessity, be taken with the footplate between the center and upper limbal area. The instrument should be lifted from the cornea and replaced twice to take 3 readings. These readings should agree within .5 on the tonometer scale. The degree of accuracy achieved in man with the use of the tonometer cannot always be attained in the dog but, with patience, a good approximation of IOP is almost always attainable. An instillation of a suitable ophthalmic antiseptic or antibiotic preparation to the tested eye is indicated, following the procedure, to forestall a possible infection from the footplate or from its abrasive action on the cornea. The tonometer itself must be cared for as a delicate instrument including cleaning following each use if it is expected to give consistent and accurate readings.

9:15 Lovekin[20] suggests that IOP be measured by rolling the dog over on its back, with its nose in the air pointing slightly to the left to take the pressure of the right eye, and then slightly to the right to take the pressure of the left eye. The third eyelid should be held gently out of the way and the tonometer placed vertically on the center of the cornea in order to achieve the most accuracy. She found the highest normal intraocular pressure to be 26 mm Hg in her series.

9:16 Applanation tonometry is a commonly used method of measuring IOP in the human. Its principle involves the measurement of the force required to flatten a standard corneal area. Applanation tonometry is more accurate in determining IOP, since it is influenced less by differences in scleral rigidity and corneal curvature than Schiotz tonometry. The MacKay Marg tonometer is probably the most accurate for the dog and cat.[11] Its use in veterinary medicine is limited primarily by the cost of the instrument.

9:17 Gonioscopy (Par. 2:10) should be confined to those veterinarians who wish to invest the time, energy, and money required for technical proficiency. It is a tool which provides information in the detection of early or preglaucomatous eyes, especially in breed predisposed dogs.[44]

9:18 Tonography attempts to assess resistance encountered by aqueous humor leaving the eye. In this procedure, an electronic indentation tonometer is placed on the eye for 4 minutes, and the change in scale values during the 4-minute period is recorded and used to determine the resistance to outflow of aqueous. We modified the technique used in man for the dog's eyes, and did demonstrate a difference in outflow between normal and glaucomatous but were not highly accurate in predicting glaucoma in a colony of Bassett Hounds.[15] Gelatt[12] devised a slightly different procedure for tonography and also demonstrated differences in outflow between normal and glaucomatous eyes.

9:19 Provocative tests have been used in man to provide information in preglaucoma patients. In breeds with a predisposition to glaucoma these tests might be warranted, although little information is available relative to their use except in research endeavors.[5,10,21,22] The water-drinking provocative test requires tonometry before and after the ingestion of large quantities of water. The dark room or mydriasis test involves this same testing before and after producing natural or artificial pupil dilatation. To date, none of the above procedures have been reported to have high predictive value.

Clinical Signs

9:20 In many instances, the diagnosis of glaucoma in the dog is relatively simple since the animal is often presented for an examination only when the clinical signs are exaggerated and visible to the owner. Important early signs of pain and of disturbance of vision go unnoticed and, undoubtedly, in many instances the dog has been subjected to transient attacks of pressure increases before a final and permanent increase manifests itself. Whereas this simplifies diagnosis, it makes adequate treatment more difficult—especially as regards the preservation of vision. Too many animals have reached the absolute (blind) stage before being examined. With proper instruction, many owners will observe the early signs, if the second eye becomes involved. Veterinarians should learn to recognize the subtle signs of early glaucoma, and should always include glaucoma in the "rule outs" for a red eye.

9:21 Wyman[45] divides the clinical signs into early, advanced, and acute congestive glaucoma:

A. Early—may be very subtle, but important to recognize for most effective management
   1. increased intraocular pressure
      a. the most important diagnostic step is tonometry
      b. cannot diagnose the disease because the eye "looks hard"
      c. Schiotz tonometry is simple to perform and should be done in all practices
      d. moderate increases—30 to 40 mm Hg
   2. epiphora
   3. mild blepharospasm
   4. conjunctival hyperemia
   5. usually no lesions demonstrable in the retina or optic nerve head
   6. intact pupillary reflex
   7. sight not clinically impaired
   8. pain—subtle to absent
B. Advanced
   1. markedly increased intraocular pressure (>40 mm Hg)
   2. fixed dilated pupil
   3. corneal opacity
      a. striae—ruptured Descemet's membrane
      b. edema (steamy cornea)
      c. disruption of stromal lamellae
      d. exposure keratopathy and associated vascularization
   4. conjunctival and episcleral vascular congestion
   5. buphthalmia
   6. insensitive cornea
   7. lens luxation or subluxation
      a. due to stretching of the lens fibers as a result of globe enlargement
      b. due to mesodermal dysgenesis, resulting in abnormal zonules
   8. blindness
   9. gonioscopic examination, if possible (often the cornea is too cloudy)
      a. goniodysgenesis
      b. narrow angle
      c. cellular debris
      d. neoplastic tissues
   10. ophthalmoscopic examination
      a. retinal atrophy—variable and multifocal
      b. cupping of the optic nerve head
      c. attenuation of retinal vessels
C. Acute congestive glaucoma
   1. most commonly observed in veterinary medicine
   2. severe pain—often causes changes in attitude
   3. all of the signs of advanced glaucoma, but accentuated

9:22 *Increase in intraocular pressure* has been discussed under tonometry (Par. 9:10).

9:23 *Pain.* Pain is produced by pressure and pull on the ciliary nerves in the eye. In obtaining case histories, some owners will volunteer the information that the dog has exhibited pain, which is often displayed by the animal rubbing the eye on the rug, against the owner's leg, or on furniture. Upon digital palpation, many dogs will wince; others appear to suffer little or no pain. Pain seems to depend somewhat upon the duration of the attack—the longer the period of increased tension, the less pain—but some dogs evidence little or no pain at any time. However, after having an increased pressure for a year or more, some dogs change completely in disposition and become extremely refractory. When the pressure is relieved, they usually again become docile—a gratifying aftermath.

9:24 *Cloudy, "Steamy" Cornea.* This is manifested most prominently in acute congestive glaucoma, less so in the chronic and absolute stages. The cloudiness has been attributed to an edema of the stroma and a collection of fluid under and between the epithelial cells.

9:25 When the pressure is decreased by medical or surgical means, the cornea quickly clears unless the eye has been under extreme pressure for a long period. In some dogs, the fundic detail is revealed on ophthalmoscopic examination; in others, because of the cloudy media, this is not possible. In several instances, increased pressure over a long period has resulted in a striate keratitis. Rucks in Descemet's membrane, due to edema and swelling of the substantia propria, causes finger-like processes or streaks in the cornea. These opacities tend to remain permanently, even after the tension has been rendered normal by surgery.

9:26 *Insensitive Cornea.* Increased pressure may cause the cornea to become insensitive from pressure upon nerve filaments. In the dog, when a glaucomatous eye is brushed with a feather or wisp of cotton, there will be no reflex blinking as in the normal eye (Par. 2:21).

9:27 *Shallow Anterior Chamber.* In acute congestive glaucoma, the anterior chamber is often shallow (Par. 2:24), due to the anterior displacement of the iris and lens. The cause of this is probably an increase in volume or swelling of the vitreous body, accompanied by an edema and swelling of the ciliary processes. Lowe[46] is of the opinion that in man increased lens thickness and a relative anterior positioning of the whole lens contribute to the shallow anterior chambers of primary angle-closure glaucoma. Increase of lens thickness may occur by three processes: (a) differences in the constitutional size of lenses within different eyes, (b) continuing growth of lens fibers throughout life, and (c) swelling (intumescence) of the lens in cataract formation caused by retention of fluid or metabolic products. The chamber depth in the dog can be approximated, and compared with the normal eye, by observing the eye from the lateral aspect with penlight and binocular loupe. When the observer's eye becomes "practiced" to depth perception, shallow chambers can readily be seen when viewing the eye from the front. Whereas a shallow anterior chamber is usually associated with primary acute attacks of glaucoma, it may be observed in instances of secondary glaucoma, *e.g.* types of lens subluxation, swelling of the lens in cataract formation (Par. 10:40), and in iris *bombé* (Par. 7:47).

9:28 *Dilatation of the Pupil* (Plate 15A). Probably the most constant and significant clinical sign of advanced or acute congestive glaucoma in the dog is full dilatation of the pupil with no response to light stimuli (Par. 7:19). This is a finding in progressive retinal atrophy and allied conditions also (Par. 11:56), and, therefore, should never be used as an independent entity to establish a diagnosis of glaucoma.

9:29 The dilatation may be caused by a pressure paresis of the ciliary nerves, a paresis of the sphincter fibers because of edematous pressure, or an irritation of the sympathetic nerves. If pressure is relieved early enough by medical or surgical intervention, the pupil may again become normally mobile and contracted. If the attack is prolonged and has produced synechiae (adhesions) at the root of the iris, or if atrophy of the iris has occurred, the pupil may remain dilated for life, even though the pressure is normalized. The pupil dilatation is often one of the first signs noticed by the owner, as it produces a peculiar greenish blue hue (especially in cocker spaniels with acute congestive glaucoma).

9:30 *Episcleral Vascularization* (Plate 15A). Episcleral vascularization, or congestion of the episcleral vessels, is a constant finding in marked pressure increase. The vortex veins within the sclera are affected by the initial increase in pressure. This makes it necessary for the anterior ciliary veins to take over their work, becoming distended in the process.

9:31 The conjunctival vessels also become injected and a mild degree of chemosis may accompany the change in the vessels. This engorgement is accentuated in the chronic and absolute stages by the inevitable globe enlargement (buphthalmos). When pressure is restored to normal, the vessels tend to return to near normal size; the smaller ones disappear but seldom do any completely revert to their original caliber. The conjunctiva becomes "thinner" and even atrophic after a sustained pressure increase.

9:32 *Loss of Vision.* Loss of vision, while due partly to failure of the owner to recognize the early stages, may also be due to failure on the part of the veterinary clinician to diagnose and treat the condition properly. If seen early, when there is little or only partial loss of vision, sight can often be preserved. When only one eye is glaucomatous, the dog may or may not show signs of blindness on the affected side. To test the ambulatory vision, a heavy black patch is placed over the normal eye (Par. 2:36) (Fig. 2–19). The dog is then observed as it moves through unfamiliar surroundings. Minimal vision (light perception) and projection should be tested (Par. 2:36) if the dog appears unable to avoid obstacles.

9:33 In the early acute congestive phase, the blindness that ensues is often transient, for when pressure is normalized, vision is restored. The initial opacification of the ocular media contributes to the reduction in the vision, but ischemic changes in the retina and ischemia of the optic nerve contribute to the permanent loss of vision.

9:34 In one instance, following normalization of pressure, 2 weeks elapsed before vision returned, although the ocular media was clear for most of that period. The return of vision was certainly dramatic, since all hope for sight had been abandoned. In other dogs, return of vision ensued within hours following pressure relief, especially when this was accomplished by medical means. As a rule, the pressure must be relieved within 24 to 48 hours following onset of acute congestive attacks and when pressure is 60 mm Hg or more, in order to prevent permanent damage and loss of vision. Although there are exceptions as cited above, some vision usually returns within 72 hours after the pressure is brought into normal range, if it is going to return at all.

9:35 *Buphthalmos (Hydrophthalmos).* The term hydrophthalmos or buphthalmos is applied to a glaucomatous eye when, under the influence of high pressure, it has increased in size. These terms are used in human ophthalmology to denote infantile (congenital) glaucoma in which, because of the softness of the tissues, the gross distension of the eyeball is the main characteristic. While this is not found in the human adult, it is a common clinical finding in advanced or acute congestive canine glaucoma, whether it be primary or secondary, probably because the canine eye stretches more easily. These terms are used synonymously, the French and English preferring "hydrophthalmos," with "buphthalmos" being more commonly used in this country.

9:36 Enlargement of the globe is usually a gradual process; however, in acute congestive glaucoma it can be fairly rapid. The full dilatation of the pupil, in the early stage of pressure increase, gives to the eye an appearance of enlargement beyond that which is actually present. However, within a few weeks the globe may increase in size, with the cornea increasing in all dimensions and the eyeball appearing exophthalmic. As the buphthalmos increases, the eye develops an unpleasant appearance and is subjected to other inflammatory processes (Fig. 9–2).

9:37 *Cupping of the Optic Disc* (Fig. 9–3A, B, Fig. 9–4) (Plate 20E). In the past it had been postulated that, since the lamina cribrosa (that portion of the sclera which is perforated by the optic nerve) is the most yielding area of the fibrous coat (Par. 6:190), it is pressed backward, producing a depression or cupping of the optic nerve head which is recognizable with the ophthalmoscope when the ocular media is clear. A study[39] proposed that the pathology of all "glaucomatous cupping" is mainly loss of tissue due to degeneration. Gelatt[13] reported loss of myelin, loss of vasculature, atrophy of the disc and infiltration with pigment accompanying glaucomatous cupping in the dog. It is now generally agreed that the cupping is due to loss of nerve tissue, not deformity of the globe.

9:38 Ordinarily, cupping is not an early finding but it has been seen distinctly in dogs a few days following an acute attack. It is most readily seen in the blind, but clear, glaucomatous eye. For the normally myopic eye, a minus 3 lens of the ophthalmoscope is used first (Par. 2:49), with changes in diopters being made to view the fundus most clearly. In the case of subluxation of the lens, when attempting to visualize the fundus around the border of the lens, a plus 7 or 8 lens is used.

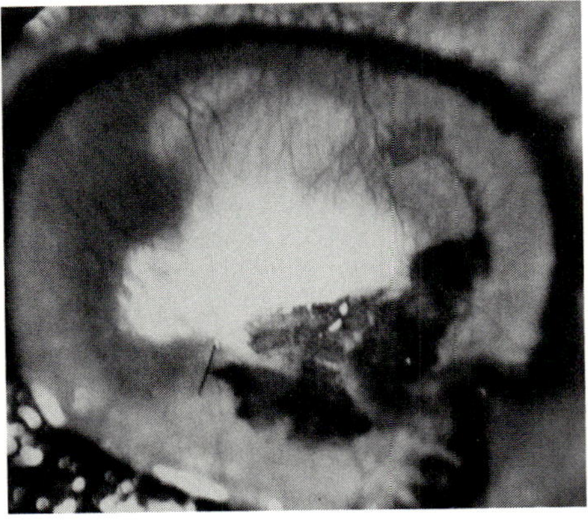

Fig. 9–2. Buphthalmic globe with glaucomatous pannus, pigment, and corneal dystrophy.

In cupping, the blood vessels appear to drop over the edge of the optic disc and are only faintly seen at the bottom of the depression.

9:39 *Atrophy of the Optic Disc and Retina* (Plate 20E). More often than not, atrophy of the optic disc accompanies the cupping. The disc becomes grayish white and few, if any, vessels can be seen emerging from it. The retina also becomes atrophic and nearly devoid of vessels. A highly reflective ring commonly develops in the tapetum around the optic disc.

9:40 *Iris Atrophy.* In the chronic and absolute types, glaucomatous changes are evident in the iris. It appears atrophic and thin, especially at the pupillary border (sphincter muscle area) (Plate 15D). In time, this area appears darker, patchy, and riddled with holes. Pigmentary deposits may be found on the anterior lens surface or free in the anterior chamber itself. In well-established cases with obscure histories, it is difficult to determine if iris atrophy is the result, or the possible cause, of the pressure increase (Par. 9:77).

Classification and General Considerations

A. Primary Glaucoma
B. Secondary Glaucoma
C. Congenital Glaucoma

9:41 Simply stated, and for all practical purposes, glaucoma may be classified as: *(a)* primary—in which the abnormal elevation of intraocular pressure occurs without other antecedent intraocular disease; *(b)* secondary—in which the abnormal elevation of intraocular pressure occurs as a complication of some other disease or damage to the eye; and *(c)* congenital—in which the abnormal elevation of intraocular pressure occurs as a result of some developmental malformation of the eye.

9:42 *Absolute* glaucoma, or blindness, is the end stage in any glaucoma. It need not be included in any classification, nor is it possible to do so in many instances in the dog for reasons previously mentioned (Par 9:20).

9:43 It is generally agreed that, in humans

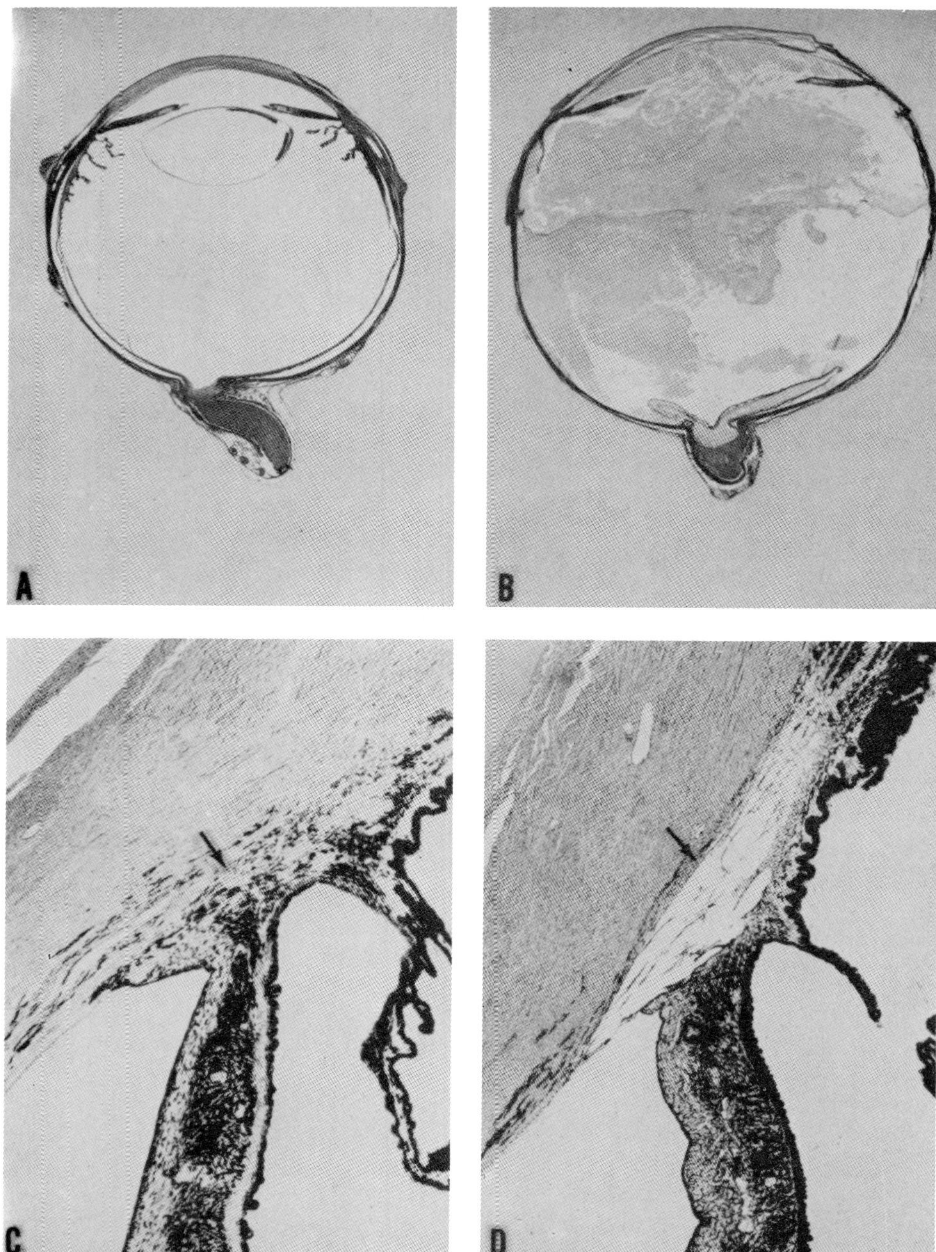

Fig. 9–3. Canine glaucoma. *A. Section* (× 2) of the left eye of a dog with moderately severe glaucoma. Note spherical outline of the eye, occlusion of the filtration angle and cupping of the optic disc. *B.* Absolute glaucoma in the right eye of the same dog as *A* (× 2). Buphthalmos, severe cupping of the optic disc, disorganization of contents of globe. *C.* Filtration angle (× 35) of same eye as *A.* Note occlusion (arrow) AFIP 717599. Contributor: Dr. Leon Z. Saunders. *D.* Normal filtration angle, eye of a dog (× 35). Compare with *C.* (Jones and Hunt, *Veterinary Pathology.* Courtesy, Lea & Febiger.)

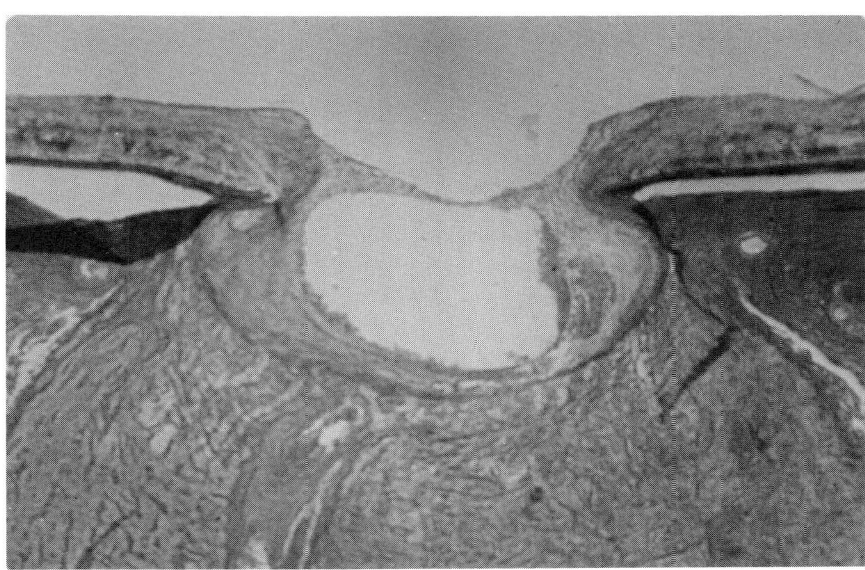

Fig. 9–4. Cupping of the optic disc.

and animals, glaucoma is due to increased resistance to outflow, rather than to increased production of aqueous. Becker and Shafer[18] have prepared a comprehensive classification of glaucoma in the human that implies *mechanisms* that impair outflow.

9:44 There is less general agreement on the mechanisms that impede outflow in the dog. Wyman[45] lists Primary (Open angle), Secondary and Congenital. Slatter[35] and Gelatt[13] list both open angle and angle closure, or narrow angle, under Primary glaucoma, as well as

Table 9–1. Classification of the Canine Glaucomas Based on Etiology (from Gelatt[13])

Type of Glaucoma	Etiology	Breed
1. Primary glaucoma	Open-angle	Beagle, Toy and Miniature Poodle
	Narrow-angle	American Cocker Spaniel, Toy and Miniature Poodle
2. Secondary glaucomas	Lens-associated luxation phacolytic lens-induced uveitis intumescent cataract Traumatic intraocular foreign bodies intraocular hemorrhage Inflammatory angle obstruction with inflammatory cells and fibrin peripheral anterior synechiae pupillary obstruction (iris bombe) Intraocular tumors	Wirehaired Fox Terrier, Sealyham Terrier
3. Congenital glaucoma	Mesodermal goniodysgenesis Other anterior segment anomalies	Basset Hound, English Cocker Spaniel

Secondary and Congenital. Table 9–1 from Gelatt[13] provides an overview of the glaucomas found in dogs. It appears that most of the secondary glaucomas in the dog, with the exception of phacolytic glaucoma and angle obstruction by hemorrhage or inflammatory cells, are caused by angle closure.

9:45 A diagnosis of primary glaucoma is made when there are no discernible secondary conditions within the eye which could lead to an increase in pressure. There is a problem in cases in which glaucoma and lens luxation co-exist. Lens luxation can *cause* angle closure and secondary glaucoma, or can *result* from glaucoma and the stress that stretching of the eye places on the zonules that hold the lens in place.

A. *Primary Glaucoma*

9:46 *Breed Incidence.* There appears to be a hereditary predisposition to an acute, angle closure glaucoma in certain breeds exhibiting narrow or anomalous anterior chamber drainage angles. In man glaucoma may be inherited as a dominant or recessive characteristic. In the study of several large series of persons with primary glaucoma that had one or more relatives affected with the disease, 13.7 to 17.8% had a hereditary history.

9:47 Evidence obtained from gonioscopic studies[20,24,25] in the cocker spaniel favors the definite possibility that a narrow iris angle predisposes to acute congestive attacks in certain individuals within the breed. A narrow or closed angle was found in both the affected and still unaffected eyes of those individual dogs in which this examination was possible. A further study[22] in cocker spaniels bred for glaucoma tends to substantiate earlier observations. The results of tests indicated repeatedly that these individuals had a poorer intraocular pressure regulatory mechanism than control dogs, and that increased pressure was more easily provoked in them than in the controls. Definite histopathologic changes were demonstrable in the eyes of cocker spaniels which had signs of glaucoma. Eyes in this state more nearly resembled human angle-closure glaucoma.

9:48 In a basset study[30] the glaucoma was attributed to a mesodermal dysgenesis of the angle (goniodysgenesis), with or without a concurrent zonular defect. Similar angle anomalies were observed in basset hounds which had normal ocular tensions. Others of the breed were found to have normal-appearing angles.

9:49 Primary glaucoma associated with an inherent ocular structural defect occurs in the dog in the United Kingdom, the disease showing some specificity toward the English cocker spaniel, the springer spaniel and the basset hound breeds, as well as exhibiting an incidence in the crossbred animal.[1] The author (Bedford) reports similar gonioscopic findings to the basset study[30] but does not agree with the interpretation of the associated histologic findings. "The undifferentiated 'sheets' and 'thick bands' of 'mesodermal tissue' are, in fact, simply dysplastic pectinate ligament, much shorter and thicker than usual but containing both iridel and corneal constituent tissues. Further, the greyish white appearance of the dysplastic ligament appears to be due to an increased thickness in Descemet's membrane. It is possible that this dysplastic structure may be the actual cause of angle narrowing in this particular breed."

9:50 *Sex Incidence.* In Magrane's cocker series[24] the ratio of females to males was 3:1. In Lovekin's series[20] the incidence was higher in males than in females, but the sample was relatively small. There was no specific sex incidence in other series.[1,30] In man primary glaucoma is reported to attack women more often than men.

9:51 *Eye Predilection.* In a series[24] the left eye was afflicted first in twice as many dogs as had an initial right eye involvement. This 2:1 ratio also resembles the ratio recorded in man.

9:52 *Age Incidence.* Primary glaucoma is a disease of middle and advancing age in the breeds mentioned and in man. In Magrane's series[24] the ages ranged from 3½ to 10 years with an average of 6 years. Lovekin[20] reports an age span of 6 to 13 in the cocker breed. The disease has been encountered in bassets ranging from 3 to 10 years of age. Bedford[1] reports an age span of 4 to 13 with an average of 9 years.

9:53 *Weather Incidence.* There appears to be a connection between weather conditions and the incidence of acute congestive attacks of glaucoma in man. Nearly twice as many attacks occur in northern cities during the cold months of October through March as in the warmer 6-month period. When the dates of acute congestive attacks in cocker spaniels in Magrane's series could be determined, a near identical ratio was discovered. In Lovekin's study[20] all acute attacks occurred between October and May.

9:54 *Second Eye Involvement.* The time interval between the attack in the first eye and that in the second varies from a few days to 2 years. Nearly all second eye involvements will take place within 1 year. It has been well established that in man the second eye is especially susceptible to an acute attack of primary, shallow-chamber angle glaucoma following such an attack in the first eye.

9:55 *Mechanism and Theory of Cause.* In a consideration of the mechanism of angle closure in the dog, two factors are proposed.[1] The first is that actual closure is an acute change, and is therefore most immediately associated with some rapid change within the eye, such as pupillary aperture variation; the second is that the disease appears to be dependent upon an age-related change, such as lens enlargement. Narrowed iridocorneal angles were observed in young dogs but the clinical manifestations of the disease were seen only in middle-aged and elderly individuals. The opinion has also been expressed[29] that glaucoma may manifest itself at middle-age in individuals with congenital angle anomalies because of exciting factors such as shallowing of the anterior chamber with age from lens growth, lens displacement, pupil size and inflammation.

9:56 Regardless of the initiating factor, closure of the angle and collapse of the ciliary cleft is maintained by the formation of peripheral anterior synechia which involves all quadrants of the angle. Aqueous humor production continues and, in the presence of the elevated pressure, structural changes occur in the sclera with closing of the aqueous drainage plexus thus adding to the dilemma.

B. Secondary Glaucoma

9:57 A classification of secondary glaucoma is made when the abnormal elevation of intraocular pressure occurs as a complication of some other disease or damage to the eye.[25]

9:58 Secondary glaucoma can affect any breed because of its multiplicity of causes. However, it is more apt to involve those breeds subjected to subluxation and luxation of the lens since this condition is the leading cause of a secondary glaucoma in the dog. Secondary glaucoma occurs more commonly than does the primary form.

9:59 *Causes.* Magrane has recognized eight causes for secondary glaucoma. It is not always possible to determine accurately the secondary cause for the increase in pressure. In many instances it become evident from the history and time element that the disease has passed through the acute and chronic phases into the absolute (blind) stage without known secondary factors affecting the pressure rise. Thus, the position and condition of the lens, intraocular adhesions, and iris pathology possibly present in the old glaucomatous eye may be the result of, rather than the cause of, the glaucoma.

9:60. 1. *Subluxation and Luxation of the Lens.* Luxation is diagnosed when the ligamentous attachment of the lens is completely disrupted and when it has vacated the patellar fossa (Plate 15C and Fig. 10–10); subluxation is diagnosed when the ligamentous breakdown is partial and displacement incomplete (Plate 15B and Figs. 10–7, 10–8, and 10–9).

9:61 In man, glaucoma secondary to lens subluxation or luxation is classified in angle closure glaucoma. It is easy to understand how a partially or completely luxated lens could act to occlude the pupil, thus causing pupillary block and subsequent forward movement of the base of the iris, producing angle closure. In other cases in which the lens luxates posteriorly, the exact pathogenesis of angle closure is less apparent. Pupillary block by vitreous has been suggested.

9:62 Secondary glaucoma resulting from subluxation of the lens is known to be familial. In man, the genealogic tree of a family in which there were many cases of glaucoma associated with subluxation of the lens has been reported.

9:63 The first significant report, from the standpoint of breed incidence, showed it to be predominantly in the pure bred wire-haired fox terrier and Sealyham.[43]

9:64 In the classical work, subluxation and luxation of the lens was encountered in only the two breeds, 90% being in the wire-haired fox terrier and 10% in Sealyhams. However, the difference between the breeds was not considered to be significant because it resembled the breed population ratios. In over 100 cases observed, no animal was under 3 years of age and the sexes were divided about equally (males, 56%; females, 44%). When first examined, 62% of the animals were bilaterally affected and 38% unilaterally.

9:65 The study indicated that lens displacement was a primary affection and was hereditable, *i.e.* certain organic defects are inherited which terminate in a defective zonule; also, that displacement of the lens is probably often precipitated by trauma but, before displacement occurs, some degree of genetic instability must be present in the suspensory apparatus.

9:66 That the disease is hereditable is presumed[6] from the following circumstances: (1) the preponderance of bilateral cases (60%); (2) the restricted and almost universal occurrence of the disease in the two named breeds of dogs; and (3) the indicated familial tendency. No figures are given as to the incidence of secondary glaucoma, but all cases, with one exception in which no trace of a lens was found at necropsy, were associated with luxation of the lens into the anterior chamber.

9:67 Our series over the years includes an equally significant number of wire-haired terriers and Sealyhams, but other breeds have been found to develop secondary glaucoma as the direct result of lens displacement. Included in this series are Welsh terriers, smooth-haired fox terriers, toy terriers, Manchester terriers, terriers of mixed breeding, Welsh corgis, Chihuahuas, basset hounds and cocker spaniels. The range in all breeds afflicted varied from 4 to 8 years of age.

9:68 In the cocker spaniel and basset breeds, it is not always possible to learn whether the glaucoma precipitates the lens luxation or vice versa. The lens displacement was known to have preceded the pressure rise in many instances. Since a primary anomalous angle glaucoma also exists in these breeds, it is possible that through long, continued tension increase, with resultant buphthalmos and stretching of the ocular structures, the lens suspensory apparatus is weakened, with a subluxation as the sequela. Primary cases of acute congestive glaucoma, which are untreated or fail to respond to treatment, can be observed to progress through stages of increased buphthalmos with eventual subluxation or luxation.

9:69 Familial glaucoma has also been reported in the beagle breed.[14] The age incidence was relatively young (9 months to 4 years: mean—2.9 years). A bilateral lens displacement was present in all cases. This often preceded any elevation in pressure. Gonioscopy revealed open angles in all eyes examined. A primary zonular defect was postulated. In other studies, Gelatt et al. found an autosomal recessive, open-angle glaucoma in the beagle. Lens luxation was not a routine finding.

9:70 *Clinical Signs.* Since patients are presented during all stages of glaucoma, the clinical manifestations may include: (1) subluxation of the lens in any direction; (2) luxation into the anterior chamber; and (3) luxation into the vitreous humor. The signs of glaucoma and the degree of buphthalmos attending tension increase will, of course, depend upon the severity and duration of the attack. In some cases there is no elevation of IOP or indication of previous elevation; however, such dogs are at high risk for glaucoma.

9:71 A corneal opacity often accompanies the lens displacement. Opacity was reported in all cases of luxation in one series.[43] In 87% of another series,[6] corneal changes varied from a slight localized opacity to a diffuse vascularized keratitis. When an opacity is localized near the center of the cornea, the anterior pole of the lens can usually be observed in contact with the endothelium of the cornea. The whole lens may be firmly adhered to the cornea in some instances. A striate keratitis has been observed in others with buphthalmos.

9:72 The ease of diagnosing lens displacement, with or without secondary glaucoma, is again dependent upon the severity of the displacement. In the early stages, the only sign may be a distinct tremor of the iris, with movement of the head or eyes. This is known as *iridodonesis* (Par. 2:25) and results when the iris no longer has a smooth resting place on the anterior capsule of the lens. If the pupil is dilated, the periphery of the lens may be readily seen as a silver gray line and the zonules may often be seen still clinging to the lens capsule. A so-called "aphakic crescent" is formed between the lens periphery and the pupillary border. Examination in a dark or semi-darkened room with magnification and focal illumination will materially aid in the diagnosis. Use of Wood's light in a dark room will effect a green fluorescence of the lens which usually makes diagnosis simple. A displaced lens will become cataractous in time and, as transparency is lost, diagnosis is simplified (Figs. 10–7, 10–11).

9:73 It must be concluded that lens displacement is by far the most important cause of secondary glaucoma in the dog. The clinician *should be highly suspicious that a subluxation is present if a middle aged dog of one of the aforementioned breeds is presented with a watery, sensitive eye.* The acute congestive symptoms of glaucoma may not be present at the initial examination, and the pressure increase may be transient, but invariably, at some time during the course of lens displacement, a secondary glaucoma will be present.

9:74 2. *Uveitis.* Glaucoma secondary to intraocular inflammation (uveitis) is probably the next most common type of secondary glaucoma.

9:75 Posterior synechiae or peripheral anterior synechiae resulting from an iritis are most frequently the cause of pressure increase. A complete adhesion of the pupillary margin of the iris to the anterior lens capsule (iris bombé) (Par. 7:47) (Fig. 7–4) will result in an absence of circulation of aqueous through the pupil, producing an increased pressure in the posterior chamber. The middle part of the iris will protrude forward, as the root and pupillary border are fixed. The lens diaphragm is also pushed forward. Due to the pressure of the iris root against the cornea, the chamber angle closes (Fig. 9–3C). Thus, what aqueous that does manage to reach the anterior chamber no longer has an exit even without iris bombé. Peripheral anterior synechiae can follow iris inflammation even without iris bombé. It can be discouraging to enjoy success in treating a severe uveitis, only to have glaucoma develop as the aqueous production returns toward normal.

9:76 Atrophy of the iris as a sequela to uveitis (Par. 7:48) can lead to a secondary glaucoma (Plate 12A). The sloughing pigment and iris debris clog the aqueous drainage through the trabeculum.

9:77 3. *Essential Iris Atrophy* (Par. 7:96). I have seen several cases in which it was believed that the iris atrophy was primary to the glaucoma. An essential progressive iris atrophy is described in man in which iris tissue is lost in all layers. Iris debris can block the angle, and as the iris atrophy becomes severe, the remaining base of the iris may come forward, causing angle narrowing or closure.

9:78 It is necessary to see iris atrophy in the early stage in the dog in order to brand the atrophy as the cause of the glaucoma. As pointed out earlier (Par. 9:40), pressure increase of some duration will produce iris atrophy. A diagnosis of essential iris atrophy will always prove difficult in the dog, but the clinician's suspicions might be aroused if an extensive iris atrophy without full pupil dilatation or without iris-lens adhesions is seen, and yet pressure is increased.

9:79 4. *Injury and Infection.* Adhesions as a sequela to trauma or endophthalmitis will, of course, block the drainage mechanism, with secondary glaucoma as the result. The trauma or infection may precede the pressure increase by some weeks. As a rule, this type of glaucoma is the most refractory to medical or surgical treatment.

9:80 5. *Postsurgical (cataract extraction).* Secondary glaucoma following operations for cataracts is common. In one series[27] approximately 13% of the dogs developed iris bombé and/or a pressure increase following extracapsular cataract extraction. In still another study[37] in which the intracapsular technique was predominant, glaucoma was also the principal postoperative complication.

9:81 There are several principal reasons for secondary glaucoma following operations for cataracts. Probably the most important factors are postoperative iridocyclitis and edema, clots and cortical lens remnants. Vitreous prolapse with blockage of the angle or production of an iris bombé as a result of any of these factors is definitely a cause. Cataract extraction in which there is vitreous presentation or loss can be followed by an especially severe glaucoma called *malignant glaucoma.* If vitreous blocks the pupil, new aqueous being formed may go behind the vitreous, pushing it and the iris forward. The anterior chamber becomes shallow, and the angle is closed. The treatment is immediate peripheral iridectomy (Par. 7:99), and restoration of the iris to its normal position. Delayed reformation of the anterior chamber which, in turn, is due to fistulization must also be included. Incarceration of the iris, lens capsule or cortical debris within the wound is most often the cause of the fistulization. Glaucoma may also occur months to years after an extracapsular cataract extraction due to low-grade uveitis (Par. 7:42).

9:82 6. *Lenticular Intumescence.* Secondary glaucoma due to lens swelling (intumescence) can occur in any eye but is more likely to occur in eyes predisposed to acute attack by virtue of a narrow drainage angle. By means of gonioscopy, it was found that the angle of the eye opposite the one with lenticular swelling was of the narrow type.

9:83 In swelling of the lens, during development of a cataract, there is a disposition to glaucoma due to the shallowing of the anterior chamber. The swelling may even press the iris against the trabecular wall.

9:84 Young cocker spaniels with a history of rapid development of juvenile cataract are the most likely candidates for this type of secondary glaucoma. Those cases seen have exhibited changes that included a "steamy" cornea, immobile iris, shallow anterior chamber, swollen cataractous lens, episcleral vessel congestion, and pressure well above normal.

9:85 7. *Hypermature Cataract and Spontaneous Lens Capsule Rupture* (phacolytic glaucoma, endophthalmitis phaco-anaphylactica). After passing through the intumescent or immature state, cataract progresses through the mature into the hypermature. In this stage, the cortex may become liquefied, as may the entire lens in a younger dog. All that remains is a sac filled with milky fluid (Morgagnian cataract) (Plate 16A). Only a thin transparent capsule is left, which may even rupture spontaneously.

9:86 As a lens beomes hypermature, some of the liquefied lens cortex escapes through the lens capsule into the posterior chamber, where it produces a macrophage response. The normal aqueous flow carries these macrophages, containing lens protein and cortical fluid itself into the anterior chamber. Here the cells may obstruct the drainage angle, causing phacolytic glaucoma.[16] The lens protein itself also may cause immune mediated uveitis (phacoanaphylaxis) which, like uveitis from any other cause, can lead to secondary glaucoma. Although these above reactions *may* occur, they certainly do not occur in every dog with hypermature cataracts. When lens induced uveitis does occur, it can most often be controlled by medical means (Par. 7:50) before it causes glaucoma.

9:87 *Intraocular Neoplasm.* Secondary glaucoma resulting from drainage angle occlusion by a uveal tract tumor may be expected in those eyes in which the growth is allowed to progress (Par. 7:91) (Plate 12F).

C. Congenital Glaucoma

9:88 Congenital glaucoma includes both cases in which glaucoma is present at birth and cases in which congenital malformation causes glaucoma to develop after birth. The former is quite rare. The latter includes mesodermal dysgenesis seen typically in the Basset Hound.

MEDICAL AND SURGICAL TREATMENT

9:89 Medical or surgical treatment should be based on goals. The goal in a case in which sight in an eye is still present or may return with treatment is to retain eyesight. The goal in a long-standing case with an enlarged blind eye is to relieve pain and prevent further enlargement and deterioration of the eye. In the first case, every effort should be made to normalize the pressure quickly and to keep it in normal range. In the second, one can take a less intense approach in trying medical management, or may wish to consider a surgical alternative, such as cyclocryosurgery (Par. 9:129) or a prosthesis (Par. 8:61).

9:90 An old adage, "An enlarged eye is a blind eye," is almost always true, but one should be cautious in assigning an eye to the irreparably blind category. Eyes of puppies stretch more easily than adult dogs' eyes, and even some adult dogs will have low-grade elevations of pressure over a long period of time that will cause the eye to enlarge but not be blind. One must also be careful not to confuse exophthalmos with buphthalmos. To be assigned to the blind category, the eye should be grossly enlarged, have no light reflex, have a cupped optic disc and retinal atrophy, if the fundus is visible. If there is any question, it is advisable to normalize the pressure by medical means for 72 hours or longer, if possible, to allow a thorough examination of the eye and to reevaluate sight before assigning it to the blind category.

Medical Treatment

9:91 If the goal is to maintain or regain eyesight, the dog should be hospitalized. Initial treatment should be a miotic (Par. 3:33), .25% Humersol or 4% Pilocarpine, repeated hourly for 3 or 4 treatments, and a carbonic anhydrase inhibitor (Par. 3:76), such as Daranide, at 2 mg/pound initially, and then 1 mg/pound BID. If the pupil is maximally dilated or the pressure is over 60 mm Hg, Mannitol 20% (Par. 3:78) should be given at 3 ml/pound, IV, initially. In any instance, Mannitol should be given if the pressure is not into normal range (12.2 to 24.4 mm Hg) within 4 hours. Water should be withheld for 12 to 18 hours after Mannitol is given, and then reintroduced slowly over the next 12 hours. CAUTION: If the cause of the glaucoma is an anterior subluxation or luxation of the lens, so that the lens is in the pupil or the anterior chamber, a miotic may be contraindicated.

9:92 The goal of medical management in primary glaucoma is to find the lowest dosage of carbonic anhydrase inhibitor that will, when coupled with a miotic, keep the pressure in the normal range. If, after 48 hours, the pressure is still in the normal range, the dose of carbonic anhydrase inhibitor can be reduced 50%, and the pressure monitored daily for 2 more days. If still under control, monitoring can be reduced to weekly or biweekly. If a miotic, alone, or a miotic and ½ dose of carbonic anhydrase inhibitor fail to be adequate for control, surgery should be considered. Primary glaucoma is a progressive disease and medication that will control the pressure, initially, will, with time, become ineffective and more intensive therapy will be required. Most cases will require surgical intervention, either initially or eventually.

9:93 In secondary glaucoma the cause should be treated, *i.e.* luxated lenses should be removed (Par. 9:133). Uveitis should be treated vigorously while the pressure is being controlled medically.

9:94 I have found epinephrine bitartrate 2% (Epitrate), 1 drop, BID is effective in treating low-grade glaucoma associated with iris atrophy in old toy and miniature poodles.

9:95 Consideration should be given to prevention of glaucoma in the fellow eye in all cases of primary glaucoma. Although gonioscopy may be helpful in predicting the likelihood of glaucoma, a normal appearing angle at one or two examinations does not rule out the possibility of glaucoma. In fact, one should assume glaucoma in the second eye is likely to occur within the next 2 years. Use of a miotic (Humersol .125%) in the unaffected eye each evening may be helpful in preventing glaucoma, and if the pressure is up in the high normal range (20 to 24 mm Hg), addition of a carbonic anhydrase inhibitor at half dosage (Daranide) 1 mg/pound daily in divided dose may also be helpful. In any instance, the owner should have a few tablets of carbonic anhydrase inhibitor on hand with instructions to give the full dose if the eye appears red, the pupil appears widely dilated, or if the dog has impairment of vision and the owner is unable to contact you.

9:96 Carbonic anhydrase inhibitors act on the eye by inhibiting the formation of aqueous humor. They have no effect on the outflow and so should be used in combination with miotics. They are synergistic with miotics since they act on the two different mechanisms producing intraocular pressure, secretion of aqueous fluid, and decreased outflow. By lowering the intraocular tension through decreased secretion, miosis is achieved more readily by miotics; thus the angle is unblocked and drainage can occur.

9:97 The importance of this combination therapy (a miotic and a carbonic anhydrase inhibitor) in normalizing tension, thus preventing further visual loss and preparing a softer eye for surgery, cannot be overestimated. If surgery is rejected or the animal is very old, the combination may be used as long as it proves effective or is without undesirable side effects. It is axiomatic that medical treatment must be tailored to the needs of the patient. There is no single drug or combination of drugs suitable for all glaucomas. Treatment is dependent upon the cause and the stage presented (Par. 9:155). In the early stages the patient should be monitored frequently to evaluate the response. In the late stages most medical and surgical attempts to maintain a normal tension will meet with failure.

Surgical Treatment

9:98 As pointed out previously, the treatment of choice for glaucoma, regardless of type, is practically always surgical. There is, however, no one surgical procedure to care for all glaucomas. A careful examination and an accurate classification are necessary in order to determine the type of procedure that is best suited for each case.

9:99 The prime objective in the surgical treatment of glaucoma is to secure a lower pressure and preserve vision; and second, if the condition be absolute, to preserve the integrity of the globe—in other words, to avoid enucleation. Since so many glaucomas in the dog are in the absolute stage before the dog is presented, pet owners are usually pleased if, through surgery, the dog's eye is rendered painless and the buphthalmos is checked. They much prefer this to enucleation and closing of the orbit, which is almost inevitable if the buphthalmos is allowed to progress. For these reasons, surgery of the blind eye is practical in the dog. Surgery on a blind eye is not commonly done in the human, for fear of producing sympathetic ophthalmia in the sighted fellow eye. We do not have this concern, since sympathetic ophthalmia does not occur in dogs (Par. 7:69). It remains, however, that corrective surgery should be done as early as possible to achieve the best results. In the advanced stages, changes secondary to the glaucoma may involve most parts of the eye precluding any attempt at correction or making a combination of procedures necessary.

9:100 Enucleation of a glaucomatous eye in the dog will not prevent glaucoma in the second eye. In the past, attacks of glaucoma in the second eye, following enucleation of the first, occurred in several instances within a matter of days and often within months. Mention has been made of involvement of the fellow eye in both primary (Par. 9:54) and lens displacement glaucoma (Par. 9:64). Continuous use of miotics will often delay the onset or reduce the incidence of glaucoma in the second eye of these individuals.

9:101 This section on surgical treatment is written only for the purpose of enumerating the procedures that have been employed in the dog and briefly describing the techniques as they apply to the various types of glaucoma. The *General Considerations for Eye Surgery* (Chapter 3) should be taken into account before the clinician makes the decision to engage in this specialized facet of canine ophthalmology.

9:102 Since the cause of primary glaucoma is decreased outflow, the ideal surgical procedures would be ones which would increase outflow by opening the narrow or closed iridocorneal angle, by creating new channels. Laser surgery, in which numerous laser "burns" are applied to the tissues in the angle, is used extensively in humans. In limited trials such surgery has not proven beneficial in the dog, probably because of the difference in the structure of the iridocorneal angle. Unfortunately, all surgical procedures that have been used to create new outflow channels in the dog have serious limitations, as will be discussed.

9:103 An alternate but less than ideal solution would be to decrease aqueous production in an attempt to match the production of aqueous to the reduced outflow capacity. Such a procedure, cyclocryosurgery (Par. 9:129), is the current surgical treatment of choice.

9:104 Iridectomy is used in iris bombé and has been used in angle closure glaucoma in an attempt to open the angle. Cyclodialysis has also been used in an attempt to improve outflow. Procedures to establish new outflow channels include filtering cicatrix, Elliot trephine, and tube or other implants. Previously cyclodiathermy was used and now cyclocryosurgery is used to reduce aqueous production. Lens ablation (intracapsular extraction) is used in cases of glaucoma in which the lens subluxation or luxation is thought to be *causing* the glaucoma.

Iridectomy

9:105 This operation was used within the first few days of an attack of primary glaucoma. If postponed, it was apt to fail because peripheral anterior synechiae had begun to develop. In primary glaucoma with a narrow or closed drainage angle the performance of a basal (iris root) iridectomy was to re-establish circulation to the trabeculum (Plate 15G). The iridectomy was sometimes combined with an electroscalpel-produced sclerotomy or sclerectomy (Fig. 9–6A) to create an additional filtering cicatrix (Par. 9:108). The procedures seemed to be beneficial, but often failed in time.

9:106 An iridectomy is the procedure of choice in the re-establishment of circulation from the posterior to the anterior chamber in an iris bombé (Plate 15H). A peripheral excision through the center and/or pupillary border of the iris will suffice, provided the drainage angle is still patent. A reverse cyclodialysis (Fig. 9–8) is needed in addition if the angle is closed, and an air bubble in the anterior chamber will not cause it to open. An iridectomy from pupillary border through the base will be indicated more often because the pupil is often small, and the iridectomy is needed to make the pupil larger as well as to treat the iris bombé.

9:107 A prophylactic basal iridectomy (Plate 15G) was occasionally performed on the normal eye in those cases of primary, closed angle glaucoma in which it was felt that the second eye would become involved in time. In our experience this prevented an attack in the second eye in several instances but has had no effect in the prevention in several others. These failures, however, may have been due to a poorly executed procedure. In any event, the decision to perform a prophylactic surgical procedure on a normal eye is a serious one.

Filtering Cicatrix

9:108 Filtering cicatrix operations have as their object the formation of a permanent filtering cicatrix at or near the sclerocorneal junction through which the excess of aqueous fluid filters out under the conjunctiva (Plate 15F). After a drainage operation aqueous humor may pass out of the eye by two major routes.[8]

1. Transconjunctival flow, in which aqueous actually passes through the epithelium of the bleb and mixes with the tears.
2. Subconjunctivally and then into the venous system.

9:109 Following iridencleisis, functional blebs may remain a long time, but the blebs usually became flat eventually. In those with flattened blebs, the pressure remained normal in some but became elevated again in others. However, in most in which the bleb appeared functional, the pressure remained normal.

9:110 The indications for filtering cicatrix procedures included: primary, closed angle glaucoma; secondary glaucoma caused by an iris bombé in which peripheral anterior synechiae had obliterated the drainage angle; and secondary glaucoma due to injury and adhesions in which the angle is closed.

9:111 When the iris becomes atrophic or degenerated, an iridencleisis is more likely than not to fail. Also, an iridencleisis is not liable to be successful in those cases in which a displacement of the lens is the cause of the secondary glaucoma.

9:112 *The Operation.* Many variations of iridencleisis or iris inclusion operations are described. Our technique has been varied to include: (1) incarceration of one tag of iris following a split of the iris from base to sphincter; (2) incarceration of both tags following the split; (3) excision of a wedge of iris before incarceration of a tag; (4) suturing the tag to the episcleral tissue; (5) incarceration of a tag through a trephine hole (sclerectomy); (6) incarceration, through the wound and into the anterior chamber, of a limbal-based half-thickness scleral flap, in addition to the iris tag inclusion; and (7) application of Gelfilm* to the incarcerated tag and incision site.

9:113 The principal steps in the iridencleisis technique which have produced the best results are:

1. The conjunctival flap is prepared, starting about 8 mm from the limbus. The incision is made only through the conjunctiva. This membrane is carefully separated from the underlying Tenon's capsule down to the limbus.
2. One mm behind the limbus a cut is made through Tenon's capsule down to the sclera. The sclera is bared for a distance of about 3 mm (parallel with the limbus). The electroscalpel is then used to remove the 3 mm by 1 mm (width) section of sclera (posterior lip sclerectomy) (Fig. 9–5A) down to Descemet's membrane. The section is completed into the anterior chamber (#65 blade) (Fig. 9–5B).
3. The iris is allowed to prolapse or is

*Gelfilm, Upjohn Co., Kalamazoo, Mich.

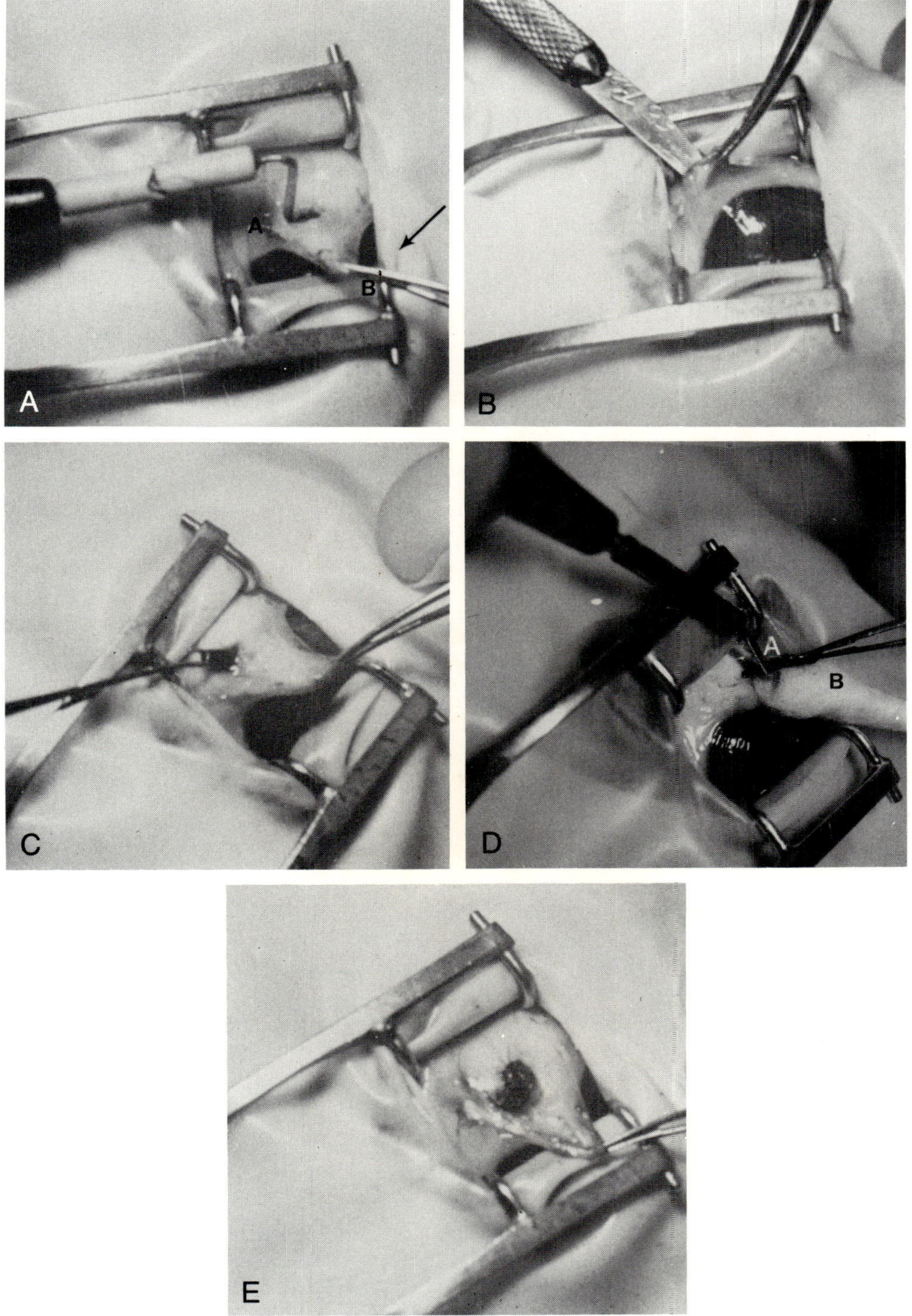

Fig. 9–5. Iridencleisis. *A*. Electroscalpel *(A)* incision and posterior lip sclerectomy (arrow). Conjunctival flap *(B)* in grasp of tissue forceps. *B*. Section completed into anterior chamber (#65 Beaver blade). *C*. Iris within grasp of blunt iris hook. *D*. Electroscalpel *(A)* splitting iris *(B)* from base to sphincter. Note how cotton tip applicator protects the underlying globe during the excision. *E*, Incarcerated iris pillar on top of Tenon's capsule.

grasped with iris forceps or a dull iris hook and brought to the outside (Fig. 9–5C). The assistant holds a cotton tip applicator to the base of the prolapsed iris to protect the cornea in preparation for the iris incision. The iris is split from base to sphincter with the electroscalpel (Fig. 9–5D).

4. One tag of iris is allowed to return to its position in the anterior chamber. The pillar to be incarcerated is turned (posterior, pigment side up), and a 6–0 chromic catgut suture is placed through the iris stroma and then to Tenon's capsule and the episclera (Fig. 9–5E). This assures maintaining its proper position as a "wick" and prevents the tag from falling back into the anterior chamber.
5. The conjunctival flap is replaced over the incarcerated tag and sutured in place with the 6–0 catgut. A drop of atropine solution (2%), an antibiotic ointment and bandaging complete the procedure.

9:114 The technique, as described, is being used because: (1) electrocautery usually prevents a complicating hemorrhage when incising the sclera and the iris; (2) electrocautery preparation of the trephine-type opening into the anterior chamber is instrumental in delaying healing and closure of the incision site around the incarcerated iris pillar; and (3) when the pillar or tag of iris is placed just under the bulbar conjunctiva, rather than under both Tenon's capsule and conjunctiva, transconjunctival and subconjunctival filtration is facilitated.

9:115 Another method employed to secure permanent filtration from the anterior chamber to the immediate subconjunctival space is utilization of a sterile, nonantigenic, absorbable film made from pig gelatin (Gelfilm*). When dry, it looks and feels like cellophane, but when wet it assumes a soft rubbery consistency which molds well to any body surface. Its absorption requires from one to three months, and an opening or "envelope" remains between the conjunctiva and sclera.

*Gelfilm, Upjohn Co., Kalamazoo, Mich.

9:116 Trephination, without incarceration of the iris, may be considered when the iris becomes atrophic or degenerated. There is a difference of opinion as to whether the results produced by trephining are due to fistulization or other factors.

9:117 Briefly, in trephining, a conjunctival flap is first prepared, extending the dissection to include the corneal epithelium for several millimeters in the center of the flap. A 2 to 3 mm trephine is then used to remove a disc which includes one-half cornea and one-half sclera. Another method is to use a scleral punch to notch the incision. A posterior lip sclerectomy constitutes trephination and is best performed in the dog with the electroscalpel (Fig. 9–5A). The conjunctival flap is replaced and sutured in the manner described for iridencleisis.

Tube Implant Filtration (Fig. 9–6)

9:118 In the search for a procedure which would maintain a patent cleft and continue filtration indefinitely, investigators have used various foreign materials for implantation. Reaction between tissues and artificial substances caused failure. With the advent of various inert substances, such as Teflon, silicone, polyvinyl and polyethylene, numerous methods of implanting these materials have been attempted. In 1963 members of the American Society of Veterinary Ophthalmology started an investigation into the use of fine gauge silastic* tubing for drainage purposes. One end of the tubing was inserted several millimeters into the anterior chamber and the proximal end was anchored to the episcleral tissue with 6–0 mersilene. Replacement of the conjunctival flap completed the procedure. Generally, a good result was obtained on a short-term basis, but latent extrusion of the tube and tissue closure on the scleral side resulted in many failures. In a similar investigation in man[32] cyclodialysis

*Medical Silastic 373, 0.025″ × 0.050″, Dow Corning, Midland, Mich.

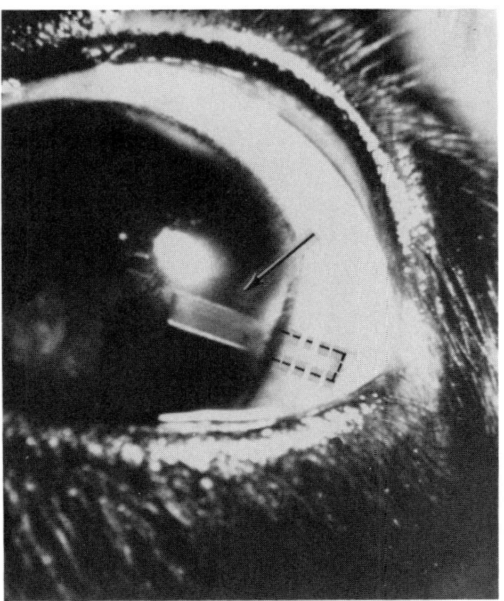

Fig. 9–6. Silastic tube extending from the anterior chamber to an area between the conjunctiva and sclera. Dotted line denotes position of the tube on the scleral side.

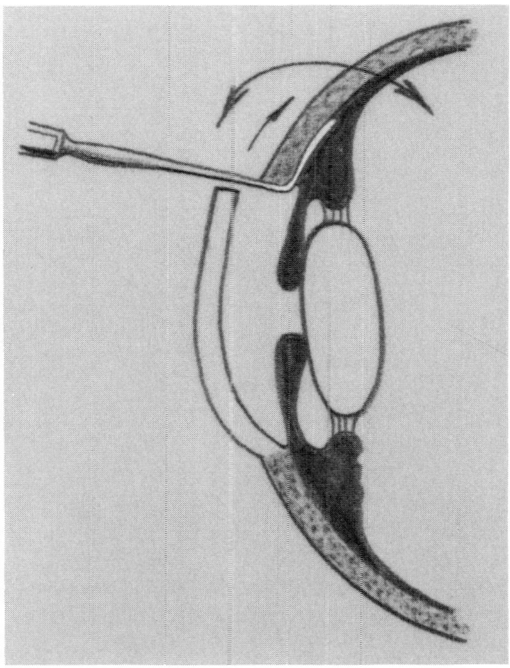

Fig. 9–7. Reverse cyclodialysis. Spatula introduced from anterior chamber to separate the iris root and ciliary body used in conjunction with removal of luxated lens or iridectomy for iris bombé to open a closed angle.

with Teflon tube implants was used 19 times for control of glaucoma. In only three was the tension controlled for longer than 6 months. Complications (erosion of the implant, infection and cataracts) occurred in eight cases. The procedure was abandoned. The use of a flat, self-retaining piece of silicone was implanted to prevent wound closing. In my experience, an hour-glass shaped silicone implant usually failed to control glaucoma in 6 to 12 months after implantation. Extrusion occurred in one eye; in others, the bleb became flat, while in a few eyes, the bleb appeared to be present, but the pressure was elevated. Newer, more elaborate implants, some with valves, are being evaluated for use in man and animals.[3]

Cyclodialysis

9:119 This operation creates an artificial communication between the anterior chamber and the suprachoroidal space, thus forming a new channel for the escape of aqueous.

9:120 A cyclodialysis spatula is introduced through an incision in the bared sclera 5 to 7 mm back of and parallel to the limbus. The blade is kept close to the sclera and advanced in a sweeping motion until its point appears in the anterior chamber. The root of the iris and ciliary body are thus detached, creating the channel. Überreiter[41] believes that this procedure was best suited to the dog, but he does not suggest the type of glaucoma in which it is indicated or most effective.

9:121 Vainisi[42] described a combined cyclodialysis iridectomy and a filtering procedure. In this operation, a 2 × 4 mm rectangular scleral 'window' was made 6 mm back of the limbus. After a cyclodialysis and peripheral iridectomy were performed through this incision, the conjunctiva was closed over the window, thus creating a filtering bleb.

9:122 My experience with the filtering and trephine operation described here, and with the Vainisi technique, indicates that nearly

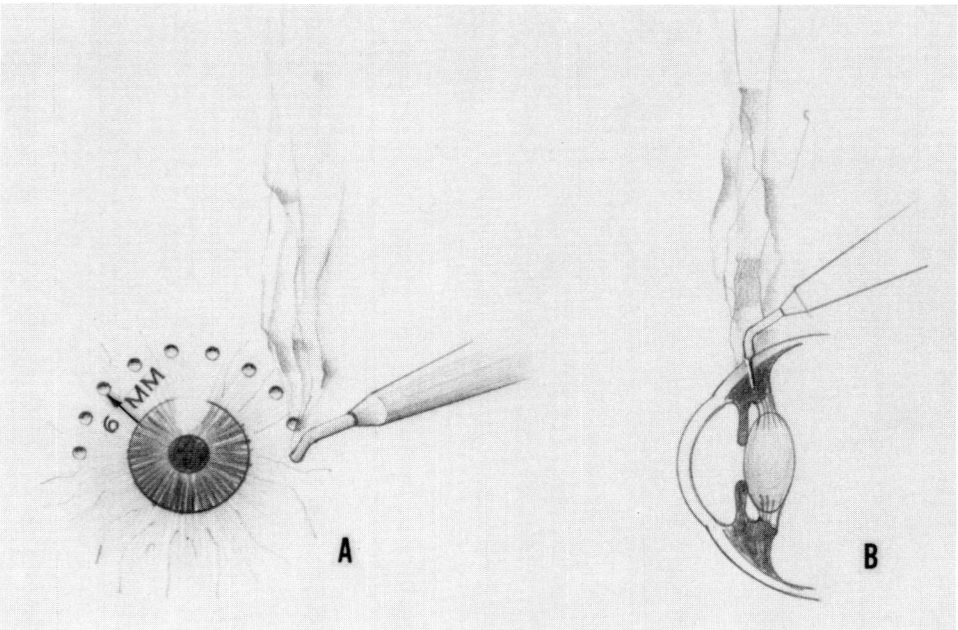

Fig. 9–8. Cyclodiathermy. *A.* Application of the electrode to the upper hemisphere of the globe. *B.* Side view showing position of the electrode in its relation to the ciliary body.

all will control pressure for several months, but that most all fail within 6 to 12 months.

9:123 We have utilized cyclodialysis to complement other procedures and when peripheral anterior synechiae are evident or suspected. The spatula may be introduced from the anterior chamber side to separate the iris root and ciliary body (Fig. 9–7). In our experience, the operation by itself often fails to afford permanent reduction in tension. Nevertheless, as a second procedure it has merit and is especially useful following displaced lens removal when the base of the iris is known to occlude the drainage angle (peripheral anterior synechia). Considerable hemorrhage can result as a complication with this procedure.

Cyclodiathermy

9:124 By definition, cyclodiathermy is application of diathermic current to the ciliary body through the sclera by means of penetrating or nonpenetrating electrodes.

9:125 The exact mechanism of action of cyclodiathermy in lowering intraocular pressure is not completely understood. Whether it acts primarily to destroy the secretory function of the ciliary body by interfering with its vascular supply, or whether it serves to stimulate the formation of a new anastomotic group of vessels and thus effect outflow of aqueous fluid has not been established. Some (in man) advocate its use primarily when all other procedures have failed, while others are of the opinion that the procedure should be reserved for cases in which filtering operations are contraindicated, or in which outflow following a filtering procedure is mildly inadequate.

9:126 We have used cyclodiathermy successfully on blind eyes after one or more procedures have already been tried and failed to normalize pressure. The patient is afforded comfort and the eyeball often returns to normal size. In other instances the procedure either failed to reduce pressure, reduced it partially, or produced a hypotony which led to a phthisis bulbi (atrophy of the eyeball). It generally is considered as "last resort" surgery. A major problem is that there is a small difference between the amount of diathermy that is effective and the amount that may result in a shrunken globe. Nevertheless, it is a possible salvage procedure applicable to the blind, buphthalmic eye. It is easily performed and may be repeated as needed.

9:127 *The Operation.* While varying techniques for applying the electrodes have been described, we employed the same one in all eyes. A Cameron-Miller electrosurgical unit (Fig. 3–4) was used. The technique follows: (1) The eye is draped and fixed below with fixation forceps so that the upper portion of the globe is well exposed and the bulbar conjunctiva taut. (2) A 2 mm or longer electrode is applied through the conjunctiva and into the ciliary body, 5 to 6 mm behind the upper limbus, and at 8 to 12 points evenly spaced to cover the upper half of the globe (Fig. 9–8). A millimeter rule may be used for the measurement. (3) With the dial set at 1 on coagulation, the electrode is held in place for 10 seconds at each application. (4) Atropine solution (2%) and an antibiotic are instilled and the eye is bandaged for 2 days.

9:128 Occasionally, there will be a loss of fluid from some of the punctures, which is desirable. In fact, for cyclodiathermy to be effective it is necessary that an electrode of sufficient depth be used so that some aqueous escapes. A moderate chemosis (edema of the conjunctiva) will be in evidence for several days following the procedure. This is alleviated by use of steroid drops or ointment. A secondary rise in tension may follow the operation but this soon subsides. The intraocular prosthesis (Par. 8:61) has replaced cyclodiathermy as the treatment of choice for blind, buphthalmic eyes. It offers a better chance for a painless, cosmetically acceptable eye.

9:129 Cyclocryotherapy (Cyclocryosurgery) is a procedure in which a probe, maintained at −70° C or colder by liquid nitrogen or nitrous oxide, placed against the sclera, is used to decrease aqueous production by destroying ciliary epithelium. Bietti[2] suggested its use in 1950, and it has been used in man to a limited extent. Smith[36] reported the effect of cyclocryotherapy on the ciliary body of the eye of humans and monkeys. It offers an attractive alternative to other surgical procedures in the dog for several reasons: (1) it is easily and quickly done, (2) it is noninvasive, thereby reducing aftercare and a chance for complications, (3) it can be repeated, if necessary, and (4) most important, it reduces intraocular pressure, at least somewhat predictably. This procedure alone, or combined with medical therapy, is, in our hands, the most successful procedure for controlling glaucoma.[4] Schmidt,[34] Wyman,[45] and others also report good results. It is not theoretically ideal, in that it controls pressure by reducing production of aqueous, rather than increasing outflow. Since glaucoma is caused by decreased outflow, the ideal treatment should increase outflow. As mentioned (Par. 9:122), most procedures to increase outflow fail, however, and repeating procedures is usually impossible.

9:130 The protocol we use is as follows: The dog is anesthetized with Surital and maintained on inhalation anesthesia. The sclera of the upper half of the globe is exposed by elevating or even proptosing the globe with a muscle hook (Par. 6:157) (Figs. 6–33, 6–34). A canthotomy is often needed in small enophthalmic eyes. The cryoprobe (3 mm or larger in diameter) (Figs. 3–18, 3–19) is placed on the conjunctiva, 6 mm back of the limbus, and held in position for a 2-minute single 'freeze' at −70° C. The procedure is repeated until 4–8 adjacent spots are similarly treated. A subconjunctival injection of 5–10 mg of Kenalog or other repositol steroid (Par. 3:65) and a temporary tarsorrhaphy (Fig. 9–14) is applied to protect the cornea. Unless the eye is especially buphthalmic or exophthalmic, the suture is removed the following day.

9:131 Aftercare consists of daily tonometry for 3 to 5 days and continuation of the carbonic anhydrase inhibitor, if necessary, for 1 to 3 days after cryosurgery. A transient rise in intraocular pressure following surgery has been reported in man and may occur in the dog. Topical steroid-antibiotic ointment is applied BID for 5 to 7 days to reduce the transient chemosis. Miotic therapy should be continued in dogs predisposed to angle closure.

9:132 Cryosurgery essentially does, on a longer-term basis, what continued carbonic anhydrase inhibitors do on a short-term basis. Tonometry should be done weekly for 2 to 3 weeks, then as indicated.

Lens Ablation

9:133 Lens extraction is recommended in glaucoma: (1) due to subluxation or luxation of the lens; (2) due to swelling or intumescence of the lens; (3) when it is producing a secondary lens-induced uveitis that cannot be controlled medically, *e.g.* capsule rupture in hypermature cataracts.

9:134 The most frequent intraocular surgical procedure to be performed in canine glaucoma is removal of a luxated or subluxated lens. Intracapsular extraction is attempted in all instances of lens displacement. Occasionally, an extracapsular extraction results when, inadvertently, the capsule ruptures during extraction. This is uncommon, but may occur when the lens is bound by adhesions.

9:135 Since lens displacement is directly responsible for a secondary tension rise, the surgery for the removal of the lens is specific for this type of secondary glaucoma. If performed properly, with meticulous attention to detail, the results achieved are generally excellent as regards affording permanent relief of pressure. The most consistent results and the highest percentage of success following surgery are encountered in this type of glaucoma. It is important, however, that surgery be performed before the eye becomes too buphthalmic, or peripheral anterior synechiae has closed the angle.

9:136 Useful vision may also be retained provided the lens ablation is performed before pressure-induced degenerative changes occur. As Knight[17] indicates, "it cannot be emphasized too strongly that if the dog with a dislocated lens is to retain useful aphakic vision, the extraction of the lens is best regarded as an operation of necessity as soon as the condition can be diagnosed; and for this reason diagnosis at the earliest stage is most important."

9:137 *The Operation.* The eye with a displaced lens of course also has a rupture of the vitreous face (hyaloid membrane). Vitreous presentation and escape are inevitable unless a maximum reduction in tension is achieved prior to the section. Intravenous mannitol offers a most satisfactory means of accomplishing a truly "soft eye" and minimizing complications attending the intracapsular extraction (Par. 3:78). If the lens is in the posterior chamber or in the vitreous and the pupil is miotic from medical treatment being given to control glaucoma, the pupil should be dilated with Mydriacyl (1 drop, 20 minutes before surgery and 1 drop during final preparation after anesthesia). Stronger and longer acting mydriatics should not be used. If the lens is in the anterior chamber, miosis should be maintained in an attempt to keep it there.

9:138 (1) *Canthotomy* (Par. 4:11) (Fig. 4–4). The necessity for performing a canthotomy depends upon the amount of buphthalmos and the size of the palpebral fissure. If the eye is well exposed, a canthotomy is unnecessary; however, if a canthotomy will reduce eyelid pressure on the globe, it should be performed.

9:139 (2) *Conjunctival Flap* (limbal based). Approximately 5 mm from the upper limbus, the conjunctiva and Tenon's capsule are incised around the upper half of the eye to the sclera, and are dissected to the limbus with knife and scissors.

9:140 (3) *Preliminary Groove.* An incision or groove is made along the line of the contemplated section about 0.5 mm posterior to the limbus and near the base of the conjunctival flap. A No. 64 Beaver blade may be used, but, to eliminate all hemorrhage, an offset electroscalpel blade (Fig. 9–9) and electrosurgery (Par. 3:84) are preferred. Ideally, the groove should be down to the depth of Descemet's membrane and should extend at least 150 degrees around the edge.

9:141 (4) *Preplaced Sutures.* Four sutures (Par. 3:108) are preplaced in the groove before the incision is made, thus eliminating the hazard of manipulating the collapsed open eye. These sutures are placed about 5 mm apart. If the incision requires more than 4 sutures, the widest space should be in the center of the incision where its post-placed suture can be easily placed. The preplacement of sutures is extremely important in this operation. When entering the anterior chamber, there is usually an immediate presentation of vitreous because the hyaloid membrane (Par. 11:2) is ruptured at the time the lens displacement occurred. The post placing of sutures following lens extraction is not only difficult, but the excessive manipulation required may result in considerable loss of vitreous.

9:142 The sutures (McLean pattern) (Fig. 9–10) do not penetrate the eye. The needle, starting at the base of the anterior (epithelial) surface of the conjunctival flap, passes through it. It is then reversed and brought anteriorly by catching the posterior scleral lip of the groove, passing in the scleral tissue to cross the groove just dorsal to its depth. The anterior scleral lip of the groove is then penetrated and the needle emerges at the limbus

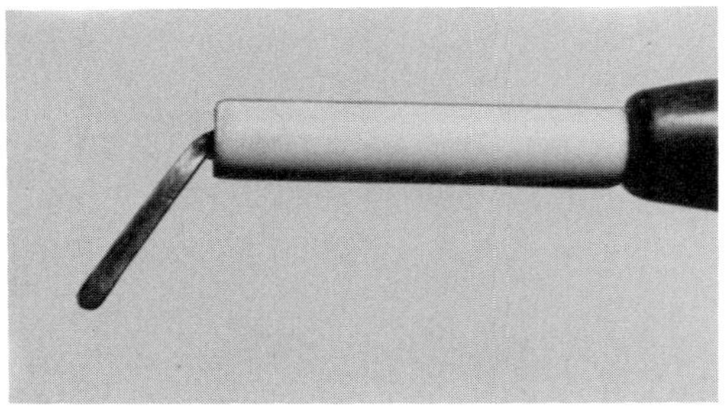

Fig. 9–9. Offset electroscalpel blade used to prepare scleral grooves.

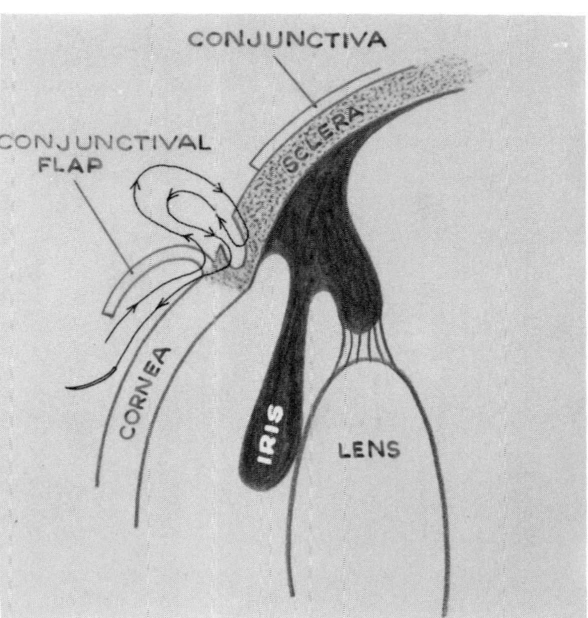

Fig. 9–10. McLean preplaced suture.

just opposite the other end of the suture (inverted mattress suture). Or, the suture may be inserted in a reverse manner by beginning at the limbus, then through the anterior to posterior lips of the groove, and reversing to finish at the base of the conjunctival flap. This reversed pattern seems easier to do. After preplacing all four sutures, each double strand of suture, where it is exposed in the groove, is picked up with an iris hook to form a loop. Each loop is separated and held away from the incision site by towel forceps or a suitable substitute (Fig. 9–11A).

9:143 (5) *Section.* While stabilizing the eyeball by holding the flap and adjacent preplaced sutures with a smooth tissue forceps, a No. 65 Beaver blade is used to enter the anterior chamber (Fig. 9–11B). The incision is then extended with corneal scissors with care being taken not to cut the preplaced sutures. The section must be as adequate as is necessary to remove the entire lens without undue pressure. An incision of at least 150 degrees of the globe is advisable. To minimize loss of vitreous there should be no pressure

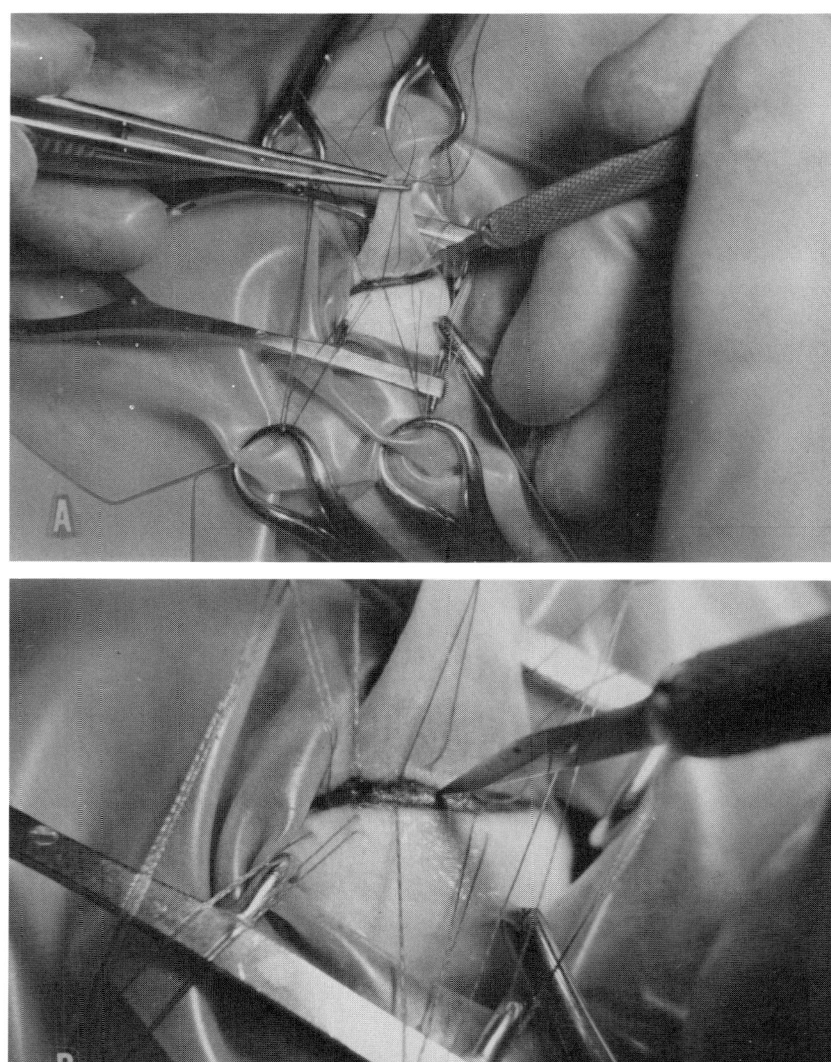

Fig. 9–11. Entry into the anterior chamber for lens ablation. *A.* Surgeon's view of the dorsal aspect of the globe. Preplaced sutures are separated and held away from the scleral groove by towel forceps. Conjunctival flap is extended perpendicularly. Eyeball is fixed with rat tooth mosquito forceps attached to the episclera. Incision is made through the center of the scleral groove into the angle of the anterior chamber. *B.* Close-up view.

on the eye; thus, the speculum tension is reduced prior to enlarging the incision. This is best accomplished by having the assistant hold and elevate the end of the speculum, thus raising the blades and lids away from the globe.

9:144 (6) *Iridectomy.* A peripheral, pupillary iridectomy may be performed to afford more working room for the extraction but this is rarely necessary. Rather, an intact iris is important to the "holding back" of the vitreous following extraction. If an iridectomy or iridotomy is performed, the use of the electroscalpel for this purpose will prevent the

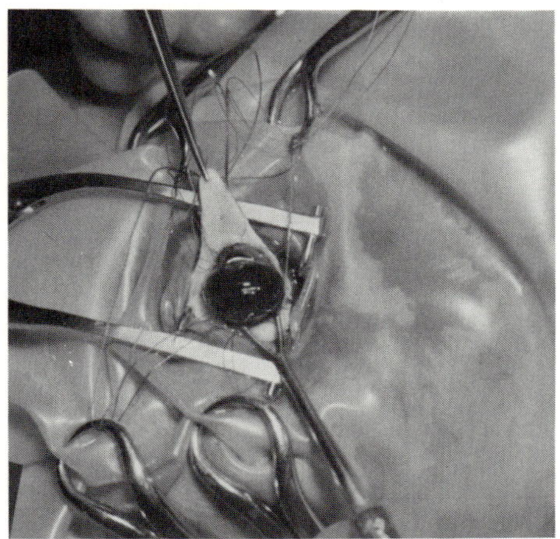

Fig. 9–12. Extraction of the lens with lens snare.

hemorrhage that accompanies the scissors method.

9:145 (7) *Extraction.* A wire lens snare is used to encompass the posterior part of the lens, thus lifting the lens forward and dorsal to and partially through the incision site (Fig. 9–12). The lens is then steadied and held with capsule forceps (Fig. 3–15M), while corneal scissors are used to cut clinging vitreous from the posterior capsule. Any vitreous is cleared from the incision site and is gently smoothed or blown into the pupillary area. Cryoextraction (Fig. 9–13) is the method of choice when

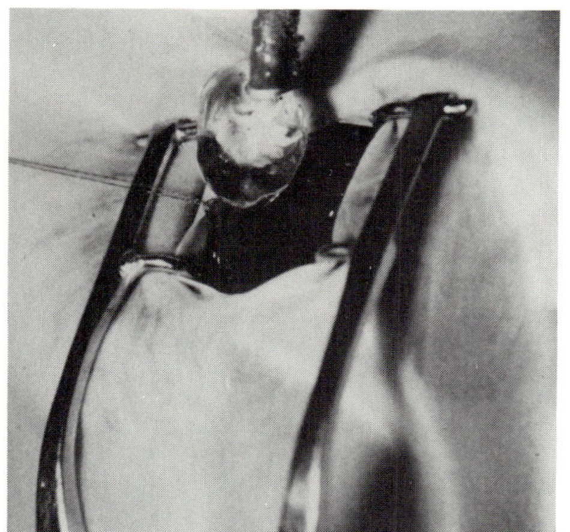

Fig. 9–13. Cryosurgical extraction of luxated lens. Note white "ice ball" adhesion between cryoprobe and lens.

the lens is partially or totally into the anterior chamber. Any formed vitreous remaining in the anterior chamber should be removed by touching it with a cellulose sponge spear, lifting it slightly and cutting it with corneal scissors at the surface of the iris and removing it. This step should be repeated until there is no vitreous protruding through the pupil. A power vitrectomy unit is ideal for this procedure if available.

9:146 (8) *Closure* (Fig. 9–14). The preplaced sutures are drawn up and held by both assistant and surgeon with sufficient tension to approximate the wound. They are not tied at this time. An air bubble is injected into the anterior chamber with an irrigating bulb and infusion needle (Fig. 3–15O, P). If the closure is secure, the air bubble will serve to "blow back" the vitreous. At this point the surgeon may choose to instil acetylcholine (Miochol*) into the anterior chamber to encourage a prompt miosis. The contracted iris acts as a protective barrier in holding back the vitreous.[33] Both good and indifferent response with this preparation have been observed. If the vitreous clinging to the iris and/or incision is freed and returned to the posterior chamber, or is carefully excised and removed, the pupil will most often constrict without Miochol (Acetocholine). Lack of response to Miochol is often a sign that vitreous is still present in the pupillary area or adherent to the iris. The sutures are tied. Tenon's capsule and the conjunctiva are replaced with a running 6–0 chromic catgut suture. If a further inflation of the anterior chamber is indicated, this is done just prior to the final tie of the catgut. A subconjunctival injection of 5 mg of a reposital-type steroid is made in the lower conjunctival cul-de-sac area. A drop of pilocarpine solution (2%) and an antibiotic are instilled, a single mattress suture is placed to close the lids (Fig. 9–15), and a bandage is applied (Par. 3:92) (Fig. 3–6). Placing the lid suture at the junction of the middle and lateral third of the eyelid, rather than cen-

*Smith, Miller and Patch, New Brunswick, New Jersey.

trally as shown in Figure 9–14, allows better observation of the eye.

Postoperative Care (all glaucoma cases)

9:147 Proper postoperative care is exceedingly important following all intraocular procedures of the eye in the dog. Bandaging is important for the reasons elicited (Par. 3:91). Dressings may be changed daily or on alternate days with instillation of a steroid-antibiotic preparation. Bandaging is discontinued on the 3rd postoperative day, to allow BID observations of the size of the pupil. About ½ dilation of the pupil is ideal. If it is ⅔ or more dilated, a miotic is used; if less than ⅓ dilated, a short-acting mydriatic (Mydriacyl) is used.

9:148 In lens ablation surgery the corneoscleral sutures are removed on the twelfth postoperative day. This is most easily accomplished by using eye tissue forceps and the tip of a No. 65 Beaver blade or a curved (No. 12) Bard-Parker blade following good topical anesthesia. Only occasionally is tranquilization and/or general anesthesia necessary for suture removal. The conjunctival suture is left to absorb. Careful handling of the patient, freedom from excitement, barking, and the use of protective collars (Fig. 9–15) for at least the first week are very important during hospitalization.

9:149 The hospitalization period will vary from 5 to 14 days depending upon the type

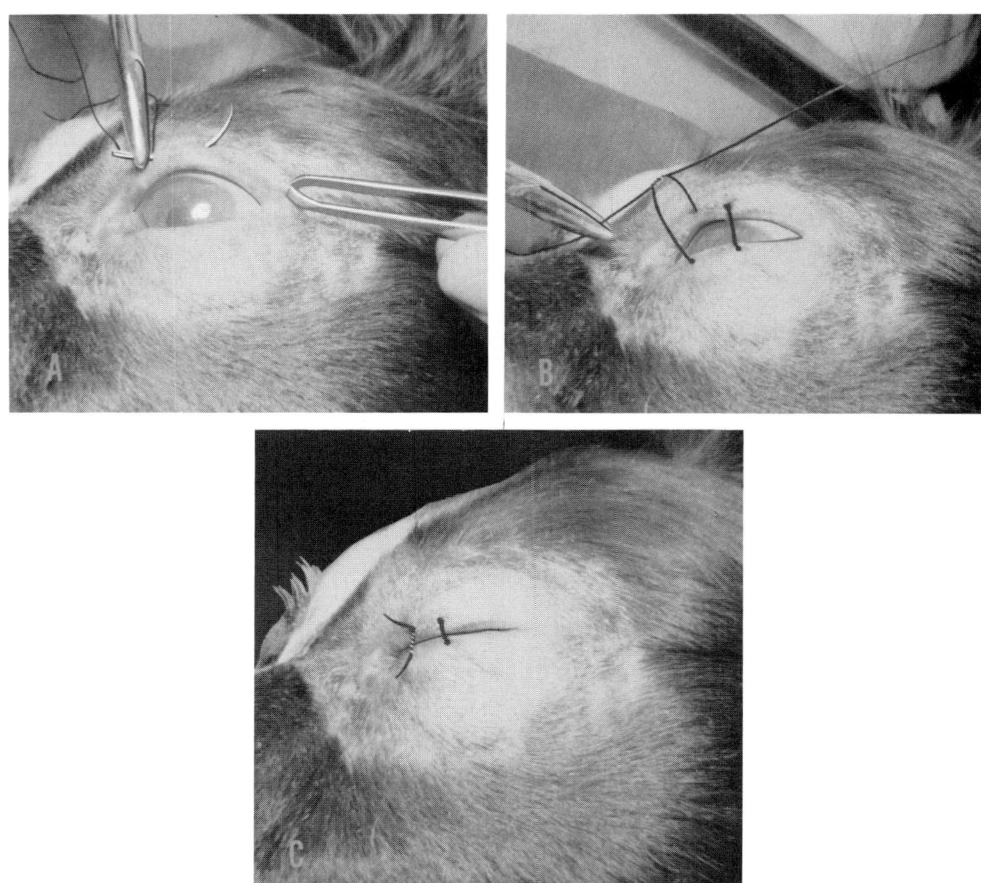

Fig. 9–14. Mode of lid closure. *A.* Needle penetrates skin only. *B.* Mattress suture is continued to the lower lid prior to the tie. C. Completed lid closure. There is no suture contact with the cornea.

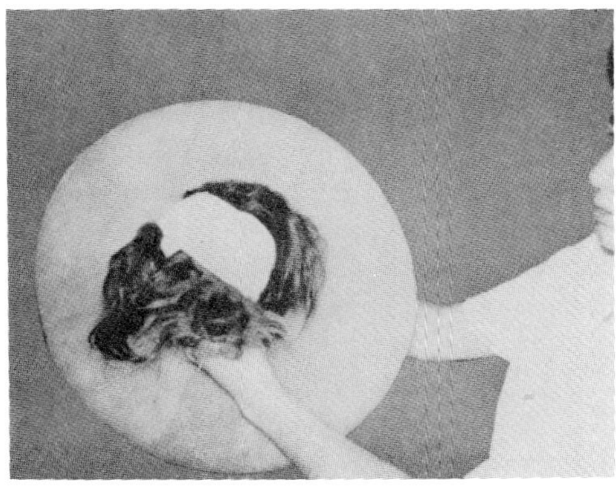

Fig. 9–15. Protection of the operated eye through use of bandaging and a plastic collar (Saf-T-Shield, Ejay International, Box 5101, Glendale, California 91201).

of surgery performed. If a simple iridectomy or filtering procedure is performed, a 5- to 7-day hospitalization usually suffices. A 2-week period is suggested following lens removal (Par. 10:118). Upon discharge the owner is instructed to continue the steroid-antibiotic preparation for about another week.

Postoperative Complications

9:150 Postoperative complications are most apt to occur as a result of faulty technique, or the selection of an improper procedure for the type and stage of glaucoma presented. However, even when the technique is apparently faultless and proper operation is selected, a certain percentage of operations are doomed to failure. Since many procedures control pressure initially, but fail to do so several months later, it is important to establish a weekly, biweekly, or monthly or bimonthly monitoring program (depending on the case) to detect slight elevations of pressure in sighted eyes, so additional medicine or surgical treatment can be instituted before sight is lost. In a blind eye it is advisable to depend on owners' observations, only, to detect impending loss of control of pressure.

9:151 One author[31] reports a minimum of 15% failure at the first operation, and at least 50% at reoperation. He cautions against repeating a procedure which has failed once. Standard surgical procedures used in man have not proved as reliable for the dog.[38] But each procedure has merit. Through proper selection and continued use these techniques will be best evaluated.

9:152 Glaucoma frequently leads to the formation of lens opacities. Cataract, however, may be hastened by operative trauma, and care must be exercised to avoid touching the lens during filtering procedures.

9:153 Other postoperative complications include: vitreous prolapse, wound separation, uveitis, late infection, filtration failures due to adhesions and fibrotic changes, lens displacement, retinal detachment, and phthisis bulbi—to name a few. Continued bleeding or large blood clots remaining in the anterior chamber may cause major complications and failure. The use of the electroscalpel for groove preparation and iridectomies, and controlling all hemorrhage attending a step before proceeding to the next, minimizes this possibility.

9:154 In summary, the surgical treatment of glaucoma in the dog is feasible provided the glaucoma is classified accurately, the proper operation is selected, and the technique is perfected. Permanent tension reduction to normal or below normal can be expected in more than half of all those operated, and a high percentage of success can be expected in certain types, *e.g.* lens displacement. The percentage of success can be expected to be the lowest in any glaucoma of long standing.

9:155 In summary one or a combination of these procedures may be applicable to these glaucoma types. As mentioned previously, cyclocryosurgery is currently preferable to cyclodialysis, cyclodiathermy, or any of the following operations currently available. The intrascleral prosthesis is preferred for grossly enlarged blind eyes.

9:156 *Criteria of control.* Glaucoma can be considered adequately controlled when the pressure stays within normal range and vision is retained in sighted eyes. In the blind eye, the criteria include relief of pain and prevention of further enlargement of the globe. Good signs include clearing of a cloudy cornea, less congestion in the blood vessels of the conjunctiva and episclera, pupil normal or near normal, buphthalmia checked or reduction in the globe size.

9:157 Happily a "burned out" glaucoma occurs in some eyes regardless of the failure of medical or surgical therapy. After so long a time ciliary body secretory function is sometimes diminished. The eye will then usually become hypotonic. It may return to normal size or eventually become phthisical.

9:158 Vainisi[48] reported use of 25 mg of gentamycin injected intravitreally to control glaucoma in irreversibly blind eyes. The gentamycin is toxic to the ciliary body and causes aqueous production to be greatly diminished or cease, resulting in a gross reduction of intraocular pressure and perhaps phthisis bulbi.

9:159 *Procedure:* After profound sedation or general anesthesia, and aspiration of 1 ml of vitreous, ½ ml (25 mg) of gentamycin mixed with ½ ml of dexamethasone is injected into the vitreous through a 22-gauge needle. (One ml of gentamycin was used if panophthalmitis secondary to blastomycosis was present.)

9:160 Moller[47] reported on the use of this technique in 16 glaucomatous blind eyes in 14 dogs. Results were generally good; however, 3 of the 16 eyes became smaller than normal within a month, and one case required a second injection. Cataract formation was observed in all eyes in which the lens was visible. The authors concluded that, although the procedure was cosmetically less acceptable than an intraocular prosthesis, it was a reasonable alternative in cases in which general anesthesia was contraindicated or client cost was a major consideration.

TYPE	*THERAPY*
Primary Glaucoma	
Acute congestive (closed angle)	Miotic; carbonic anhydrase inhibitor Iridectomy (basal) Cyclocryotherapy
Chronic congestive (closed angle)	Miotic; carbonic anhydrase inhibitor Filtering cicatrix Cyclocryotherapy
Secondary Glaucoma	
1. Subluxation and luxation	Miotic; carbonic anhydrase inhibitor Lens ablation
2. Uveitis (adhesions)	Carbonic anhydrase inhibitor Iridectomy Cyclodialysis Filtering cicatrix Cyclocryotherapy
3. Essential iris atrophy	Miotic; carbonic anhydrase inhibitor Epinephrine ophthalmic drops Cyclocryotherapy
4. Injury and infection (adhesions)	Carbonic anhydrase inhibitor Iridectomy Cyclodialysis Filtering cicatrix Cyclocryotherapy
5. Postsurgical (cataract)	Carbonic anhydrase inhibitor Iridectomy; break adhesions; removal of lens debris
6. Lenticular intumescence	Miotic; carbonic anhydrase inhibitor Lens ablation
7. Hypermature cataract	Miotic; carbonic anhydrase inhibitor Lens ablation
8. Intraocular neoplasm	Enucleation
Absolute (blind) *Glaucoma*	Cyclocryotherapy; cyclodiathermy; intrascleral implant

REFERENCES

1. Bedford, P.G.C.: The Aetiology of Primary Glaucoma in the Dog, J. Sm. An. Pract., *16*:217–239, 1975.
2. Bietti, G.: Surgical Intervention of the Siliary Body, J.A.M.A., *142*:889–897, 1950.
3. Boldy, K., Baerveldt, G., and Minckler, D.: Molteno Filtration Implants in Canine Glaucoma, Proc. ACVO, 1986.
4. Brightman, A.H., Vestre, W.A., Helper, L.C., et al.: Cryosurgery for the Treatment of Canine Glaucoma, J.A.A.H.A., *18*:319–322, Mar/Apr 1982.
5. Brounley, D.W.: A Comparison of Pilocarpine Hydrochloride and Epinephrine Bitartrate, Ann. Ophth., *3*:9, 1971.
6. Formston, C.: Observations on Subluxation and Luxation of the Crystalline Lens in the Dog, J. Comp. Path. & Therap., *55*:168, 1945.
7. Friedenwald, J.S. and Pierce, H.T.: Circulation of the Aqueous, Arch. Ophth., *7*:538, 1932; *8*:9, 1932.
8. Galin, M.A., et al.: The Mechanism of External Filtration, Am. J. Ophth., *61*:63, 1966.
9. Gelatt, K.N., *et al.*: Glaucoma in the Beagle, Trans. Am. Acad. Ophthalmol. Otolaryngol., *8*:636, 1976.
10. Gelatt, K.M., et al.: *Consecutive Water Provocative Tests in Beagles Bred for Glaucoma,* Proc. Am. Coll. Vet. Ophth., 1974.
11. Gelatt, K.N., Gum, G.G., Barrie, K.P.: Tonometry in Glaucomatous Globes, Trans. ACVO, pp. 228–229, 1980.
12. Gelatt, K.N., Gwin, R.M., Peiffer, R.L., et al.: Tonography in the Normal and Glaucomatous Beagle, Am. J. Vet. Res., *38*(4):515–520, 1977.
13. Gelatt, K.N.: *Veterinary Ophthalmology,* Philadelphia, Lea & Febiger, pp. 393–394, 401, 1981.
14. Gelatt, K.N.: Familial Glaucoma in the Beagle Dog, J.A.A.H.A., *8*:23–28, 1972.
15. Helper, L.C., Magrane, W.G., et al.: *Preliminary Studies of Tonography in the Dog,* Proc. ACVO, 1974.
16. Hogan, M.J., Zimmerman, L.E.: *Ophthalmic Pathology. 2nd Ed.*, Philadelphia, W.B. Saunders Co., 1962.
17. Knight, G.: The Indications and Technique for Lens Extraction in the Dog, The Veterinary Record, *74*:1065–1069, 1962.
18. Kolker, A.E., Hetherington, J. Jr.: *Becker and Shafer's Diagnosis and Therapy of the Glaucomas,* St. Louis, C.V. Mosby Co., pp 16–20, 1976.
19. Leber, T.: Cited by Troncoso, M.U.: *Gonioscopy,* Philadelphia, F.A. Davis Co., p. 57, 1948.
20. Lovekin, L.G.: Primary Glaucoma in Dogs, J.A.V.M.A., *145*:1081–1091, 1964.
21. Lovekin, L.G.: Water Provocative Test for Glaucoma: Range of Normal Tonometric Responses of the Canine Eye, Am. J. Vet. Res., *29*:1179–1183, 1971.
22. Lovekin, L.G. and Bellhorn, R.W.: Clinicopathologic Changes in Primary Glaucoma in the Cocker Spaniel, Am. J. Vet. Res., *29*:379, 1968.
23. Magrane, W.G.: Canine Glaucoma I—Methods of Diagnosis, J.A.V.M.A., *131*:311–314, 1957.
24. Magrane, W.G.: Canine Glauoma II—Primary Classification, J.A.V.M.A., *131*:372–374, 1957.
25. Magrane, W.G.: Canine Glaucoma III—Secondary Classification, J.A.V.M.A., *131*:374–378, 1957.
26. Magrane, W.G.: Canine Glaucoma IV—Medical and Surgical Treatment, J.A.V.M.A., *131*:456–464, 1957.
27. Magrane, W.G.: Cataract Extraction: A Follow up Study (429 cases), J. Sm. An. Pract., *10*:550, 1969.
28. Martin, C.L.: Development of Pectinate Ligament Structure of the Dog: Study by Scanning Electron Microscopy, Am. J. Vet. Res., *35*:1433, 1974.
29. Martin, C.L.: Scanning Electron Microscopic Examination of Selected Canine Iridocorneal Angle Abnormalities, J.A.A.H.A., *11*:300–306, 1975.
30. Martin, C.L. and Wyman, M.: Glaucoma in the Basset Hound, J.A.V.M.A., *153*:1320, 1968.
31. Meyer, S.J.: The Physiopathology and the Technique of Iridencleisis, Am. J. Ophth., *35*:78, 1952.
32. Pinnas, G., and Boniuk, M.: Cyclodialysis with Teflon Tube Implants, Am. J. Ophth., *68*:879, 1969.
33. Rizzuti, A.B.: Acetylcholine in Surgery of the Lens, Iris and Cornea, Am. J. Ophth., *63*:484, 1967.
34. Schmidt, G., Vainisi, S., West, C., et al.: Retrospective Survey of Cyclocryotherapy for the Control of Canine Glaucoma, Proc. ACVO, p. 55, 1983.
35. Slatter, D.H.: *Fundamentals of Veterinary Ophthalmology,* Philadelphia, W.B. Saunders Co., p. 473, 1981.
36. Smith, R.S., Boyle, E., and Rudt, L.A.: Cyclocryotherapy. A Light and Electron Microscopic Study, Arch. Ophthalmol., *95*:284–288, Feb 1977.
37. Startup, F.G.: Cataract Surgery in the Dog, J. Sm. An. Pract., *8*:677, 1967.
38. Symposium on Glaucoma, Proc. Am. Soc. Vet. Ophth., Dallas, Texas, 1967.
39. Teng, C.C.: Glaucomatous Cupping, Am. J. Ophth., *58*:379–407, 1964.
40. Troncoso, M.U.: *Gonioscopy,* Philadelphia, F.A. Davis Co., 1948.
41. Überreiter, Von O.: Examination of the Eye and Eye Operations in Animals, *Advances in Veterinary Science,* Vol. 5, New York, Academic Press, Inc., p. 67, 1959.
42. Vainisi, S.J.: The Diagnosis and Therapy of Glaucoma, Vet. Clin. No. Am., *3*: 1973.
43. Wright, J.G.: Clinical Case Records, Beaumont Hospital, Royal Veterinary College, 1937.
44. Wyman, M.: Applied Anatomy and Physiology of the Anterior Chamber Angle, Symposium on Ophthalmology, Vet. Clin. No. Am., *3*:439–451, 1973.
45. Wyman, M.: *Manual of Small Animal Ophthalmology,* New York, Churchill Livingstone, pp. 217–225, 1986.
46. Lowe, R.F.: Causes of Shallow Anterior Chamber in Primary Angle Closure Glaucoma, Am. J. Ophth., *67*:87–92, 1969.
47. Moller, I., Cook, C.S., Peiffer, R.L., Nasisse, M.P.,

Harling, D.E.: Indications for and Complications of Pharmacological Ablation of the Ciliary Body for the Treatment of Chronic Glaucoma in the Dog, J.A.A.H.A., 22:319–326, May/June, 1986.

48. Vainisi, S.J., Schmidt, G.M., West, C.S., et al.: Intraocular Gentamycin for the Control of Endophthalmitis and Glaucoma in Animals, Trans. ACVO, p. 134, 1983.

10

DISEASES AND SURGERY OF THE LENS

Embryology, Anatomy, and Physiology

10:1 Anderson and Shultz[2] have observed that the stages of lens development in the dog are similar to those of man. The dog embryo at 23 days is 5 mm long, and at this stage the lens pit is formed. At 27 days (15 mm) a well-developed lens vesicle containing lenticular fibers is evident. It is not until the fetus is 24 to 25 mm long (mid-gestation) that the secondary lens fibers begin to form. These proliferate from the equator of the lens toward the posterior and central portions, forming the lens suture lines. It is during this stage of development that epithelial cells at the periphery of the lens secrete the lens capsule. Cells of secondary lens fibers remain at the equator as the so-called lens bow. This stage of lens development is of concern since inherited (congenital) cataract has its beginning as a capsular lens defect.

10:2 The crystalline lens is a transparent body suspended in the anterior portion of the eyeball between the aqueous and vitreous chambers. The depression in the anterior surface of the vitreous humor into which the lens is set is called the *patellar fossa*. Anteriorly the iris rests on the lens surface.

10:3 Prince's[27] measurements show that the lens is usually about 9 to 11.5 mm in diameter (most frequently about 9.5 mm) and 7 mm thick in the anteroposterior direction. Its volume is about 0.5 ml. Its surfaces are more similarly curved than the lens in man and the lens is biconvex in shape.

10:4 The lens is completely enclosed within an elastic *capsule* which varies in thickness. The posterior capsular thickness is seldom more than 7% of the anterior thickness, the two thicknesses being 3.5 and 50 μ, respectively. Unlike man, there is little variation in thickness in the anterior capsule.

10:5 The lens is held in position by its *suspensory ligaments* (zonules). The zonular ligaments are numerous and dense. They insert on a narrow area of the lens capsule near its equator, but they insert widely in the opposite direction, covering the ciliary processes both posteriorly and anteriorly.

10:6 The lens consists of a peripheral portion, the *cortex*, and a central part, the *nucleus*. The cortex is semi-solid and softer than the nucleus.

10:7 All the lens fibers are bound together with an amorphous medium which appears to be most noticeable just under the capsule.[27] Lens fibers are formed by epithelial cells near the equator (lens bow) and extend toward the anterior and posterior pole of the lens. They are tapered, and join at a Y at the anterior pole and as an inverted Y at the posterior pole. The sheets of amorphous material receive and bind the ends of the lens fibers.

10:8 The lens is devoid of blood vessels except in fetal life, its nourishment being derived from the intraocular fluids. Being a living structure with definite metabolic needs, it must be supplied with nourishment, and the end products of metabolism must escape from it. These functions must be carried on without interfering in any way with the transparency of the lens.

10:9 The formation of new lens fibers takes place throughout life. As the formation of new lens fibers takes place, the older fibers are compressed and pushed in toward the center. This results in an increasing density of the lens from the surface to the center. The increasing density of the center, or nucleus, with increasing age is also the result of a loss of water, as well as compression of the lens fibers. If it were not for this process of sclerosis, the lens would soon grow to a size incommensurate with the eyeball. With this compensating sclerosis a dense, hard nucleus is formed.

10:10 Therefore, after attaining maturity, when ablation of a cataractous lens is contemplated, it is important that the nucleus be removed in its entirety.[23] It cannot be broken up and expected to be absorbed by the aqueous humor, as is the case in the younger animal when discission of the lens, or surgical procedures of a like nature, will bring about absorption of any lens debris remaining in the anterior chamber. In addition, in a young lens the albuminoids are low, so it is possible to get absorption, whereas as the lens becomes older the albuminoids increase in quantity and absorption is rendered nearly impossible.

10:11 The function of the lens in man is to focus rays so that they form a perfect image on the retina. To accomplish this, the refractive power of the lens must change with the distance of the object (accommodation), and is produced by a change in shape of the lens.

10:12 In the dog this function of the lens becomes relatively unimportant. So far as focusing range of the lens is concerned, the dog has distinct limitations. The poor accommodation (ability to focus) is the result of a weak ciliary muscle and a firm lens (Par. 1:3).

Diseases

Congenital Anomalies

10:13 Congenital anomalies of the lens are few in type. A number of small congenital lens opacities exist, but most do not cause visual impairment and go unnoticed. *Persistent* remains of the *hyaloid artery* (embryologic) may be seen occasionally with magnification as a small dot (Mittendorf's dot) on the posterior capsule, sometimes with an attached strand hanging in the vitreous. *Microphakia* is a rare condition in which the lens is unusually small and spherical. With dilatation, the edge of the lens is clearly seen within the circumference of the pupil. The lens may easily subluxate or luxate with a secondary glaucoma resulting. This has been encountered in the St. Bernard. *Posterior lenticonus* is a congenital defect of the posterior lenticular surface.[1] The posterior cortical and capsular regions of the lens have a circumscribed cone-like or globular protrusion of variable size. Opacities may be present in the region of the conus.

Cataract

10:14 *Cataract,* from Latin *cataracta,* means a waterfall; from Greek *kataractis,* meaning to break down or to strike. Medically, it refers to *any opacity of the lens or of its capsule.* It is due to a breakdown of the normal structure of the lens.

10:15 Opacification of its fibers and alteration in water content are the only pathologic changes the lens can undergo, since it has no blood supply after birth. It cannot react to deleterious physical and chemical agents by an inflammatory process, as is true with other tissues. The transport of nutrients and waste products to and away from the lens takes place by an exchange between the lens substance and the aqueous humor. Any changes in the composition of the aqueous, or in its rate of formation, might be expected to influence the metabolism of the lens. Further, since the lens is enclosed in a capsule, changes in the permeability of this membrane are important in the maintenance of a normal metabolism. Loss of transparency (cataract formation) may then be a sequela to this disturbance in metabolism.

10:16 Numerous theories have been advanced as to the cause of cataract formation, but each form is probably due to interference with some specific physiochemical mechanism, this probably being different in each of the different types seen clinically. The loss of any one of these mechanisms is sufficient to produce opacification of lens fibers. The pathophysiology of diabetic cataracts is probably the best understood (Par. 10:31). In a study[18] of dogs with cataracts, the authors proposed that the cataracts might be connected with a parathyroid failure.

Varieties and Classification. Cataracts are classified in various ways and this multiplicity leads to confusion. They have been classified as to how they occur, location of the opacity, rate of development, consistency of the lens, and stage of development. Generally, and in the interest of simplification, cataracts may be classified under two main divisions: developmental and degenerative.

10:17 1. *Developmental Cataracts.* The normal development of the lens fibers and epithelium is affected during growth by heredity, nutritional, or inflammatory changes. This group includes *congenital* and *juvenile* cataracts. Congenital cataracts are cataracts that are present at birth. Juvenile cataracts are ones that are not present at birth, but develop at a young age; in dogs, by 4, or perhaps 6 years of age.

10:18 True *congenital* cataracts are not commonly recorded. They may be first noticed by an observant owner as a peculiar reflection in the eye of a young puppy. The clinician, in conducting a complete physical examination in the puppy, may ascertain its presence. Or, it may be much later in life or never noted, depending upon the degree of opacity. Most congenital cataracts remain stationary for life and many do not interfere, noticeably, with vision.

10:19 In examining 1200 dogs at the age of 4 weeks to 8 years with the ophthalmoscope, Westhues[45] observed this type of cataract in 34 dogs in the form of a disc-shaped opacity in the posterior half of the lens. He also found the opacities to be stationary and concluded that they develop during fetal life or in the first days postnatum.

10:20 Szutter[40] found that these opacities do not extend from the anterior half of the lens to the posterior, but lie at the depth of the posterior lenticular star, *i.e.* parallel to the equatorial plane of the lens. He feels they might be an abnormality acquired at some time during fetal life as a local loosening of the lenticular fibers with formation of fissures, which, in turn, results in the opacities. He describes congenital cataract as "being characterized by sharp contours, a silver-wire glittering, and visible in incident light."

10:21 Andersen and Shultz[2] believe this form of cataract may best be explained as a defect in the development of the secondary lens fibers, apparently as the result of incomplete lens capsular continuity. The etiology of congenital cataracts is obvious if associated with a specific syndrome or when there is a definite hereditary pattern, such as a dominant gene, passing through several generations. Congenital anterior subcapsular cataract of a non-progressive nature with an apparent hereditary factor has been reported in the red cocker spaniel.[26] A congenital autosomal recessive cataract has been reported in the miniature schnauzer.[8,32] Barnett[4] suggests that congenital and acquired (juvenile) posterior subcapsular and cortical cataracts of Golden Retrievers are dominant with incomplete penetrance and variable expression. Rubin[31] suggests that perhaps the posterior polar and the diffuse cortical forms in the Golden Retriever are present in the heterozygous and homozygous states respectively. Curtis[7] suggests that the congenital and acquired cataracts in the Golden and Labrador Retrievers are identical. But in many cases these cataracts seem to be sporadic and are not of hereditary origin. It must be postulated that an intrauterine inflammatory process, toxic, metabolic, or infectious maternal influence can cause lens changes. In one study[16] congenital cataracts were observed in 30 of 38 pups in four different litters. Repeat breedings of the unaffected sires and dams in each instance did not produce the disease entity. Observations suggested that factors other than simple genetic principles were involved.

10:22 We have noted that congenital lens opacities may disappear, remain stationary, or that eventually the remainder of the lens becomes opaque. Szutter,[40] too, reports of the transient nature.

10:23 Another form of stationary congenital cataract may be caused by persistent pupillary membrane (Par. 7:26). Persistent remnants of the membrane originate from the collarette and course in varying numbers toward the anterior surface of the lens (Fig. 7–3). In the area of insertion on the lens there is often a circumscribed opacity (anterior polar cataract) and pigmentation. Varying degrees of opacity are seen in congenital cataract associated with persistent hyaloid (Par. 10:13).

10:24 *Juvenile* cataracts are not uncommon (Plate 17A), and it is with this group we need be most concerned. There is apparently a heredofamilial predisposition to lens opacity, ranging from small opacities to complete involvement and blindness in a number of breeds. Many congenital cataracts of the nucleus or the lens capsule are non-progressive, but most juvenile cataracts progress to complete lens opacity. Both eyes are involved in most dogs; however, this rate of progression is extremely varied. Whereas developmental cataract may afflict any individual within a breed, the fact remains that certain strains within breeds are prone to this affliction. The mode of inheritance of juvenile cataract has not been firmly established in any breed.

10:25 Early (juvenile) cataract development (1 to 6 years of age) occurs most often in poodles, cocker spaniels, wire-hair terriers, miniature schnauzers, Boston terriers and Afghan hounds.[22] Breed popularity and geography will, of course, have a direct bearing on the number seen. Smythe[39] has seen the greatest percentage of cataracts, in proportion to the number of individuals, in the Sealyham breed. When family backgrounds have been made available, it has often been ascertained that a parent or grandparent on either side also had early cataract. Cataract has been reported as a familial trait in golden retrievers,[11] old English sheepdogs,[17] beagles,[13] Afghan hounds,[28] and standard poodles.[33]

10:26 *Genetic Implications.* Not all congenital or early onset acquired (juvenile) cataracts are hereditary, and it is often impossible to distinguish by examination between cataracts that are inherited and ones due to other causes. It is, therefore, best to advise dog breeders to eliminate all dogs with cataracts from their breeding programs, but not incriminate the sire or dam on finding one dog, even several pups, in one litter affected. The exceptions to this general rule include the finding of a cataract that is due to some other obvious cause, such as a penetrating wound to the eye, or finding cataracts in offspring of test breedings in a breed in which the genetics are well established. Although juvenile cataracts appear to be familial in many breeds, the exact mode of inheritance is clear only in the Miniature Schnauzer, and perhaps in the Golden and Labrador Retriever.

10:27 Nutritional (deficiency) cataract is rare in dogs except when produced deliberately in experimental animals. It can be caused by a deficiency of certain essential amino acids and vitamins, especially of the B complex. Barnett[4] describes foxhound puppies with cataract born of mothers fed large quantities of potato chips and little protein. Cataracts developed in all wolf puppies born to a sire and dam with cataracts that were taken from the dam, and fed a commercial milk replacement. No cataracts developed in the wolf pups that nursed the dam. The development of cataracts was attributed to a deficiency in the amino acid arginine.[42]

10:28 2. *Degenerative Cataracts.* The normally developed lens substance loses its transparency as a result of degenerative changes from various causes. In this group are placed senile nuclear and cortical cataracts, diabetic cataracts, traumatic cataracts, radiation cataracts, and cataract associated with systemic disease or poisoning (toxic cataract).

10:29 True *senile* cataract (Plate 17C) with loss of vision is not encountered nearly as often as is the juvenile type. A dog must live to a "ripe old age" before lens changes exert a demonstrable effect on vision. Rather, examination of most middle age to aged dogs reveals a bluish-grey haze back of the pupil which is often erroneously referred to as senile cataract.

10:30 In reality, this apparent loss of translucency is due to *nuclear sclerosis* (Par. 10:9) (Plate 17H). Because the lens fibers have increased in density some rays entering the lens are reflected back, giving the impression that a cataract is present. When ophthalmoscopy is used for the purpose of examining the lens (Par. 2:27) and fundus, it will be noted that the fundus is clearly visible.

10:31 *Diabetic cataracts.* Diabetes mellitus cannot be considered a major cause of cataracts in dogs because the disease is of low incidence. Diabetes, however, whether it is treated or not, will predispose to cataract formation. In those instances when the diagnosis has been made and the dog is under treatment, it may be concluded that sudden cataract development is due to the disease. It is axiomatic that if a middle age dog is presented with only a history of *rapid* bilateral cataract development and a sudden loss of vision, diabetes should be suspected. In the absence of the usual systemic clinical signs of diabetes, urine and blood sugar tests will most often confirm the suspicion. It is also noteworthy that juvenile cataracts usually develop earlier than middle age and seldom with "overnight" suddenness, and that senile cataracts are even slower and in very old age. This places diabetic cataract in a fairly distinctive age group.

10:32 The pathogenesis of diabetic cataracts is fairly well understood. In general, the high level of glucose in the aqueous, acted upon by the enzyme Aldose reductase forms sorbitol, dulcitol and other sugar alcohols which accumulate in the lens. This higher level of sugar alcohols causes an increased osmotic gradient, and causes water to be drawn into the lens from the aqueous. The lens fibers absorbing this increased water, at first swell, causing a clouding of the lens, then rupture, causing irreversible cataract formation. Aldose reductase inhibitors, which decrease the formation of sugar alcohols, will prevent cataracts in diabetic rats, and seem promising for prevention of cataracts in humans and dogs.

10:33 *Traumatic* cataracts (Plate 17F) can occur as a result of a perforating wound of the lens capsule or from a blow to the head. Within a few hours to a few days after a perforating injury, the lens becomes cloudy from the absorption of aqueous. Soon the entire lens becomes opaque. Contusion cataract may not develop for many weeks after an injury. Traumatic cataracts are almost always unilateral.

10:34 *Radiation* induced cataracts must be considered rare in the dog, but should be remembered if radiation therapy is being considered for tumors of the head or neck area.

10:35 *Complicated* cataracts can occur secondary to another ocular disease such as uveitis or in cases of lens luxation, retinal detachment, intraocular tumors, and glaucoma.

10:36 *Toxic* cataract may result from circulation of disease toxins or poisons (*e.g.* naphthalene). Smythe[39] lists distemper-like diseases and uremias as possible causes. Cataract formation is a most important sign to the veterinary ophthalmologist evaluating the safety of drugs in toxicological trials.

10:37 *Secondary (hereditary) Cataract* (Plate 17E). It is not uncommon for the lens to become gradually opaque in association with or following progressive retinal atrophy (Par. 11:66). This may occur at any age. Although the pattern of development is usually consistent, the pathogenesis is not understood. It is unclear whether this type of cataract should be considered developmental or degenerative, so it is placed in a separate category.

10:38 Barnett[3] describes it thusly, "The first signs are usually of cortical cataract, frequently posterior, rarely anterior, sometimes both. The cataract often appears in the form of marks or lines on the faces of the lens and never completely obscures the lens in its early stages. These marks may take the form of a posterior polar cataract or, far more frequently, appear as lines crossing radially from the lens periphery toward its center. As development proceeds the lens substance becomes involved, taking on the appearance of a soft granular diffuse cataract. Later this cataract becomes dense and total and may show the typical "Y" suture marks on its anterior face. At this stage it is quite impossible to examine the retina and the cataract may be mistaken for a primary cataract suitable for operation. The absence of a pupillary reflex in the secondary cataract will distinguish it from a primary one obscuring a healthy retina, as however dense the cataract may be in these latter cases, a brisk pupillary reaction to light will be seen."

Stages of Cataract

10:39 1. *Incipient Stage* (Plate 17A and Fig. 11–4). The opacity frequently begins as streaks or vacuoles extending from the nucleus or just inside the posterior lens capsule, near the suture lines or near the equator. There is no noticeable loss of vision.

10:40 2. *Immature Stage* (Plate 17B). The lens becomes cloudy throughout with an actual increase in the total size of the lens. In this stage a "fundic reflex" (reflection of light from the tapetum) will be still discernible and portions of the fundus may still be seen, though hazily. If both eyes are similarly involved, the dog will experience some difficulty in getting around.

10:41 3. *Mature Stage* (Plate 17C). In this stage the lens shrinks somewhat and becomes completely opaque. A "fundic reflex" cannot be discerned. In this stage the cataract is often referred to as being "ripe" since it can be extracted by extracapsular means without leaving much cortex behind. The dog becomes blind if both eyes are involved.

10:42 4. *Hypermature Stage* (Plate 17D). A cataract may progress from the mature to the hypermature stage slowly or quite rapidly. Progression is more often rapid in young dogs, noticeably in breeds like Schnauzers and Afghans that develop cataracts before 2 years of age. The lens becomes still smaller in size, the cortex liquefies and may become milky or "speckled" in appearance. Finally, the nucleus may sink to the bottom of this fluid (Morgagnian cataract, Plate 16A). There may be a return of vision (second sight) due to the "clearing" of the lens.

Symptoms and Diagnosis

10:43 Ordinarily a case is not presented for diagnosis until an owner notices that the dog is becoming a bit insecure, is missing a tossed ball, or occasionally hits a table leg. Or, the owner may attribute these changes in behavior to clumsiness until such time that the dog experiences real difficulty in getting around. Cataracts resulting in sudden loss of vision (Par. 10:30), on the other hand, will initiate a quick request for an examination.

10:44 As Knight[15] has indicated, "a remarkable feature of cataracts in dogs is the degree of vision retained in spite of their diffuse bilateral formation, providing the retinae are healthy. The lenses have to lose considerable transparency before vision is seriously impaired or lost."

10:45 Therefore, it becomes relatively simple to make a diagnosis of cataract by the method suggested (Par. 2:5 and 2:27). To determine the extent of lens involvement, dilatation of the pupil is necessary (Par. 3:28). A number of tests have been suggested[41] for the locating of opacities and the depth of opacities of the lens. The use of depth perception in the gross examination, with a focal light source and binocular loupe, and proper use of the ophthalmoscope, especially using the slit of light (Par. 2:24, 2:27) obviate the need for employing these tests.

10:46 There are no inflammatory symptoms except when cataract is associated with intraocular disease (Par. 7:46) or with intumescence and secondary glaucoma (Par. 9:84). Hypermaturity may also provoke inflammatory symptoms (Par. 9:85).

10:47 *Predilection.* As has been noted in glaucoma (Par. 9:51), a predilection for an initial left eye involvement in cataract has been reported.[22] Usually the right eye exhibits an incipient stage, but it may well be several months before an opacity is noted in the second eye. In any event, with the exception of traumatic cataract, it is rare when the fellow eye is not soon similarly affected, with blindness resulting.

Treatment

10:48 Medical treatment of cataracts has always appealed to the general practitioner in veterinary medicine. It would be preferable since lens extraction techniques and postoperative care are difficult. Yet there is nothing now known which significantly influences the progression of lens changes in cataract or prevents their formation. Claimed success for any treatment has been based on untrustworthy evidence or advanced by charlatans. Studies[47] related to previous claims of medical success rather conclusively proved that any apparent improvement in vision was not due to medication[25,46] but probably to spontaneous cataract resorption. In the eye undergoing cataract resorption, without an associated reaction (Par. 10:65), atropine (1 to 2%) can be used twice a week for a limited time to increase the pupil aperture and enhance vision. Surgery is the only reliable method for improving the vision in a blind or nearly blind eye. The need for surgery depends upon the vision of the fellow eye and the maturity of the most mature cataract.

Rationale[24]

10:49 Simply stated, cataract extraction is performed in dogs to restore vision, or prevent blindness in dogs in imminent danger of going blind. A cataract is not removed simply because it is there. Without some knowledge of the existing differences in the physiology and optics of man and dog, the veterinarian has assumed that, since strong, convex lenses and a proper refraction are requisites in order for man to obtain useful vision following a successful extraction, surely the dog will not benefit unless a corresponding refraction and an artificial lens also are used postoperatively.

10:50 This would be true, and would render the operation useless in the dog, except that some optical differences do exist. The requirements for visual acuity do differ; primarily, the dog does not need the vision required for the reading of a newspaper nor does it need to pursue an occupation dependent on reasonably good vision. It is important only that this restored vision will enable the animal to live out a normal life, free from the dangers and insecurity associated with bumping into furniture, being struck by a car, or stumbling up and down stairs.

10:51 Briefly, *aphakia,* or absence of the lens following surgical removal, is marked by a change in the focus of the dioptric system, or, simply, insufficient refracting power and loss of accommodation. The point of focus is considerably behind the retina, and convex lenses must be used, in man, to correct the ametropia.

10:52 Without correction, a blurred image is seen and the edges of objects appear wide and indistinct, but the object can be seen. Without a lens, the object also appears smaller. One can appreciate the approximate vision that is present after lens removal by holding a −10 to −14 trial frame lens in front of one eye and looking at objects. The minus lenses compensate for the plus lens in the observer's eye, and give the view one would have without a lens. A common misconception is that a person or animal without a lens would see images upside down and backward. This is not true, because other structures of the eye, especially the cornea, account for most of the refracting power, and the lens provides only the fine focus. As mentioned above, the animal sees a blurred image, but it is erect, not inverted.

10:53 There are, perhaps, other differences with which we are not familiar and which might well have a bearing on the fact that the blind dog sees so well following a successful cataract extraction. Almost unbelievable results have been achieved in a consequential number of dogs which were nearly or totally blind before undergoing surgery.[21,22] Whereas the owner would have been happy to note return of ambulatory vision, many animals were, in addition, again able to run and play without any hesitancy. They were even able to follow and catch a bouncing ball. The splendid natural "motion vision" of the dog is certainly a factor important to the end results achieved (Par. 1:5).

10:54 The success rate in cataract extraction has steadily improved over the years. Whereas restoring sight in about 50% of the cases operated was reported in the late 1960s,[35] the overall success reported by some is well over 80% now and over 90% in select groups of dogs.[29] Success rate is, of course, related to the surgeon's experience,[29] but also to factors such as previous ocular inflammation.[19]

10:55 It is interesting to note also that when Magrane had two postoperative patients refracted by retinoscopy and "fitted" with an appropriately ground contact lens by a specialist in this field, the animals wore and tolerated these lenses and did not object to their daily removal or reinsertion. This bit of investigation was still more gratifying, however, in that, although vision appeared to be improved through use of the lenses, it was satisfactory enough without them to preclude the routine use of artificial lenses on practical and economic grounds. The use of intraocular lens implants in dogs is being investigated by several veterinary ophthalmologists. A lower success rate and the expense of the lenses preclude widespread use at present, but as techniques improve and prices come down, use may become commonplace.

General Considerations; Selection of Cases[21]

10:56 It is not the intent to leave the impression that results following surgery are 100% or that every blind animal with cataracts should be placed on the prospective operative list, or that even when good results are obtained they are to be expected at once. Neither can the results be expected to be constant in a series of the same breed or age group. Some animals will have better close vision, others better far vision, and many will have an adjustment period to pass through before a final evaluation can be made.

10:57 In removing the lens in cataract surgery, we have altered the lens system and the size of the image which falls upon the retina. When the signals thus elicited are transmitted to the brain and to consciousness, they are misinterpreted, especially as to localization. The conscious mind must relearn a skill and interpret the retinal stimuli on a new basis. Fortunately, this adjustment takes place rather rapidly in most instances, but then again "tincture of time" must be prescribed.

10:58 Although all of these considerations are important, they are of little consequence unless the proper preoperative preparation and evaluation of each case are carried out, and unless a good surgical technique is employed, with postoperative care receiving its just due. The optical and physiologic differences discussed mean nothing if the operator is not prepared to devote an unusual amount of time to the perfection of one of the accepted techniques employed in human cataract surgery. There is no "short cut" to successful cataract surgery, and until this fact, well known to the ophthalmic surgeon, is accepted by his veterinary counterpart, he will be discouraged constantly by the results obtained. It is unfortunate that, for the most part, techniques previously described in veterinary literature have not fulfilled this criterion, and the reader has employed procedures which are too often doomed to failure even before they are attempted. Startup[35] sums it up, ". . . the many failures experienced by veterinary surgeons over the past 75 years have been due, in part at least, to the limited facilities and instrumentation available at the time, the lack of suitable anesthesia, and a lack of knowledge of the anatomy and physiology of the canine eye."

10:59 Age of the dog, degree of preoperative myopia, absence of complications, and other unexplained factors have a bearing on the degree of vision return. Failures cannot be attributed to the operation in principle, but rather to poor technique or improper selection of cases. A good basic knowledge of ophthalmology is essential to success. It is not sufficient simply to be an accomplished surgeon. An understanding of the macroscopic and microscopic anatomy and of the physiology of the eye is the first requisite. In addition, a knowledge of ophthalmic pathology is a most important aid in the proper selection of cases. Some lens extractions, even though properly executed, are doomed to failure without this knowledge. It is of no use to remove the cataract from an eye in which the retina has been destroyed by glaucoma (Par. 9:39) or progressive retinal atrophy (Par. 11:66).

10:60 The steps which should precede endorsement of a cataract operation include: examination of the adnexa for infection, determination of intraocular pressure by tonometry, a general physical examination, including urine and blood analysis, in the middle aged and older patient, and above all a *check of the pupillary response to light stimuli*. The pupil must react promptly and normally. Interference or absence of this reflex is indicative of a retinopathy. Even in the presence of an apparently normal reflex, however, it is possible for the eye to be in the throes of a retinopathy which would preclude eventual success as regards return of vision. When the lens is so cloudy that the retina is invisible, the age of the patient, breed, history concerning the loss of vision, and pupillary light response are important to the evaluation. If the history and pupil response is in doubt, electroretinography assumes an important role (Par. 2:64). Unless a preoperative determination of retinal viability is assured, the prognosis must remain in doubt. Otherwise, as the eye clears in the postoperative period, ophthalmoscopy reveals the retinal changes and the reason for the failure of vision return is apparent.

10:61 Other considerations which are important to the degree of success achieved are: adequate practice surgery, a sufficient number of cases for perfection of a technique, and religiously adhering to the time-proven procedures of preoperative care, surgical technique, and postoperative care practiced by ophthalmologists in human medicine (Par. 3:98).

10:62 Those who have performed intraocular surgery without the assistance of veterinary ophthalmologists almost invariably have widely solicited the aid of an M.D. ophthalmologist for their initial attempts. It is then that both the veterinarian and the medical doctor learn that the dog's eye presents a more difficult surgical field than does the human eye. Proper exposure of the eye is sometimes difficult, the structures through which incisions must be made are tougher, more hemorrhage is encountered, and the lens itself is more firmly attached.

10:63 Cataract extraction is not usually performed unless both eyes are similarly involved and/or unless total or imminent blindness is evident. On a number of occasions, I have operated one blind eye at the owner's request, but only if it was apparent that cataract was starting in the second eye. This routine offers the advantage of restoring vision to one eye as the second goes blind. Admittedly, however, the results are not as dramatic since the owner and patient are never exposed to the trials attending total blindness.

10:64 It is not necessary, as it was once advocated, to wait until a cataract is "ripe" (Par. 10:41). Conversely, it is often to the surgeon's advantage to remove the cataract before hypermaturity occurs (Par. 10:42). This often takes place rapidly and unbeknown to the owner and surgeon. The advantage to the patient and owner in performing surgery as soon as blindness ensues is apparent.

10:65 In addition, there is a distinct danger in allowing cataract in the young dog to progress through hypermaturity in the hope that some resorption of the lens will occur, with some vision regained (Par. 10:42). Leaking of lens protein through the capsule or even spontaneous rupture of the lens capsule is not an uncommon sequel to cataract hypermaturity. In this stage the lens cortex escapes through the capsule into the chambers and provokes a macrophagic response. The liberated lens material may be absorbed spontaneously with little or no inflammation or it may result in severe inflammation and even loss of the eye. In most cases, the liberation of cataractous lens material results in lens-induced uveitis and occasionally a subsequent secondary phacolytic glaucoma (Par. 9:85).[10]

10:66 Paulsen et al.[19] report that previous lens-induced uveitis resulted in a marked reduction in the success rate for extracapsular cataract extraction in the dog.

10:67 With these things in mind and, certainly, in deference to the existing blindness, we are reluctant to endorse postponement of cataract extraction in a blind dog for upward of a year as advocated by others[31] unless there is strong evidence that reabsorption is beginning. Nor is the average owner willing to "gamble" on resorption with the possibility of no return of vision or even the loss of an eye or eyes. In any event, if surgery is not performed, it is imperative that the cataractous eye be kept under close surveillance—else there remains no opportunity to intercede and restore vision before irreparable damage is done.

10:68 In conclusion, spontaneous cataract resorption is possible, especially in those breeds so predisposed and between the ages of 1 and 3 years. The resorption process, if extensive, will restore vision but medical control of the lens-induced uveitis by use of mydriatics and corticosteroids is essential. The main potential complications, severe medically nonresponsive uveitis and glaucoma, necessitate immediate cataract extraction.[12]

Surgery of Cataract

10:69 The type of operation needed for removal of a cataract depends upon the consistency of the cataract (stage), the age of the patient, and the presence of intraocular complications such as adhesions.

10:70 The two methods of lens removal are:

1. *Extracapsular.* The anterior capsule of the lens is opened by means of a cystitome or capsule forceps and the lens content is expelled, leaving the posterior capsule and zonular attachments intact.
2. *Intracapsular.* No opening is made in the lens capsule. The zonular attachments are severed and the lens is delivered enclosed within its capsule.

10:71 Variations employed with either the extracapsular or intracapsular extraction include:

(*a*) *combined* extraction—in which an iridectomy, including the pupillary border (sphincter), is performed.
(*b*) *round pupil* extraction—in which one or more peripheral iridectomies or iridotomies, away from the sphincter, is performed.
(*c*) *simple* extraction—in which the extraction is performed without iridectomy or iridotomy.

10:72 There are, of course, advantages and disadvantages pertinent to the two methods and their variations. It remains for the surgeon to evaluate these procedures as they apply to the case at hand and as to his ability to execute the technique.

10:73 Extracapsular lens extraction is preferred in most instances. This is especially true in juvenile cataract surgery. It has proved the safest procedure because of the difficulty and danger attending the breaking of the tough lens attachments (zonules) and posterior vitreous attachment inherent to the young dog. Since loss of vitreous is one of the most important complications in cataract surgery, every effort is made to avoid this complication. The use of intraocular alphachymotrypsin to aid in the lysis of the zonules for the purpose of performing an intracapsular extraction has not proved advantageous in the dog. This is not so much because zonular lysis fails to take place, but the posterior capsule of the lens is attached firmly to the face of the vitreous (Par. 11:3) and separation of the two (intracapsular extraction) will allow the escape of some portion of the vitreous.

10:74 In humans the concentration of alphachymotrypsin used is 1:5000. This concentration produces luxation of the lens within 3 minutes. Stronger concentrations have resulted in significant postoperative complications and there have been reports of adverse reactions at even the 1:5000 concentration. Startup[35] concludes that such a concentration will not produce any apparent digestion of the zonule in the dog. In further trials with concentrations of 1:2500 to 1:500 he noted a definite increase in postoperative complications when the enzyme was used at a strength that would produce some zonulolysis.

10:75 Überreiter[41] is convinced, after large-scale comparative trials in the dog, that the extracapsular technique is far less dangerous. Vierheller[43] has found that the pressure required to tumble or express the lens from the eye within its capsule is often enough to create disastrous vitreous prolapse. Knight[15] attempted intracapsular extraction, but confessed that in only a few instances had he been fortunate enough to find a hyaloid membrane intact after an uncomplicated extraction. His results and percentage of success reported by this method are not encouraging. Startup[35] records a splendid review of the literature, results obtained by others and himself, and factors responsible for failure. Reports of success attending the intracapsular procedure range from 20 to 30% with an additional 20% included in a somewhat obscure "fair result" category.

10:76 Disadvantages of the extracapsular approach are: (1) fragments of lens tissue in the eye which may result in various grades of inflammation. This condition has been attributed to an allergic reaction of the eye to the lens tissue; (2) the presence of capsular and lens debris in the pupillary area predisposes to iris adhesions with a small or occluded opening resulting.

10:77 These pupillary adhesions constitute the most vexing complication attending the extracapsular extraction. Mydriatics and cycloplegics, even when used early, frequently, and in high concentration, have been of questionable value in preventing occlusions when debris is present in appreciable amounts. However, in the young dog these complications occur infrequently if care is taken to keep debris and blood clots at a minimum. The use of the operating microscope to visualize lens cortex, and the use of phacoemulsification and irrigation-aspiration units in cataract surgery, have greatly reduced the presence of lens debris and accompanying inflammation, following extracapsular cataract extraction.

10:78 In one series[21] it was concluded that results attending the iridectomy group versus the non-iridectomy group were about the same. In a later series[22] far fewer iridectomies were performed because improved methods of achieving pupil dilatation obviated the need. Thus, an iridectomy is not now performed unless more working room is needed for placement of the capsule forceps and for the extraction.

10:79 Degenerative cataracts (senile and diabetic) may be extracted by the extracapsular method with good results. We have found, however, that any remaining lens debris in the older or diabetic patient is apt to create more intraocular reaction. To minimize this reaction a non-steroidal, anti-inflammatory agent, usually banamine (Par. 3:66), is used preoperatively and again postoperatively if needed.

10:80 Due to the nature of the cataract (Par. 9:85), a hypermature lens should ideally be removed by the intracapsular method whenever possible. If the capsule should rupture during extraction, it is important that its liquefied content be irrigated from the anterior chamber and that steroids be used in the manner described. I feel certain, however, that the extracapsular approach is still preferable if excessive manipulation, with the danger of vitreous loss, is needed to accomplish the intracapsular extraction.

10:81 The percentage of success could certainly be increased were an uncomplicated intracapsular extraction possible in every instance. The advantage of a clear pupil area and relative freedom from intraocular reaction and adhesions are apparent. But the disadvantage of vitreous prolapse, with its multiple complications, is not to be taken lightly. In a review of the published works on cataract surgery in the dog, we learned that:

1. Everyone agreed that the vitreous is found to be adherent to the posterior capsule of the lens;
2. That loss of vitreous is almost inevitable when an intracapsular extraction is attempted;
3. That loss of vitreous does not necessarily result in loss of an eye, but may result in other complications leading to failure in restoring vision.

10:82 A relatively poor percentage of success has been reported by those using the intracapsular method (Par. 10:75). In Magrane's series[21,22] twice as many extracapsular extractions were successful as compared with the intracapsular type. It is certain that the percentage of intracapsular success would be even lower if this method were routinely employed in the juvenile type of cataract. This type of extraction was used only in certain older animals and in selected cases when it was felt that it might prove advantageous. A success ratio of 80% was achieved on a long-term study[22] (6 months to 6 years) when the extracapsular technique was employed.

10:83 Criteria for success must be based on the knowledge that:

1. The unoperated eye is blind;
2. The fundus of the operated eye is discernible (clearly or hazily) upon ophthalmoscopic examination;
3. The patient has a return of ambulatory vision, can negotiate an obstacle course, and can get along well in strange surroundings.

Failure simply means that the patient's vision has not been improved following surgery. It is usually quite apparent to the surgeon why this is so. Admittedly, some dogs will see better than others and will be able to resume all or nearly all of their former activities. But all should conform to the criteria to be considered successful. If there are those in which the surgical and optical results have been marred by some postoperative complication sufficient to restore good vision, then that eye should be reoperated in an attempt to correct this complication. They then again are either considered a success or failure depending upon the outcome of this corrective procedure.

10:84 *Discission or needling* is a method for correction of cataract that can be used only in very young dogs, preferably under 6 months of age. The cases presented are usually of the congenital type with bilateral, diffuse lens opacity and loss of vision. Discission is usually combined with aspiration of lens content, but the consistency of lens cortex in the puppy often precludes complete aspiration. In one series[22] of 10 eyes in which discission or discission and suction was employed, a 100% success ratio was achieved. These cases were carefully selected and included animals 4 to 9 months of age.

10:85 Essentially, discission constitutes an extracapsular approach. The operation consists of invading the anterior chamber by one of several means, incising the anterior capsule, aspirating and irrigating as much lens content as can safely be removed from the eye, and leaving the remainder to absorb. The entry into the anterior chamber can be made through clear cornea near the limbus with a Graefe knife or Beaver knife with a #65 blade. The lens capsule is punctured with a capsulotomy knife or blade and the contents broken by stirring. An aspiration needle, connected to silastic tubing and a hypodermic syringe (Fig. 10–1) completes the irrigation-suction system required to remove some of the lens content or to expel it into the anterior chamber. One or two 6–0 chromic catgut sutures are sufficient to close the small knife wound. An air bubble is injected aside the suture to reform the anterior chamber. Or, entry can be made under a conjunctival flap on the scleral side (Par. 10:99), and the required sutures pre- or postplaced. A mydriatic-steroid-antibiotic combination is continued for about one month. The aqueous eventually absorbs most of the remaining lens content.

10:86 Discissions can be followed by severe intraocular reaction or even infection if a large amount of lens matter is left behind. Lens cortex is an ideal medium for the growth of organisms.[9] The source of this infection may be the patient's own organisms. Postoperative infection has not been a problem in my experience; however, inflammation and pupil occlusion has been a common problem in small eyes. I will no longer perform the procedure on micro-ophthalmic eyes or ones in which good preoperative pupil dilation cannot be obtained. The use of a Girard or similar phacoemulsification unit, a Peyman or Frigitronics vitreophage or another irrigation aspiration unit will allow more complete removal of the lens cortex and nucleus. Such units are superior to the simple needle irrigation aspiration technique, but are quite expensive.

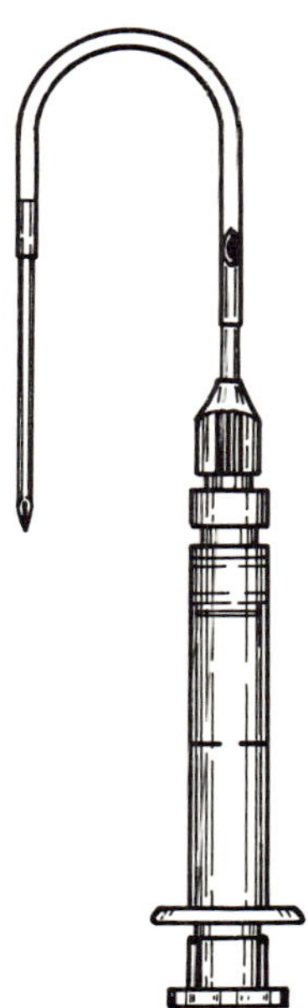

Fig. 10–1. Irrigation-suction apparatus, 1½″ filed 16 g needle and silastic tubing.

10:87 Rapid and extensive swelling of the lens that has only been incised may also cause a secondary pressure rise requiring immediate lens ablation. Severe anterior uveitis following discission is also a possibility. For these reasons, simple discission is not recommended. Discission should always be accompanied by aspiration. The complications following discission and aspiration can be minimized by the pre- and postoperative use of steroids (Par 10:94). But the most important single factor contributing to success is to limit the procedure to the puppy. After 6 to 9 months of age the standard extracapsular procedure is preferred.

Extracapsular Extraction

10:88 It is beyond the scope of this chapter to enumerate and describe all of the variations in technique employed by ophthalmic surgeons. A myriad of books and papers have been written on the subject of human cataract surgery and the interested reader should seek further knowledge in this specialized field by reference to these publications. The principle of cataract surgery, as developed for the human, should certainly be employed in canine cataract surgery. However, certain individual techniques are not applicable to the dog because of differences already alluded to.

10:89 The following is a technique applicable to the dog which has produced gratifying results. Also, instead of giving a complete discussion of operative complications which may preclude success, attention is drawn to important considerations which will prevent these complications.

Steps

10:90 The preoperative preparation of the patient, suitable operating area, positioning of the patient for surgery, instruments needed (with the exception of special ones), and anesthesia required are all enumerated in Chapter 3—General Consideration for Eye Surgery. Mannitol is used routinely just prior to or as an infusion during the procedure (Par. 3:78).

10:91 In addition, it is most important that good mydriasis be obtained and that an adequate preoperative steroid blood level is established. A phenylephrine hydrochloride (10%) and scopolamine hydrobromide (0.3%) combination* instilled the day before and 3 times at 30-minute intervals prior to surgery, is superior to atropine for achieving and maintaining mydriasis during the extraction.

10:92 A frequently encountered problem in the dog is constriction of the pupil when the anterior chamber is entered. This miosis has been attributed to the combination of iris and corneal trauma, causing release of histamine; however, a series of experiments in dogs demonstrated that histamine causes little if any miosis. Rather, the loss of aqueous humor, with subsequent decrease in intraocular pressure, precipitates the miosis.[34] Any preparation that will aid in maintaining mydriasis should be used. Whereas our topical instillations are effective, a subconjunctival injection of a combination of 10.0% phenylephrine and 2.0% homatropine 10 to 15 minutes prior to surgery, has been recommended by others.[37]

10:93 One of the most significant findings to evolve from Magrane's study[22] was the result attending the use of steroids. It was our practice for many years to use topical antibiotic-steroid combinations from the day of surgery and for at least a month thereafter. In the majority of these cases a subconjunctival injection of a prednisolone preparation was also made immediately following the surgical procedure. There remained no doubt but that the use of steroids postoperatively increased the chances for eventual success.

10:94 In view of this finding, the last 89 cases of the total 429 in one series received preoperative steroid administration in addition to the postoperative administration and instillation. Twenty-four hours prior to surgery, 1 mg per pound body weight of prednisone was given by intramuscular injection. At the completion of surgery 5 mg of a repositol type steroid were injected subconjunctivally. In most instances it was apparent at the unveiling on the fifth or sixth day that the eye was "quieter" by following this regimen. In addition, there were fewer postoperative complications.

10:95 There was an increase of 12% in the success in those cases receiving both pre- and postoperative steroids as opposed to postoperative administration only. It is felt that the preoperative use of steroids is instrumental in preventing much of any intraocular inflammation and, especially, fibrin formation that attends and complicates the usual cataract extraction.

10:96 At one time it was generally supposed that the immediate postoperative use of the steroids would be detrimental to wound healing. In my experience this has not been the case. Hubner[14] conducted an experiment on 20 dogs in which he concluded that delay in healing of corneal incisions resulting from use of corticosteroid-antibiotic preparations was of little significance. In another trial[5] the administration of topical corticosteroid ointment twice daily, even when started immediately postoperatively, did not affect the tensile strength of corneal wounds in rabbits tested 21 days after surgery.

10:97 For the last several years, we have been using prostaglandin inhibitors almost routinely, preoperatively and occasionally

*Murocoll #2. Muro Pharmacal, Tewksbury, MA 01876.

postoperatively, since it is known that prostaglandins are major mediators of inflammation in the eye. Aspirin, at 10 mg/pound was helpful, but flunuxin meglumine (Banamine) at .5 mg/pound at the time of induction of anesthesia (Par. 3:66), produced more profound anti-inflammatory effect. The disadvantage of aspirin was that it caused nausea and vomiting in some dogs. The disadvantage of Banamine is that, when combined with deep general anesthesia, it can produce kidney failure, 3 to 4 days postoperatively, probably by blocking prostaglandin regulation of blood pressure in the kidneys. We therefore consider the depth and duration of anesthesia, and monitor kidney function.

10:98 1. *Canthotomy* (Par. 4:11) (Fig. 4–4). Elongation of the palpebral fissure is usually necessary in poodles, schnauzers, and wirehair terriers. It is seldom required, for example, in cocker spaniels, but is of value in any breed if it improves exposure of the eye.

10:99 2. *Conjunctival flap* (Par. 9:139). Advantages:

(*a*) As a solid tissue with Tenon's capsule, it is used as partial fixation support for preparing the groove and making the section.
(*b*) Acts as a mechanical covering for the wound, preventing further access of conjunctival secretions into the wound.
(*c*) Its continuity with the superficial cornea assists in sealing the lips of the wound and keeping them from separating.
(*d*) Prevents the epithelium from entering the anterior chamber.
(*e*) The exudate of plasma and fibrin found from severed conjunctival vessels binds or seals the wound completely. Infection is inhibited, repair promoted.

Disadvantages:

(*a*) The flap may tend to obstruct the surgeon's view of the chamber and act as a hindrance in making the section (easily overcome by holding the flap perpendicularly).

10:100 3. *Preliminary groove* (Par. 9:140). Preparation of the groove with the electroscalpel eliminates hemorrhage, presenting a clear dry field for the placing of sutures. There has been no noticeable retardation in wound healing. Disadvantage—possibility of burning the conjunctival flap.

10:101 4. *Preplaced sutures* (Par. 9:141). Four sutures are usually sufficient for the extracapsular extraction, five for the intracapsular method. An alternative is to always preplace four, and use post-placed catgut if additional sutures are needed.

Advantages:

(*a*) Easier to place in the formed eye.
(*b*) Eliminates the hazard of manipulating the opened eye.
(*c*) Assures exact wound apposition when properly placed.
(*d*) Reduces incidence of shallow anterior chamber, iris prolapse and hyphema.[38]

Disadvantages:

(*a*) Increases the complexity of making and enlarging the section.
(*b*) Loops of suture to contend with (moistening with saline solution keeps loops in place).

10:102 Considerable research[30] has been conducted in the use of absorbable sutures for wound closure. Although chromic catgut continues to be advocated and used by many who are loath to the removing of non-absorbable sutures, the advantages of the latter are established. Non-absorbable sutures (silk, mersilene) produce less reaction, fewer wound infections, and can be counted on to hold the wound firmly closed until healing is well established. Catgut is stiff and more difficult to handle than silk; its knot is less secure and firm; and its tensile strength and absorption may vary so much with the degree of reaction as to render it unreliable for the important 10- to 12-day period of wound healing. Mersilene and newer synthetic nonabsorbable and absorbable sutures often create less tissue reaction than silk but are usually harder to handle because of kinkiness (Par. 3:108).

10:103 5. *Section* (Par. 9:143). The incision and enlargement of the incision throughout should be made in a moderately beveled manner. Beveled wounds have a valve-like action which prevents aqueous leakage. The bevel may be increased or decreased with corneal scissors by tipping the blades. By making the section under the flap and on the scleral side as opposed to through clear corneas, scarring of the cornea is avoided. Very little hemorrhage accompanies a scleral incision, especially when the preliminary groove has been prepared with the electroscalpel.

10:104 6. *Iridectomy.* An iridectomy is not performed unless more working room is needed for the extraction. If dilatation is not adequate or the eye is quite small, it is best to remove a portion of the upper pupillary aspect of the iris to allow for a good grasp with the capsule forceps and extraction of the lens content, rather than traumatize the iris and risk excessive manipulation within the anterior chamber. Startup[36] advocates performing a small sphincterectomy at the 6 o'clock position to prevent an up-drawn pupil. In my experience this procedure did not appear to be helpful.

10:105 Regardless of the mydriatic effect obtained in an eye preoperatively, there is a tendency toward pupil contraction following anesthesia and especially after entering the anterior chamber. This, in my opinion, can only be minimized by the repeated preoperative use of the aforementioned mydriatic (Par. 10:91) and employment of steroids (Par. 10:94). Use of a local anesthetic in the anterior chamber and the pre-warm irrigating solutions advocated by others have not been of much help to me in preventing this miosis. The degree of contraction also differs considerably in individuals, making it almost mandatory that an iridectomy be performed in the patient whose pupil dilated poorly prior to surgery.

10:106 If the iridectomy is performed with the electroscalpel (Fig. 10–2) (moderate current setting), a clear, blood-free field may be obtained for the extraction.

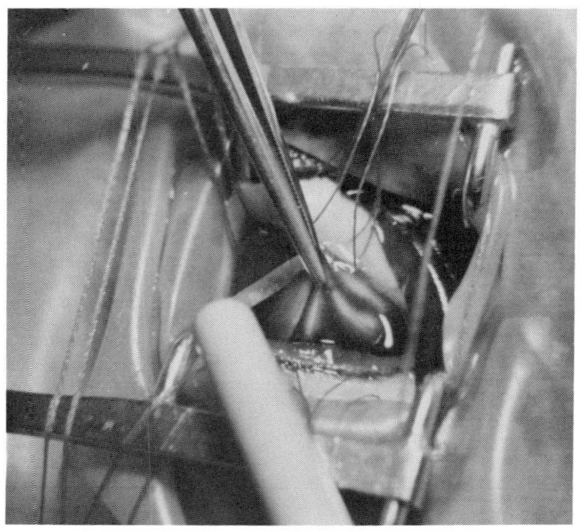

Fig. 10–2. Iridectomy using the offset electroscalpel blade.

10:107 7. *Extraction. Extracapsular*—several ways are used to open the lens. A cystitome may be used to tear the anterior capsule before removing some of it with forceps. In the dog, however, the capsule tends to "spring back" after being cut, making it difficult to find and extract. In an extracapsular extraction it is important that the surgeon removes a large piece of anterior capsule to prevent formation of a secondary membrane and to facilitate removal of the nucleus and as much cortex as possible. In performing the capsulectomy care must also be taken to preserve the capsulozonular barrier and avoid dislocation of the lens. Thus, I prefer the use of capsule forceps (Fig. 10–3) for tearing and removing the anterior capsule. They are introduced into the section, rested lightly on the lens, spread for a distance of 3 to 5 mm, pressed gently but firmly against the lens, and closed so as to grasp a large portion of the capsule, while backward pressure is being exerted. Counter pressure, or a steadying effect on the lens, can be achieved by holding the capsule at the top of the lens or down near the 6 o'clock position with Colibri forceps held in the opposite hand. The capsule will often split at or near the vertical equator of the lens; thus most of the anterior capsule will be removed within the grasp of the for-

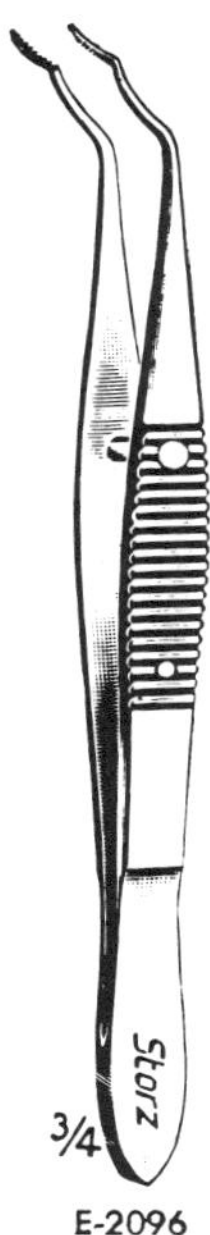

Fig. 10–3. Extracapsular capsule forceps. Storz (E-2096. 3365 Tree Ct. Industrial Blvd., St Louis, Mo. 63122.)

ceps. It is helpful if the assistant holds the conjunctival flap perpendicularly while the capsule is being viewed, grasped and extracted.

10:108 When the capsule has been opened and a sizable "chunk" of anterior capsule has been removed, the lens content is ready to be expressed. In soft cataract (Par. 10:40) some of the cortex will begin to spill out. Irrigation with a bulb of balanced salt solution or saline and curved irrigating needle worked between the cortex and posterior lens capsule of the lens will loosen and dislodge the content. Considerable irrigation is required to remove all of the cortex and nucleus in a soft cataract, and care must be taken that the irrigation process is slow and gentle to avoid endothelial damage (Par. 6:12). Cortical debris may be removed with Weck-cel cellulose spears.

10:109 In mature cataract the mass is first "floated" forward from the posterior capsule with the irrigating bulb and needle. A lens loop is then used to encompass the content just anterior to the intact posterior capsule. A forward and upward movement will bring the solid mass to the incision site. Subsequent irrigation is needed to remove residual cortex. But overzealousness on the part of the surgeon to remove the last bit of cortex may lead to complications. It is better to permit some cortex to absorb rather than use too much force and thus increase the danger of vitreous loss or permanent damage to the endothelium.[44] When a fundic reflex is discernible and/or a fairly clear black pupil is established, the lens content removal can be considered adequate. Weck-cel cellulose sponges can be used to gently sweep the posterior capsule and equator area for fragments of cortex.

10:110 When the anterior capsule has been ruptured in a hypermature cataract a milky, fluid cortex will pour into the anterior chamber. The remaining shrunken nucleus can be removed with the lens loop. Gentle irrigation is then used to cleanse the anterior chamber of the potentially irritating hypermature cortex. At this point the surgeon must be certain that the posterior capsule is relatively clear and that a fundic reflex is discernible. In cataracts of long standing the posterior capsule may be partially or entirely opaque, necessitating the removal of a portion or all of it. If this appears necessary a prick is made in the capsule, it is grasped and lifted with the Colibri forceps, and a section is carefully cut out with the corneal scissors. On occasion I have carefully "stripped" the entire posterior capsule from the vitreal face without complication and with an excellent operative result. Although it is sometimes necessary, I try to avoid breaking or cutting the posterior capsule, as this seems to increase the chance for complication, especially retinal detachment.

10:111 8. *Closure.* The preplaced sutures are drawn up with sufficient tension to approximate the wound. They are not tied at this time. An air bubble is injected into the anterior chamber with an irrigating bulb and infusion needle (Fig. 3–15N,O). This reforms the anterior chamber immediately, thus preventing the eventual formation of anterior synechiae. Reforming the anterior chamber with air also serves to test the integrity of the closure. All lens debris should be cleared from the lips of the wound before the ties are made. A triple tie is recommended. Following the first tie the wound opposition should be checked before securing the knot. This applies to each of the sutures.

10:112 Tenon's capsule and the conjunctiva are replaced and sutured with 5–0 or 6–0 chromic catgut, depending on the tissue thickness. The two layers may be sutured together with a continuous running suture tied on both ends. If a further inflation of the anterior chamber is indicated, this is done just prior to the final tie of the catgut. A subconjunctival injection of 5 mg of a repositol-type steroid is made in the lower conjunctival cul-de-sac area. A drop of the mydriatic (Par. 10:88) and an antibiotic ointment is instilled. The canthotomy wound is closed, a single mattress suture is placed to close the lids (Fig. 9–15) and a bandage is applied (Par. 3:92) (Fig. 3–6).

Intracapsular Extraction

10:113 This method of extraction is reserved for subluxated and luxated lenses and is described (Par. 9:138–9:146). An intracapsular extraction may be attempted in the older dog with hypermature cataract and weakened zonular attachments. A combination of slow torsion and sliding, with stripping of the zonules as needed, are methods commonly employed. Zonulolysis with the aid of alphachymotrypsin has been found wanting (Par. 10:74).

10:114 A study by Magrane to determine the uses and limitations of cryosurgery in lens extraction led to several conclusions. An uncomplicated intracapsular lens extraction with the aid of three types of cryoprobes and two sources of intense cold was attempted in the normal, cataractous, and misplaced lens categories.

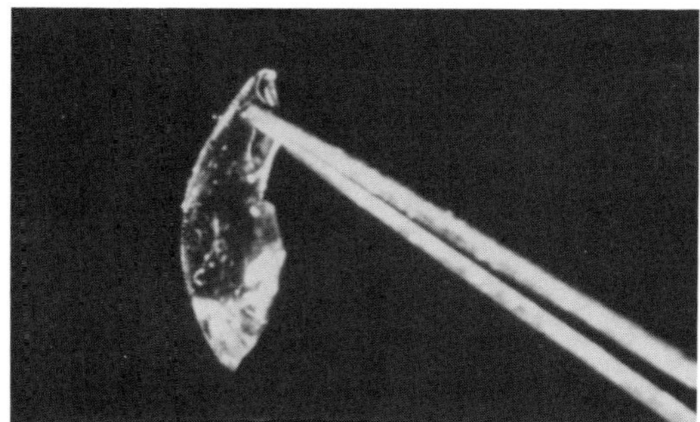

Fig. 10–4. Anterior capsule of the lens separated from the thinner posterior capsule at the vertical equator.

10:115 In those dogs with normal, intact lenses or with uncomplicated juvenile or senile cataract the anterior capsule ruptured at or near the vertical equator leaving the lens content behind (Figs. 10–4, 10–5). An extracapsular extraction was then required. In hypermature cataract extraction the results varied. In some, the capsule tore, even when enzymatic zonulolysis was employed, with the fluid contents spilling into the anterior chamber. In others, without the use of zonulolysis, a successful intracapsular extraction of the collapsed, Morgagnian lens was accomplished (Fig. 10–6). Nevertheless, careful

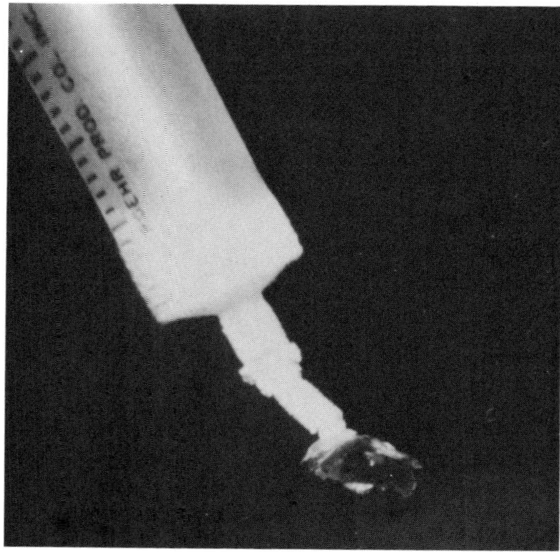

Fig. 10–5. Cryoprobe adhered to and removing only the anterior capsule of the lens.

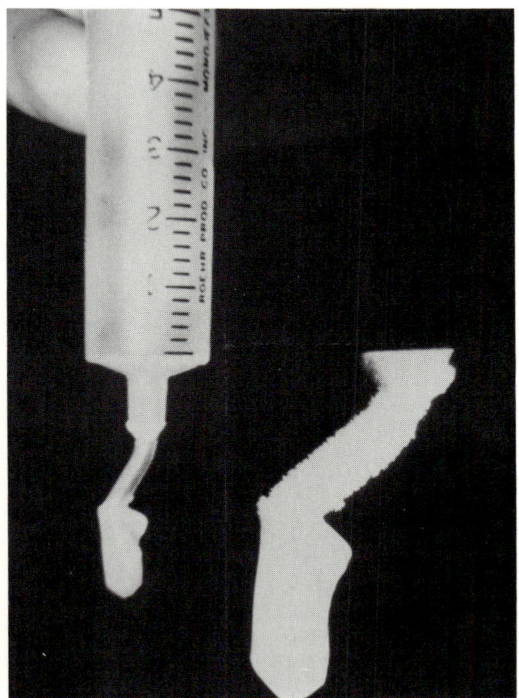

Fig. 10–6. Cryoprobe adhered to capsule and collapsed lens content (Morgagnian cataract) achieving an intracapsular extraction. *Inset,* Close-up of the frozen lens.

stripping of the vitreous attachment with a sable brush or spatula was required.

Postoperative Care

10:116 This is similar to that recommended following glaucoma surgery (Par. 9:147). Bandaging is important for the reasons elicited (Par. 3:91). Dressings should be changed daily with instillation of the mydriatic and the antibiotic used following surgery. Bandaging may be discontinued after 4 or 5 days. In a series by Magrane in which comparisons were made between bandaged and unbandaged eyes, the eyes bandaged for 4 to 6 days "quieted" down and presented fewer complications than the unbandaged eyes.

10:117 The lid suture is removed 5 days following surgery. Atropine and a steroid-antibiotic are used several times a day and for as long as 1 month postoperatively. The corneoscleral sutures are never removed before the twelfth postoperative day (Par. 9:148). The conjunctival suture is left to be absorbed.

10:118 Careful handling of the patient, freedom from excitement, and the use of protective collars (Fig. 9–15) for at least the first week are important during hospitalization. I am not in accord with the practice of routinely sending a cataract case home several days after surgical procedure, even if the patient could be kept quiet at home. Daily checks are important for the first 2 weeks to ascertain possible complications which would go unnoticed by the owner. Insistence on hospitalizing a cataract case for a minimum 2-week postoperative period has allowed recognition of the complications that can occur during that period and to reoperate those eyes before it is too late. *Most postoperative complications occur between the seventh and tenth days.*[22] A few dogs that just will not tolerate hospitalization and bark continually, if not tranquilized, are kept sedated for 5 days and sent home then, if the eye appears to be doing well.

Complications

10:119 *Complications During Surgery.*[22] Of the seven major complications occurring during or immediately after surgery, vitreous loss or, worse, vitreous loss and hemorrhage in the anterior chamber account for a high percentage of failure. This again points out the importance of avoiding a break in the posterior lens capsule and hyaloid membrane, thus eliminating the danger of vitreous presentation or loss Vitreous should be carefully removed from the anterior chamber (Par. 9:145) if vitreous presentation or loss occurs.

10:120 *Postoperative Complications.* The most frequent complication following an extracapsular extraction will be formation of pupillary adhesions (Par. 10:76). Adhesions are unimportant, however, provided the opening is sufficient for light to reach the retina and the aqueous circulation is free. Whereas a large pupil free of adhesions is always desirable, a small pupil and a clear opening to the fundus are often sufficient to allow adequate vision.

10:121 Iridocyclitis is more likely to occur following extracapsular extraction with posterior synechiae and dense secondary membranes a possibility. This usually follows extractions in which considerable cortical debris has been permitted to remain within the eye. In the series reported,[22] failures over the long term were due largely to iris bombé and/or loss of the pupil (massive intraocular adhesions). Other causes included latent glaucoma, retinal detachment (as long as 4 years later), phthisis bulbi, self-mutilation, opaque cornea, after cataract, and endophthalmitis.

10:122 In man, complications secondary to intraocular surgery accounted for 17% of 739 enucleated eyes accessioned at The Armed Forces Institute of Pathology in 1968.[6] Surgical trauma ranked second as a cause of enucleation. Most complications were due to corneal trauma, loss of vitreous or faulty closure of the wound.

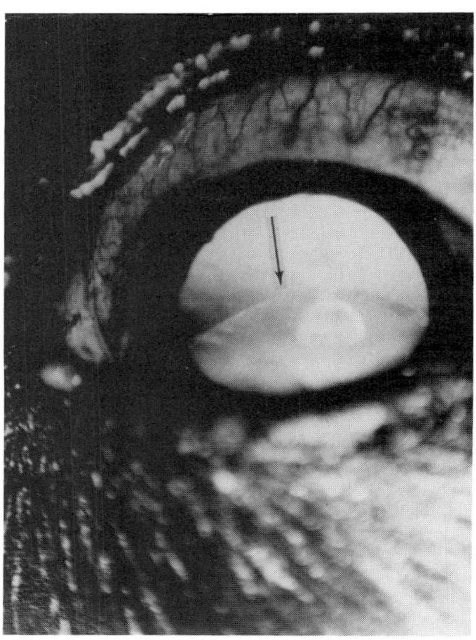

Fig. 10–7. Subluxation of the lens to the inferior position. Lens is becoming cataractous. Note congestion of conjunctival vessels and dilatation of pupil (secondary glaucoma).

Dislocation of the Lens
(Plate 12B and C)

10:123 Dislocation of the lens may occur as a result of injury, from a hereditary predisposition, or from a combination of the two. Increased intraocular tension over a long period can result in lens displacement (Par. 9:68). Dislocation may be partial (subluxated) or complete (luxated).

10:124 Subluxation may consist of a tilting of one edge of the lens or of displacement to a superior, inferior, nasal (medial), temporal (lateral), or anterior position (Figs. 10–7, 10–8 and 10–9). Luxation occurs when the zonular attachment of the lens is completely disrupted and when it has vacated the patellar fossa (Par. 10:2). The lens is then usually displaced anteriorly into the anterior chamber in front of the iris (Fig. 10–10) or posteriorly into the vitreous.

10:125 Traumatic dislocation is generally the result of a blow to the eye or it may occur following rupture of a corneal ulcer and sud-

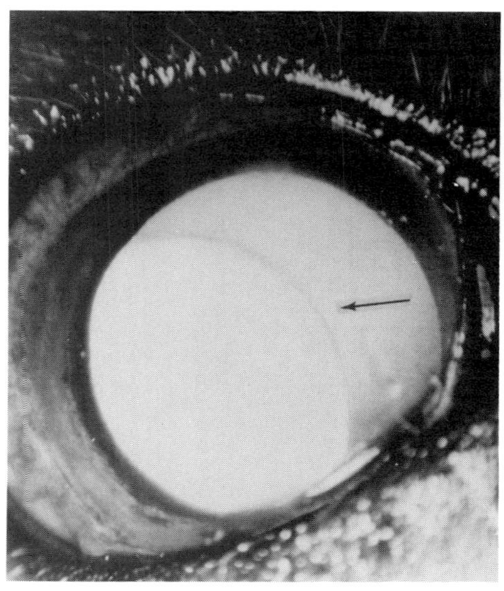

Fig. 10–8. Subluxation of the lens to the temporal position.

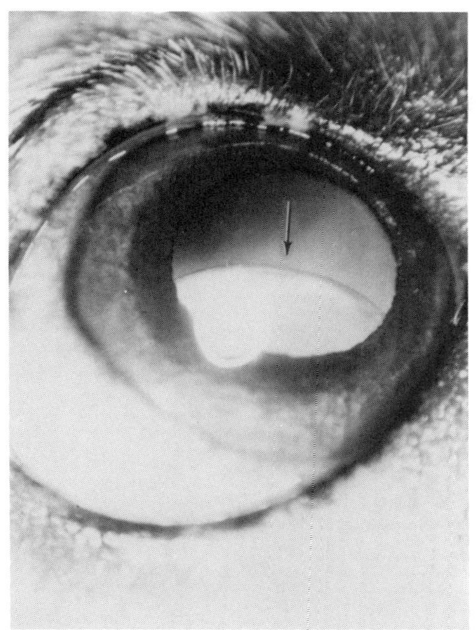

Fig. 10–9. Subluxation of the lens to the inferior position. Note near normal pupil and absence of congestive signs of secondary glaucoma.

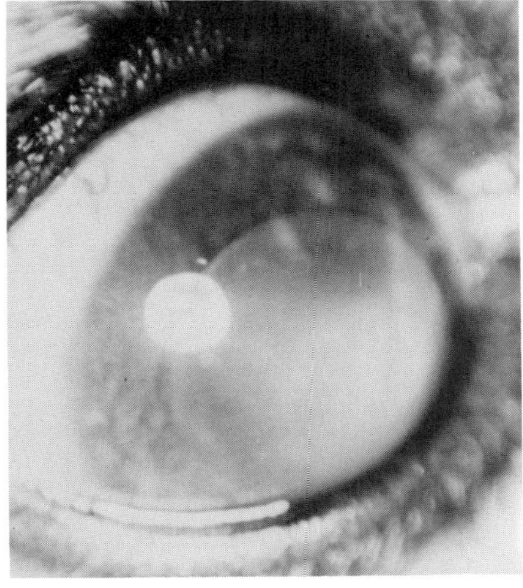

Fig. 10–10. Luxation of the lens into the anterior chamber with adhesion to the corneal endothelium.

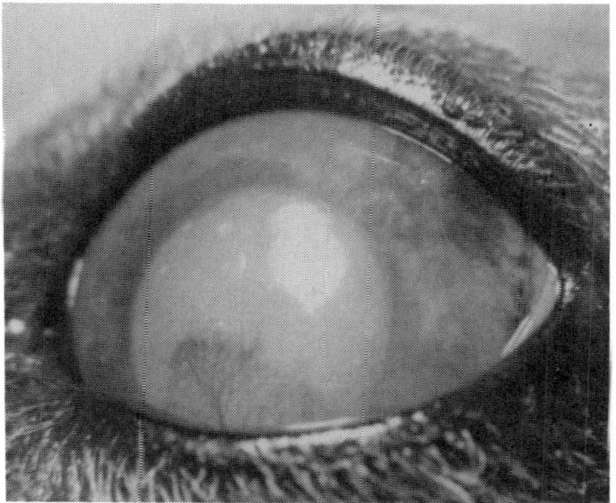

Fig. 10–11. Luxation of the lens into the anterior chamber. Note opaqueness of lens and superficial vascularization of the cornea.

den loss of the anterior chamber. By far the most important cause of lens dislocation in the dog is genetic instability in the suspensory apparatus (Par. 9:65).

10:126 *Clinical Signs.* If the IOP is not increased, the only signs may be iridodenesis (quivering of the iris), and possibly an aphakic crescent (Figs. 10–7, 10–8, 10–9) (Plate 15B) in which an area of increased light reflection in a part of the pupil area is evident. This denotes displacement of the lens from that area. If the pressure is elevated, the signs will be any or all of those of glaucoma described previously (Par. 9:21). Briefly, they are red, watery, sensitive, sometimes painful eye, reduced or absent light reflex, corneal haze, congestion of conjunctival and scleral blood vessels, and increased pressure, as determined by tonometry. Loss of vision on the affected side or sides may be present.

10:127 When the lens luxates completely into the anterior chamber (Fig. 10–10) or into the vitreous, the tension may return to normal with alleviation of the inflammatory symptoms. The completely dislocated lens soon becomes opaque (Fig. 10–11) and is then easily seen, regardless of its position.

10:128 In the early stages use of the Woods light (ultraviolet) is often helpful in diagnosing subluxation or luxation. The clear lens appears opaque and its borders are more easily discerned.

10:129 *Breed incidence* and age (Par. 9:64) are important considerations to the establishment of a diagnosis when the clinical signs are not immediately discernible or prominent.

10:130 *Treatment*. The medical and surgical treatment of lens displacement has been discussed (Chapter 9). In summary, it is imperative that an early diagnosis be made if vision in an eye or eyes is to be retained by medical or surgical means.

10:131 *Prevention*. Involvement of the second eye in the heredofamilial type of lens displacement can be expected, therefore at least an effort should be made to prevent its occurrence. We caution owners to discontinue throwing balls, to discourage violent exercise, and not to allow the patient to pull hard on collar and lead. Daily use of a miotic that will keep the pupil in a partial state of miosis is sometimes helpful. This allows for additional support of the iris to the lens upon which it rests. The owner is asked to present the animal immediately at the first sign of irritative symptoms in the "good" eye. The owner should also have a small supply of carbonic anhydrase inhibitor with specific instructions to give it in case there is any sign of glaucoma and they are unable to contact the ophthalmologist (Par. 9:95).

REFERENCES

1. Aguirre, G. and Bistner, S.: Posterior Lenticonus in the Dog, Cornell Vet., *63*:455–461, 1973.
2. Andersen, A.C. and Shultz, F.T.: Inherited (congenital) Cataract in the Dog, Am. J. Path., *34*:965–975, 1958.
3. Barnett, K.C.: Hereditary Retinal Atrophy in the Poodle, The Vet. Record, *74*:673, 1962.
4. Barnett, K.C.: Types of Cataract in the Dog, J.A.A.H.A., *8*:2–8, 1972.
5. Beams, R., et al.: Effect of Topical Corticosteroids on Corneal Wound Strength, Am. J. Ophthal., *66*:1131, 1968.
6. Bettman, J.W., Jr.: Pathology of Complications of Intraocular Surgery, Am. J. Ophthal., *68*:1037, 1969.
7. Curtis, R.: Hereditary Cataract in Golden and Labrador Retrievers in the United Kindgom, Trans. ACVO/ISVO, pp. 23–29, Nov., 1986.
8. Donovan, R.: *Congenital Cataracts in the Miniature Schnauzer*, Proc. Am. Coll. Vet. Ophth., 1971.
9. Fasanella, R.M.: *Modern Advances in Cataract Surgery*, Philadelphia, J.B. Lippincott Co., 1963.
10. Flocks, M., Littwin, C.S., and Zimmerman, L.E.: Phacolytic Glaucoma. Clinicopathologic Study of 138 Cases of Glaucoma Associated with Hypermature Cataract, Arch. Ophth., *54*:37, 1955.
11. Gelatt, K.N.: Cataracts in the Golden Retriever Dog, VM/SAC, *67*:1113–1115, 1972.
12. Gelatt, K.N.: Spontaneous Cataract Resorption and Lens-induced Uveitis in the Dog, MVP, *56*:331–335, 1975.
13. Heywood, R.: Juvenile Cataracts in the Beagle Dog, J. Sm. An. Pract. *12*:171–177, 1971.
14. Hubner, L.: Effects of Corticosteroids on Healing of Corneal Incisions, Wiener tierarztl. monatss., *53*:75–89, 1966.
15. Knight, G.C.: Canine Intraocular Surgery, The Vet. Record, *72*:644, 1960.
16. Koch, S.A. and Rubin, L.F.: Probable Nonhereditary Congenital Cataracts in Dogs, J.A.V.M.A., *150*:1374, 1967.
17. Koch, S.A.: Cataracts in Interrelated Old English Sheepdogs, J.A.V.M.A., *160*:299–301, 1972.
18. Lapolla, L., and Mastronardi, M.: La Cataratia Nei Giovani Cani, U. of Naples, Italy, Institute of Pathology, 311–320, 1966.
19. Paulsen, M.E., Lavach, J.O., Severin, G.A., et al.: The Effect of Lens Induced Uveitis on the Success of Extracapsular Cataract Extraction: A Retrospective Study of 65 Lens Removals in the Dog, J.A.A.H.A., *22*(1):49–56, 1986.
20. Lescure, F.: L'Examen Ophthalmologique de L'Oeil En Clinique, Actes de la Conference Nationale des Veterinaires Specialistes de Petits Animaux, 37–44, 1965.
21. Magrane, W.G.: Cataract Extraction: An Evaluation of 104 Cases, J. Sm. An. Pract., *1*:163–168, 1961.
22. Magrane, W.G.: Cataract Extraction: a Follow-up Study (429 cases), J. Sm. An. Pract., *10*:545, 1969.
23. Magrane, W.G.: Ocular Physiology—Clinical Application, No. Am. Vet., *36*:563, 1955.
24. Magrane, W.G.: Rationale of Cataract Surgery, No. Am. Vet., *35*:759, 1954.
25. MacMillan: A Comparison of Zinc Ascorbate vs Saline Placebo in the Treatment of Canine Cataracts (Eye of Newt, Wing of Bat—Medical Treatment of Cataracts), Trans. ACVO/ISVO, p, 484, Nov., 1986.
26. Olesen, H.P., Jensen, O. and Norn, M.: Congenital Hereditary Cataract in Cocker Spaniels, J. Sm. An. Pract., *15*:741–750, 1974.
27. Prince, J.H., Diesem, C.D., Eglitis, I. and Ruskell, G.L.: *Anatomy and Histology of the Eye and Orbit in Domestic Animals*, Springfield, Charles C Thomas, p. 82, 1960.
28. Roberts, S.R. and Helper, L.C.: Cataracts in Afghan Hounds, J.A.V.M.A., *160*:427–432, 1972.
29. Rooks, R.L., Brightman, A.H., Musselman, E.E., et al.: Extracapsular Cataract Extraction: An Analysis of 240 Operations in Dogs, JAVMA, *187*(10):1013–1015, 1985.

30. Roper, K.L.: *The Cataract Operation—A Study of Details*, Manual Am. Acad. Ophth. & Otol., 1961.
31. Rubin, L.F.: Cataract in Golden Retrievers, J.A.V.M.A., *165*:457, 1974.
32. Rubin, L.F., Koch, S.A., and Huber, R.J.: Hereditary Cataracts in Miniature Schnauzers, J.A.V.M.A., *154*:1456, 1969.
33. Rubin, L.F. and Flowers, R.D.: Inherited Cataract in a Family of Standard Poodles, J.A.V.M.A., *161*:207–208, 1972.
34. Silvera, C.: Cause and Prevention of Miosis as Related to Cataract Surgery in the Dog, Thesis, Texas A. & M. University, 1971.
35. Startup, F.G.: Cataract Surgery in the Dog, J. Sm. An. Pract., *8*:667–699, 1967.
36. Startup, F.G.: *Diseases of the Canine Eye*, London, Bailliere Tindall and Cassell, 1969.
37. Szymanski, C.M., Koch, S.A. and Silvera, C.E.: Effective Mydriasis for Cataract Surgery in the Dog, J.A.V.M.A., *163*:260–261, 1973.
38. Singh, D.: Pre-placed versus Post-placed Corneoscleral Sutures in Cataract Surgery, Brit. J. Ophth., *47*:116–122, 1963.
39. Smythe, R.H.: *Veterinary Ophthalmology*, London, Bailliere Tindall & Cox, 1956.
40. Szutter, L.: Ophthalmoskopische Und Lupenspielgelunter-suchungen An Neugeborenen Haustieren. II, Acta Veterinaria, Academiae Scientiarum Hungaricae, *11*:issue 2, 1961.
41. Überreiter, Von O.: Examination of the Eye and Eye Operations in Animals, *Advances in Veterinary Science*, Vol. 5, New York, Academic Press, Inc., 1959.
42. Vainisi, S.J.: Nutritional Cataracts in Timber Wolves, Report at ACVO Ninth Annual Scientific Program, Kansas City, MO, Oct. 22, 1978.
43. Vierheller, R.C.: Canine Cataract Surgery, Vet. Med., *52*:487, 1957.
44. Weiner, M. and Scheie, H.: *Surgery of the Eye*, 3rd ed., New York, Grune & Stratton, 1952.
45. Westhues, M.: Arch. Tierheik, *54*:32–83, 1926.
46. Winston, S., Wyman, M., and Martello, M.: Superoxide Dismutase Treatment of Cataracts in Miniature Schnauzers: A Double Blind Study, Trans ACVO, pp. 155–162, Nov., 1979.
47. Yakely, W.L. and Tilby, R.H.: Selenium in the Lens of the Dog, J.A.V.M.A., *158*:1561–1564, 1971.

11

DISEASES OF THE VITREOUS, RETINA AND OPTIC NERVE

VITREOUS

Anatomy

11:1 The vitreous is a transparent, colorless, jelly-like mass filling the chamber of the eye behind the lens. It constitutes 75% of the ocular volume and is composed of 99% water and 1% solids. The primary vitreous is formed during embryogenesis, and the secondary vitreous is secreted by the inner limiting membrane of the retina. It is attached to the pars plana of the ciliary body, the lens and around the optic disc. The vitreous has no blood vessels, but receives its nourishment from the surrounding tissue, the choroid, ciliary body and retina. Formed vitreous is a colloidal gel of high viscosity, as well as some rigidity and elasticity. It contains highly-hydrated, minute fibrillae held in position by the semi-solid nature of the gel. The framework is a collagen-like protein filled with molecules of hyaluronic acid. The gel formation is an interaction between the hyaluronic acid and the protein framework. It is thought that, if water passes out of the minute fibrillae and they become less hydrated, the vitreous changes from a colloidal gel to a colloidal sol, and the fibrillae may coalesce in aggregates to form fibers of microscopic size or a coagulate or curd.[20] One of the principal functions of the vitreous is to hold the retina smoothly in place.

11:2 The outer surface of the vitreous presents a thin condensation, the so-called *"hyaloid" membrane*, which serves to contain the vitreous and separate it from the posterior aqueous chamber. Electronmicroscopic studies[21] of the human vitreous showed that the framework of interconnecting filaments end abruptly in an interwoven net to form the *face* or anterior border layer. No specialized limiting membrane that could be called a hyaloid membrane was observed. Thus, vitreous *face* might be a better term than hyaloid membrane.

11:3 In any event, the lens is cradled on this anterior condensation of the vitreous in what is known as the patellar fossa (Par. 10:2). In the dog the lens is somewhat firmly attached to this "face of the vitreous" (Par. 10:73). When the lens has been removed, the normal anterior membrane is pressed forward by the vitreous. This membrane then becomes more cloudy, seems to increase in tensile strength, and holds the vitreous back, forming a retaining wall between it and the aqueous. I have repeatedly observed this phenomenon following removal of a displaced lens. In spite of the rupture of the vitreous face, a second condensation, which serves to divide the aqueous and the vitreous, appears to form in 4 to 5 days.

Diseases

11:4 *Congenital* abnormalities of the vitreous include persistent hyaloid artery (Par. 10:13) and persistent hyperplastic primary vitreous (PHPV). This refers to the persistence of the fibrovascular tunic of the lens and part of the hyaloid vascular system. It is manifested by a white reflex behind the pupil (leucocoria) or a reddish hue to a cataractous lens (Fig. 11–1). In one report[11] the primary

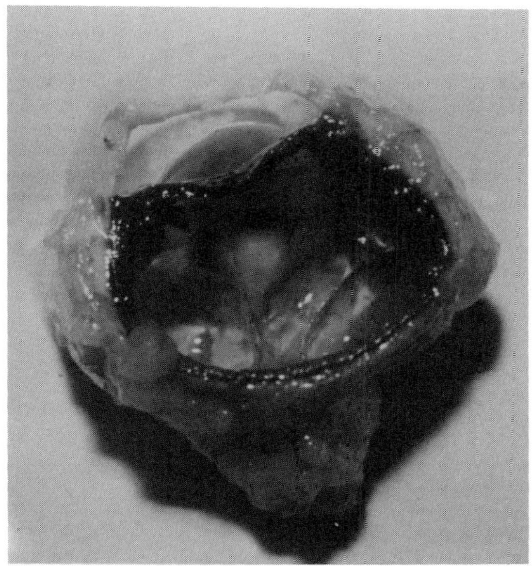

Fig. 11–1. Gross specimen (with calotte removed) from a 6-month-old Great Dane puppy with bilateral persistent hyperplastic primary vitreous (PHPV) and congenital cataracts. There is a stalk extending from the optic disc to a fibrovascular mass on the posterior lens capsule. Blood in vessels in the posterior lens capsule give the cataractous lens a reddish hue.

ocular finding was a posterior capsular cataract, the cataractous material being invaded by fine bright red blood vessels which radiated out into the vitreous.

PHPV appears to be a hereditary anomaly in the Doberman Pinscher[62] and the Staffordshire Bull Terrier.[18,34] The signs include persistence of the hyaloid vasculature, including the tunica vasculosa lentis, at the equator and anteriorly, lenticonus (Par. 10:13), a fibrovascular plaque on the posterior lens capsule, intralenticular hemorrhage, secondary cataracts and persistence of all or any part of the hyaloid artery. In mild cases, the only sign was foci of pigment on the posterior lens capsule.[34] The mode of inheritance is unclear.

11:5 Affections of the vitreous include: (1) degenerations; (2) opacities; and (3) abscesses.

11:6 *Asteroid hyalosis* (Fig. 11–2) (Plate 20B) is a rather common degenerative change occurring in middle age to older dogs. In one series of 300 dogs (beagles) between the ages of 8 and 10, a 10% incidence was noted (one or both eyes). Within this same group the incidence rose to 30% when they reached the age of 11.[35]

11:7 It is characterized by minute solid bodies *suspended* in a substantially normal vitreous. These bodies are of different sizes and shapes with no orderly arrangement and resemble a galaxy of stars. They are seen to move upon motion of the head, but return to their original position in the vitreous. The condition does not appear to cause reduced visual acuity or other symptoms in the dog and will usually go unnoticed unless the eye is examined for some other reason.

11:8 Rubin[48] examined the vitreous bodies of some representative cases of asteroid hyalosis and found them grossly normal. Tests also showed that the asteroid bodies were composed of a calcium lipid complex, similar chemically to that of man.

11:9 *Synchysis scintillans* (fluidity of the vitreous) is an alteration in consistency occurring as a senile change (degeneration) or, secondarily, to disease of its neighboring parts, the choroid, ciliary body, and retina. The vitreous becomes fluid and cholesterol crystals are present. These crystals move as a shower of glittering particles on quick movement of the globe, but settle down to the floor of the vitreous chamber after movement has stopped.[33] Magrane[36] reports having encountered it in dogs from middle to old age, sometimes without any accompanying lens involvement, but in others with cataractous changes beginning. With movement of the eyeball, synchysis scintillans can be likened in appearance to the snow-filled, crystal-ball paperweight when it is turned end for end. Vision is not always appreciably impaired, but with the condition there is a predisposition to detachment of the retina, often diminished tension in the eyeball, and more likelihood of lens subluxation. Synchysis is encountered far less frequently than asteroid hyalosis.

11:10 *Opacities* of the vitreous are not un-

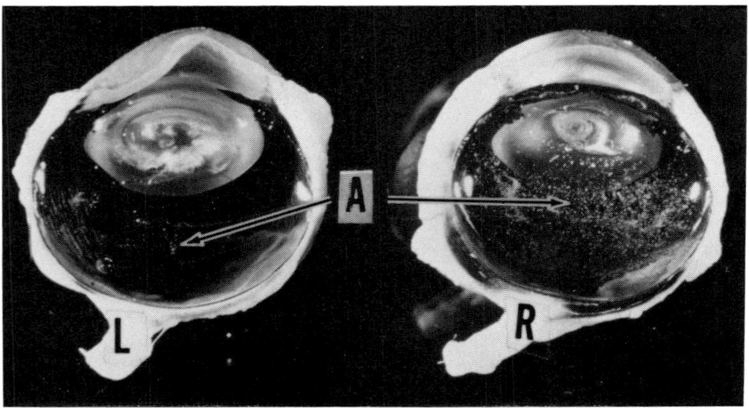

Fig. 11–2. Asteroid hyalosis. Gross specimens of eyes (with calottes removed). Asteroid bodies (A) are numerous in right eye (R). Few are seen in the left eye (L). (Courtesy of Dr. Lionel Rubin, Philadelphia, Pa.)

common. They may occur as a consequence of the changes mentioned (synchysis, asteroid hyalosis), but usually they are the result of disease or of hemorrhages from the neighboring structures, commonly from the retina. A cloudy haziness often accompanies or follows uveitis (Par. 7:46). Hemorrhage into the vitreous may be diffuse or may occur in strands. Vision will generally be affected. A diagnosis is made with the ophthalmoscope or pen-light held at a distance. For a detailed study the ophthalmoscope is used at the proper setting (Fig. 2–20).

11:11 Determining the cause of an *intravitreal hemorrhage* (Plate 20A) is often difficult. Contusion or perforating injury must certainly be considered. Certain systemic disorders (Chapter 12), including bleeding disorders, clotting defects and hypertensive retinopathy, may be held responsible. Strands of blood can be seen in the vitreous associated with retinal detachment. The vitreous may also contain blood when a hemorrhage into the anterior chamber is noted, but this cannot be verified unless the anterior chamber clears. Hemorrhage into the vitreous and anterior chambers has been noted following lens removal for glaucoma. In these cases it is thought that the bleeding is from a retina that had been previously damaged by the glaucoma, and bleeds as a consequence of the lowering of pressure to a state of hypotony.

11:12 Regardless of cause, the blood may be absorbed completely over a 3- to 6-week period. If absorption does not occur, there is danger of organization and retraction of the clot with the risk of a subsequent detachment of the retina.

11:13 *Treatment* consists of giving attention to any possible predisposing systemic disorder, to prevent further bleeding. CVP with K* and Adrenosen† 25 mg, one tablet of each daily for a 25-pound dog, were used with what appeared, empirically, to be favorable results. The value of these products is now questioned. There is no effective treatment for bleeding that occurs following reduction of pressure in a glaucomatous eye. If the owners find the eye objectionable, an intraocular prosthesis (Par. 8:61) should be recommended.

11:14 *Abscess of the vitreous* denotes suppurative endophthalmitis in which the exudate remains confined to the vitreous (Par. 7:63). Treatment is that recommended for endophthalmitis (Par. 7:65).

11:15 Inflammatory debris may, commonly, accumulate in the vitreous in endophthal-

*U.S. Vitamin Corp.
†Massengil, Bristol, Tennessee.

mitis or chorioretinitis due to fungus diseases, such as blastomycosis or cryptococcosis, or bacterial infections. A vitreocentesis revealed the causative agent in 13 of 20 eyes in which it was used in one study, and proved more reliable as a diagnostic aid than a paracentesis of the anterior chamber.[14]

11:16 *Procedure.* After giving a short-acting general anesthesia or profound sedation and several instillations of topical anesthetic, a 1 inch, 22-gauge needle is inserted through the conjunctiva and sclera about 8 mm back of the limbus on the dorso-lateral aspect of the globe (Fig. 11–3). The needle is directed posteriorly, toward the center of the vitreous cavity, to avoid the lens. About ½ ml of vitreous is aspirated for cytologic examination and culture. In these cases, the vitreous is usually liquefied and can be easily aspirated. If not, we should remember that the non-formed secondary vitreous is located peripheral to the formed primary vitreous, and the needle should be carefully directed into a more peripheral area. If the ocular media is clear enough, the pupil should be dilated prior to the procedure, so that the location of the needle in the vitreous can be observed through a monocular indirect ophthalmoscope.

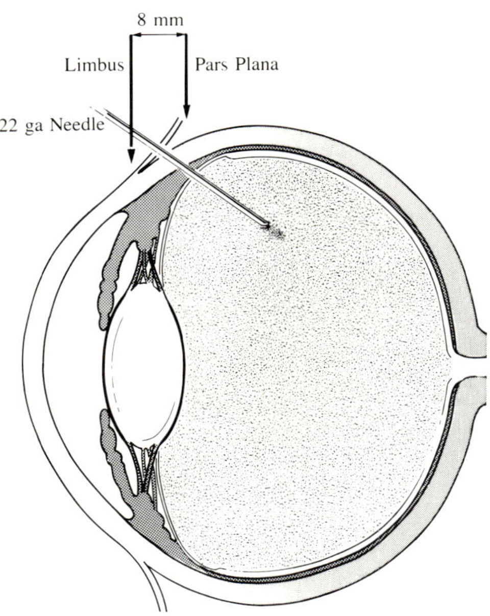

Fig. 11–3. Vitreocentesis, using a 22-gauge needle inserted to penetrate the globe about 8 mm back of the limbus, will help establish the etiology of endophthalmitis.

RETINA

Anatomy

11:17 The retina is a thin, delicate transparent membrane which is really an invaginated extension of the brain (the optic cup) (Fig. 11–2) to which it is connected by the optic nerve and its ramifications (Par. 1:9) (Fig. 1–3). The retina extends forward to the ciliary body, terminating at the *ora ciliaris retinae* (analogous to the *ora serrata* in man) where it becomes continuous with the epithelium over the inner surface of the ciliary body. The retina consists of 10 layers (Fig. 11–4). The outer layer, the retinal pigment epithelium (RPE), originates from the outer layer of the optic cup (Fig. 11–5). The term *pigment epithelium* is somewhat a misnomer in the dog and other animals with a tapetum, because there is no pigment in the RPE over the tapetum. The RPE extends continuously over the ciliary body as the inner pigmented epithelial layer, and onto the posterior surface of the iris to become modified and form the dilator pupillae muscle. The other 9 layers enumerated in Figure 11–4, which make up the sensory retina, originate from the inner layer of the optic cup. Whereas the RPE is firmly attached to the Bruch's membrane and underlying choroid, the inner 9 layers, although attached to one another, are not firmly attached to the pigment epithelium. The sensory retina is essentially attached only at the ora ciliaris retina and at the optic disc. The optic disc attachment is, by far, the strongest. The sensory retina is held in contact with the pigment epithelium by the pressure of the vitreous (Par. 11:1).

11:18 The retina of the dog is about 0.24 mm thick where there is a tapetum behind it, but tapers to 0.12 mm at the periphery, the dimensions being shared by all of its ten layers.[46] Two forms of light-sensitive cells are

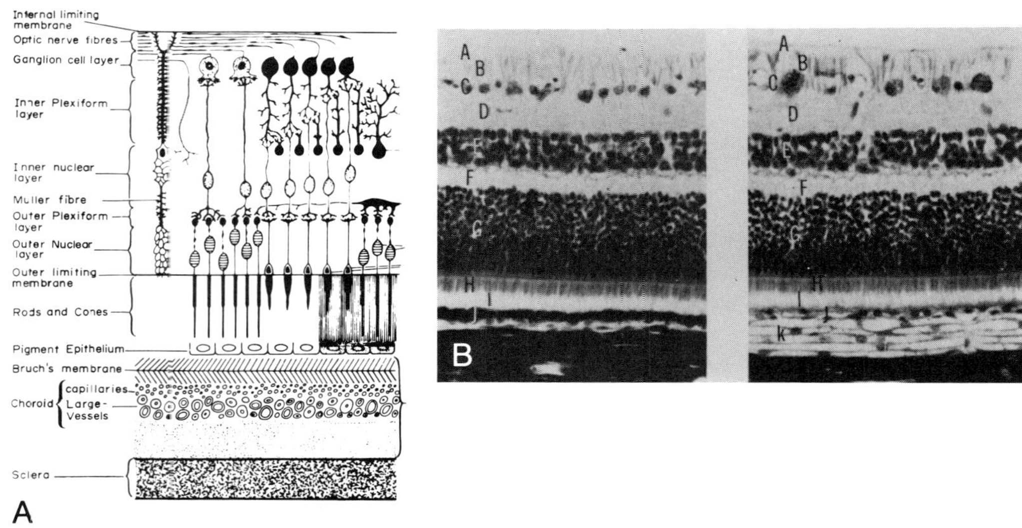

Fig. 11–4. Layers of the retina over the non-tapetal area on the left over the tapetal area on the right. (Note the tapetal cells (k) in the choroid.) (A) inner limiting membrane, (B) nerve fiber layer, (C) ganglionic layer, (D) inner plexiform layer, (E) inner nuclear layer, (F) outer plexiform layer, (G) outer nuclear layer, (H) outer limiting membrane, (I) rods and cones, (J) pigment epithelium, (K) tapetal cells. (Part A from Slatter, D.H., Fundamentals of Veterinary Ophthalmology, Courtesy of W.B. Saunders Co.) (Part B from Anderson, Allen C. with Lorraine S. Good, Technical Editor, The Beagle as an Experimental Dog, Courtesy Iowa State Press.)

found in the layers of the retina: *rods* which are exceedingly sensitive and are used for vision in low illumination and at night; and *cones* which function at higher levels of illumination. Of these retinal receptors the rods predominate, the cones comprising little more than 5% of the total receptors (Par. 1:4). There is no part of the retina actually free of rods in the dog as there is in man. There is, however, an area of greatest sensitivity, an area centralis (Par. 2:52) about 3 mm lateral to the optic nerve. It can be recognized by its freedom from large blood vessels and this is the area in which sharpest vision and discrimination are enjoyed. The cone population of the retina is most dense in that portion.[29] Prince[46] prefers to use the term "macula" for this area because it relates this area to the terminology used for a similar area in the human eye; whereas, "area centralis" only denotes its position, not its function. Most agree, however, that the dog does not have true macula.

11:19 The blood supply to the retina is via the short posterior ciliary arteries, which originate via the long posterior ciliary arteries from the anastomosis of the internal and external ophthalmic arteries (Par. 1:25). There is no large artery corresponding to a central retinal artery, but rather about 20 cilioretinal arterioles that radiate from the periphery of the optic disc, in a holangiotic pattern, to provide a direct blood supply to the entire surface of the retina. Most arterioles lie deep in the nerve fiber layer. The veins also in the nerve fiber layer are larger and darker in color than arterioles. They often join to form a network around and over the optic disc (Plate 1,A–F).

11:20 Pulsations of the veins may be observed, and are related to changes of pressure in the eye caused by eye movements or other externally applied pressure. Modest pressure on the globe by the examiner will often cause the veins to blanch completely. See Par. 1:25 and Par 2:56 for further information.

11:21 Hypoplasia of the tapetum occurs not infrequently in miniature breeds, especially

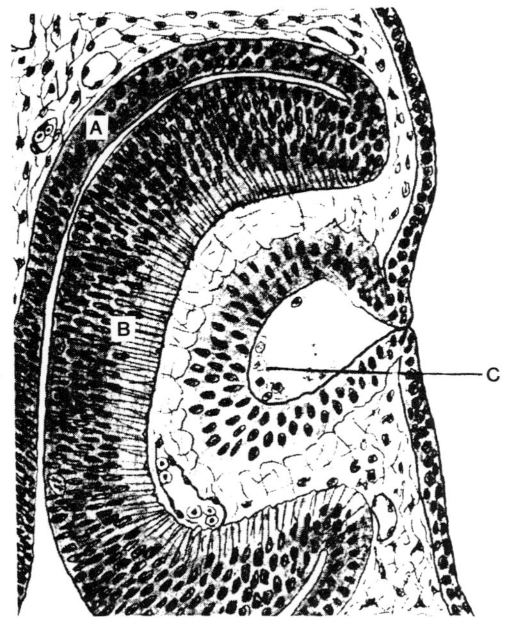

Fig. 11–5. Section through the optic cup and lens vesicle of a 7-mm human embryo. (A) outer layer of optic cup, (B) inner layer of optic cup, (C) the lens vesicle, an invagination of the surface ectoderm, just prior to being separated from it. (After Bach and Seefelder in Mann, *Development of the Human Eye*. Courtesy Grune and Stratton, Inc.) Note that the outer surface of the ectoderm forms the inner surface of the lens vesicle.

the Chihuahua. The tapetum is markedly reduced in size and the underlying choroidal vessels may be observed through the hypoplastic tapetal fundus. Subalbinism of the fundus is often seen in those with heterochromia irides. The nontapetal fundus is usually reddish-brown and the underlying choroidal vessels can be observed through the incompletely pigmented retinal pigment epithelium and choroid. The yellow tapetum may be normally developed or may be absent. In dogs with color dilution, such as the buff American cocker spaniel and the German short-haired pointer, the nontapetal fundus may have radiating red lines representing the choroidal vasculature. This "tigroid" nontapetal fundus is normal for the color diluent dogs. The canine fundus will occasionally be totally pigmented and appear brownish-black with total ophthalmoscopic absence of the tapetum.

Diseases of the Retina

11:22 *Affections of the retina* may be divided into: (1) congenital anomalies; (2) injury; (3) circulatory disturbances; (4) inflammation; (5) detachment; (6) tumor; and (7) degenerations.

11:23 *Congenital anomalies* are uncommonly observed or recorded unless there is an associated loss of vision. Those reported include hypoplasia, coloboma, and retinal dysplasia.

11:24 A congenital hypoplasia of the optic nerve and retina in collie puppies, with blindness, has been described by Saunders.[58] In his series the vasculature of the retinas appeared grossly normal but on histopathologic examination it was apparent that the ganglion cell layer was involved. Our findings in similar cases of near or total blindness included collies with microphthalmia, lens opacities and no visible retinal blood supply or optic disc. Other collies and several poodle puppies exhibited choroidal and retinal circulation, but very small discs. An optic nerve hypoplasia was confirmed in all cases that came to necropsy. Wyman[69] has documented the heritability of an optic nerve hypoplasia in miniature poodles. The mode of inheritance is unknown.

11:25 A congenital posterior ectasia (coloboma) of the sclera (Par. 11:86) may result in retinal detachment and intraocular hemorrhage as sequelae.[55] Rubin[49] describes coloboma of the choroid in a coonhound, in which the veins and arteries emanating from the optic disc coursed around the crater of the coloboma, and small vessels, branches of the major retinal vasculature, dipped into the ectatic area. Histologically, the retina was completely disorganized in the depths of the ectatic area. Colobomas are a common feature of collie eye anomaly (Par 11:84).

11:26 Retinal dysplasia is abnormal retinal development. It is characterized histologically by folds in the retina and rosette formation in the least dysplastic retinas, and by complete disorganization of the retina and often detachment in the most severe cases. Only retinal folds and associated defects in the pigment epithelium have been reported in the American Cocker Spaniel[40] (Plate 18E). The dysplasia in English Springer Spaniels[31] and Beagles[26] commonly appears as folds or patches (Plate 18F) with no other associated eye defects. That of the Bedlington[50] and Sealyham[6] terriers, Australian Shepherd,[24] and Labrador Retriever[4,15,30] is commonly characterized by more severe retinal disorganization, detachment and other eye anomalies, such as microphthalmus and congenital cataracts. Associated skeletal anomalies have also been reported in some Labradors.[15] Dysplasia is transmitted as a simple recessive trait in the Bedlington terrier and Labrador Retriever, and is thought to be recessive in the Sealyham terrier and American Cocker Spaniel. There is usually a normal pupillary light reflex and frequently there is an intermittent and rapid form of nystagmus in severe cases. Although the condition is present at birth, it may not be suspected in affected puppies until they are several weeks old and are noticed blundering into objects. The less severe forms, as seen in Cocker Spaniels, Beagles, and Springer Spaniels usually cause no clinical signs.

11:27 *Injury* of the retina may occur as the result of contusion of the eyeball or luxation of the globe (Par. 8:74). There is usually impaired vision, and a milky edema of the retina and hemorrhages within the layers will often be discernible. Treatment consists of rest and treatment of concurrent traumatic anterior uveitis.

11:28 A transient blindness may result from injurious exposure of a dog's eyes to sunlight reflected from snow (snowblindness). This type of photoretinitis has been observed primarily in out-of-doors farm dogs exposed to rather long periods of brilliant sunlight and heavy snow cover. An accompanying conjunctival chemosis and catarrhal discharge (Par. 5:28) may be noted. The symptoms will disappear upon change of environment.

11:29 *Circulatory disturbances* of the retina, while common to man, are seldom encountered in the dog. Catcott[16] concludes "the fact that retinal vascular lesions are seldom observed and are difficult to produce in the dog is attributed to the resistance of this species to vascular hypertension." However, it must be presumed that cyanosis, anemia, and hemorrhages of the retina occur as the result of systemic disease, but go unnoticed by the clinician unless subjective symptoms of impaired vision are prominent. Hemorrhages of the retina do occur as the result of trauma, blood dyscrasia, lymphosarcoma, septicemia, leptospiral infections, diabetes, heart conditions, poisoning, and in terminal nephritis (uremia). Rubin[52] reports severe and recurrent retinal hemorrhages in older dogs in which blood pressure was elevated. In those which were autopsied, arterial and/or arteriolosclerosis was found and was accompanied by thyroid atrophy. Retinal and preretinal hemorrhage is not uncommon in dogs with prolonged renal hypertension associated with chronic kidney failure. Although retinal hemorrhage, associated with renal hypertension and with hypothyroidism, seems to be more common in the cat, it is being observed more often in dogs, as more dogs with these and other diseases are being examined.

11:30 The shape and size of retinal hemorrhage can localize the lesion within or beneath the retinal layers.

1. Pre-retinal hemorrhage—blood originates from the superficial retinal vascular network and lies in the vitreous on top of the retina, often large and of a "keelboat" shape.
2. Superficial retinal hemorrhage—blood is confined within the nerve fiber layer and hemorrhage is "flame-shaped."
3. Deep focal retinal hemorrhage appears compact and "round" because free blood accumulates in cellular nuclear layers and plexiform cells.
4. Subretinal hemorrhage is characterized

by dull red hemorrhage within and beneath the retina with the vasculature elevated.

11:31 *Inflammation* (retinitis) is seldom limited to the retina but is commonly associated with disease of the choroid (Par. 7:46). It is commonly bilateral. Retinochoroiditis describes inflammation with a primary focus in the retina, but spreading to the choroid. Canine distemper, toxoplasmosis, cryptococcosis and, possibly, toxocara larvae migrans are the more common causes. Chorioretinitis describes inflammation starting in the choroid and spreading to the retina, such as caused by blastomycosis or any other disease that produces uveitis (Par. 7:24).

11:32 *Signs of Retinitis**

ACTIVE

1. Cellular infiltration
   Tapetum—dark-colored; shows dull gray areas with indistinct borders (Plate 20G).
   Nontapetal fundus—gray or white areas with indistinct borders. Nontapetal retina appears dull. Perivascular sheathing of vessels gives a white appearance.
2. Edema
   Tapetum—focal gray areas, often well demarcated.
   Nontapetal fundus—gray.
3. Retinal exudates or focal granulomas
   Tapetum—focal gray areas (Plate 18G).
   Nontapetal fundus—focal white areas.
   "Cotton wool spots" (infrequently seen) are areas of ischemic necrosis in the inner retinal layers.
4. Retinal hemorrhages. Appearance depends on depth within the retina (Par. 11:30) (Plate 19A).
5. Retinal detachment. Cystic spaces between retina and pigment epithelium.
6. Progressive enlargement of lesion or satellite lesion.
7. Haziness of adjacent vitreous (Plate 19A).
8. Defective vision.
9. Uveitis frequently concurrent.

INACTIVE

1. Retinal atrophy
   Tapetum—tapetal hyperreflectivity (Plate 20D).
   Nontapetal fundus—pale, light-brown areas of depigmentation.
2. Pigment epithelial hypertrophy, hyperplasia, and migration.
   Tapetum—focal, multifocal, or diffuse pigmentation, usually within hyperreflective areas (Plate 18H).
   Nontapetal fundus—focal, multifocal, or diffuse pigmentation within pale or pigmented areas.
3. Vascular thinning; sclerosis.
   Tapetum—decrease in size of blood vessels.
   Nontapetal fundus—decrease in size of blood vessels. Sclerotic choroidal vessels show as radiating thin white lines through a depigmented retina and choroid.

*From Slatter,[60] as modified after Aguirre[4] and Blogg.[13]

11:33 *Detachment* of the retina (Plate 18A and B) is a separation of the rods and cones from the retinal pigment epithelium (RPE). It may be partial or complete (except where it is attached at the optic disc) (Par. 11:15), and may affect one or both eyes. Detachments are classified as rhegmatogenous (with holes or tears) or non-rhegmatogenous (without holes or tears). An extensive separation at the ora ciliaris retinae is called dialysis or disinsertion (Plate 18A).

Causes

11:34 Rhegmatogenous detachments

A. Congenital anomalies, such as retinal dysplasia or Collie eye anomaly.
B. Vitreous movement or loss following surgery, injury or luxated lens. Vitreous attachments to the retina produce traction on the retina and tears in the retina. Vitreous goes through the hole or holes, and dissects the sensory retina from the pigment epithelium.
C. Traction by the vitreous following vitritis, vitreous hemorrhage or shrinkage of the vitreous.

D. Following retinal atrophy or other retinal degeneration.
E. Other.

11:35 The hole or holes in the retina are often superior to the area of detachment. In long-standing cases, dialysis or extensive disinsertions are not uncommon.

11:36 Non-rhegmatogenous detachments
A. Congenital anomalies—In Collie eye anomaly and retinal dysplasia, non-rhegmatogenous detachments may occur in the affected area. Tears or holes may develop later.
B. Subretinal masses (neoplastic or inflammatory, such as a blastomycosis granuloma)—solid detachments.
C. Exudate—associated with choroiditis or chorioretinitis.
D. Serous or bullous detachments may be due to hypertension associated with chronic renal failure. Retinal hemorrhage (Par. 11:29) may or may not be present. Spontaneous bullous detachments of unknown etiology may also occur.
E. Other

11:37 *Clinical Signs of Detachment.* Unless or until a loss of vision is apparent, a dog will not be presented for examination. Small detachments do not markedly impair vision and thus will go unnoticed. The dog is presented only when the detachment progresses, or when a sudden, complete detachment occurs. Opacities of the ocular media may make it difficult or impossible to diagnose detachment. An inflammatory, exudative type of bilateral retinal detachment with sudden blindness is occasionally encountered. There usually is no history or findings suggestive of a systemic cause. In some instances there is an associated uveitis. In others the surrounding structures are clear.

11:38 In retinal detachment, the eye usually becomes hypotensive and on gross examination the pupillary response to light stimuli may be normal, incomplete, or absent. During this part of the examination, a detachment may be noted if it is extensive and central (Plate 18B).

11:39 The ophthalmoscopic appearance differs from case to case. The detached portion usually appears grey and silvery. This part may undulate with movement of the eye. A detached portion may be seen as a billowing "cumulus cloud-like" mass which usually has a sharply defined edge on to the normal fundus. The retinal vessels are tortuous and can be seen to run up and down in the "hills and valleys." They may disappear beneath folds of detached retina. The ophthalmoscope setting must be changed constantly during the examination in order to visualize clearly the normal and abnormal zones (Par. 2:38).

11:40 Unless the retina "settles back" and reattaches, a progressive atrophy takes place with eventual obliteration of all normal retinal architecture (Fig. 11–6). Late changes may include secondary cataract (Par. 10:37), uveitis, secondary glaucoma or phthisis bulbi.

11:41 *Treatment.* In man, early operative treatment is essential to success in treating rhegmatogenous detachments. These procedures include: perforating diathermy; electrolysis; coagulation; scleral buckling; laser and photo-coagulation and "vulcanizing" by cryo (freezing) methods. Because of the extent of the lesion in the dog, when first presented, and the special skills and equipment required, surgical correction of congenital or traumatic detachment is seldom possible.[53]

11:42 We have experienced a relatively high rate of success in treating a specific type of bullous or exudative type of nonrhegmatogenous detachment. This typical history is one of sudden blindness, usually in a middle-aged to older dog, otherwise in apparent good health. Examination reveals complete bilateral retinal detachment with no holes in the retina. Retinal blood vessels are often visible just behind the lens. The light reflex is often absent or reduced and the pupils dilated. Renal disease and elevated blood pressure have been found in some cases, but no cause was found in others.

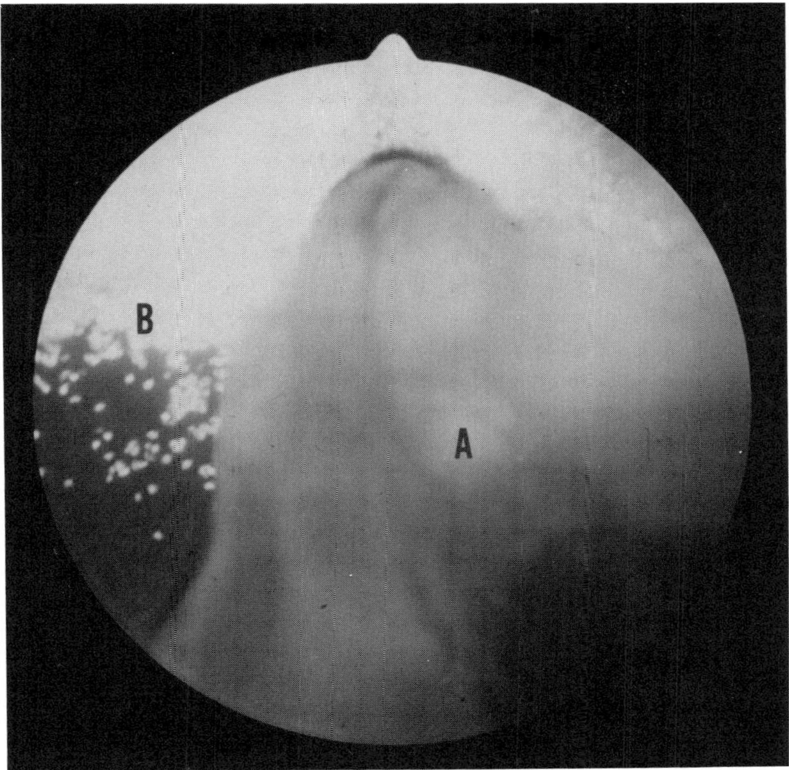

Fig. 11–6. Retinal detachment and disinsertion (A). Note absence of vessels in area detached (B). (Courtesy of Keith C. Barnett, Cambridge, England.)

11:43 Treatment with furosemide (Lasix) for 3 to 5 days accompanied by prednisolone at 1 mg/pound/day for 3 days, ½ mg/pound/day for the next 3 days, then ½ mg/pound/every second day for 2 weeks has given good results. Chloramphenicol at 50 to 100 mg/pound/day in divided dose is usually given for the first 5 days. The retina usually settles back to normal position, and sight returns in 7 to 10 days. Treatment should be continued for at least 2 weeks before a hopeless prognosis is given. Rest and confinement may improve recovery rate. Use of systemic enzyme therapy in the initial treatment has been reported to be helpful, but I doubt its value. If thyroid disease, renal disease or hypertension is thought to be the cause, the prednisolone and antibiotic may not be needed, but dietary and other management of the underlying disease should be initiated.

Tumors

11:44 Tumors of the retina will usually occur secondarily to uveal tract neoplasia (Par. 7:81). Grice and Hutchison[25] described a retinoblastoma, a congenital malignant tumor arising from the nuclear layers of the retina.

Degenerations (Plate 18C, D, E, F)

11:45 The most common affection of the retina is degeneration in its varying forms. Generally, we recognize two types of retinal degeneration: primary (hereditary) form and a secondary form. There is, additionally, a degenerative process of the retina due to probable independent senile changes. Secondary retinal degenerations occur as sequelae to *systemic* disease such as distemper (Par. 12:31) or toxoplasmosis (Par. 12:35), and probably toxocara larvae migrans (Par. 12:56), glaucoma (Par. 9:39), deficiencies (Par. 12:64), injuries (Par. 11:27) and toxins (Par. 12:67).

11:46 In order to differentiate the hereditary form of retinal degeneration from that which may be the sequela to systemic disease, the following diagnostic criteria are suggested: (1) one owner possession since early puppyhood; (2) no history of previous illness of any importance; (3) loss of vision noted to be gradual by the owner; (4) no accompanying neurologic signs; and (5) owner aware of "increased tapetal reflectivity" for some time. In addition, one should find light reflexes that are similar in both eyes, and the lesions characteristic of retinal atrophy should be bilaterally similar.

11:47 In contrast, the retinopathy associated with or following distemper or other systemic disease is diagnosed on a basis of: (1) history; (2) sudden blindness; and (3) light reflexes that may not be the same in both eyes, or marked differences in degree of retinal degeneration. Parry[43] has concluded that the dog distemper virus can cause serious damage to the dog retina, either during the acute phases of the disease, or as a delayed sequela to the infection with a chronic generalized primary retinopathy which may develop slowly one to two years after the primary infection. He has reported[44] cases also of generalized progressive atrophy of uncertain etiology which are very similar to hereditary atrophy but with an onset later in life.

11:48 Thus, because of the difficulty in eliciting accurate histories, the possibility of systemic and local diseases influencing vision may have gone unnoticed, it always will remain difficult to classify the atrophies accurately as to cause. The differentiation is not so difficult by histologic examination. It has been shown[28] that a virus infection is characterized by necrosis of the ganglion cells, whereas in the various hereditary atrophies it is not unusual to find intact ganglion cells in retinas which are atrophic and in which all semblance to normal layer organizations has been lost. It is sometimes possible to clearly differentiate progressive retinal atrophy from other degenerative changes by electroretinography, if the retinas still produce some response.

11:49 The hereditary form, progressive retinal atrophy, has been reported in the literature as occurring in primarily the hunting breeds: the Gordon setter,[39] Irish setter,[27] Labrador retriever,[59] miniature poodle,[9] English setter, English pointer, Norwegian elkhound, English springer spaniel, beagle, and American and English cocker spaniels. But scattered cases of what appeared to be true hereditary, bilateral progressive retinal atrophy have been encountered in other breeds and in dogs of mixed breeding.[37] Barnett[7] has encountered the disease in an additional number of breeds.

11:50 These primary tapeto-retinal degenerations have been classified as *abiotrophies*. Francois[23] describes an abiotrophy as a progressive, partial or complete destruction of a tissue which has begun to develop normally. The destruction is not brought about by inflammation or trauma but by hereditary causation of premature tissue death. An ocular abiotrophy has a number of distinctive characteristics and all of these occur in both the generalized and the central progressive retinal atrophies in the dog.[10] The term dystrophy, which implies progressive weakening or atrophy of a part, is more commonly used now. A rod-cone dysplasia (abnormal development) has been found in some breeds, making the term *abiotrophy* inappropriate for those breeds.

Types

11:51 Initially, progressive retinal atrophy (PRA) was thought to be one hereditary disease. Then, central retinal atrophy (CPRA) was split off as a separate clinical entity. More recently, several mechanisms of degenerative change have been enumerated, and we realize that PRA is really a series of diseases with similar clinical signs. Slatter[60] in 1981 proposed the following classification of retinopathies (Table 11–1), and primary retinal degenerations (Table 11–2). Although the

Table 11–1. Classification of Retinopathies (From Slatter, *Fundamentals of Veterinary Ophthalmology)*

Retinopathy	
Dystrophies	Atrophies
(Primary Retinal Degeneration)	(Acquired Retinopathies)
Generalized progressive retinal atrophy (PRD type I)	Nutritional
Central progressive retinal atrophy (PRD type II)	Traumatic
	Postinflammatory
	Toxic

proposed nomenclature has not gained common acceptance, the tables illustrate well the complexity of the syndrome.

11:52 The following further illustrates the complexity of these diseases. When a Collie with rod-cone dysplasia was bred to an Irish Setter with rod-cone dysplasia, the puppies did not develop clinical signs of retinal atrophy[66,67] indicating that the disease in these two breeds, although morphologically similar, is not identical. Another study[1] demonstrated that, although the early onset of retinal degeneration in Collies, Elkhounds, and Irish Setters appear similar, they are genetically and biochemically three different diseases. This is in contrast to late onset PRA in poodles and American and English Cocker Spaniels in which the defect is carried on the same gene and cross-breeding will result in affected offspring.

11:53 Progressive retinal atrophy (PRA) [Slatter classification Type I (PRD 1)] can be categorized by age of onset and rate of progression, according to Wyman:[69]

A. Early onset, rapidly progressive (onset to blind <1 year of age)
   1. Collie
   2. Irish Setter
   3. Cardigan Corgi
B. Early onset, slowly progressive (onset <1 year of age, blind by 2 years of age)
   1. Miniature Schnauzer
   2. Norwegian Elkhound
C. Late onset, slowly progressive (onset >2 years of age, blind by 4 years of age)
   1. Afghan Hound
   2. Border Collie
   3. Cocker Spaniel—English and American
   4. Collie
   5. Dachshund
   6. English Springer
   7. Gordon Setter
   8. Labrador Retriever
   9. Miniature Poodle
   10. Poodle
   11. Saluki
   12. Samoyed
   13. Shetland Sheepdog
   14. Cross breeds

11:54 1. *Generalized Progressive Retinal Atrophy.* Since, in the early stages, the disease involves primarily the rod cells, inability to dark-adapt is one of the first symptoms to appear. The *subjective symptoms* follow a remarkable pattern of regularity. The dog is shy and exhibits defective vision at dusk, at night, or in dimly lighted places, bumping into objects and moving with caution. The animal is usually in the finest health. The owner may note the pupil dilatation and increased tapetal reflectivity so evident when the dog faces lights at night.

11:55 Electroretinography (Par. 2:64) may be used to advantage in the early stage of this type of retinal atrophy. There is an early loss of the ERG, because of poor rod function and inability of the rods to become dark adapted. No positive b-wave or negative potential can be obtained in cases with good day vision but defective night vision. These cases have a fair pupillary light reflex although the ERG is extinguished.[10]

11:56 *Gross and ophthalmoscopic* findings vary from case to case but, generally, are as

Table 11–2. Types of Primary Retinal Degeneration (From Slatter, *Fundamentals of Veterinary Ophthalmology)*

Primary Retinal Degeneration (Progressive Retinal Atrophy Syndrome)		
Progressive Retinal Degeneration Type I (PRD I)	*Progressive Retinal Degeneration Type II (PRD II)*	*Progressive Retinal Degeneration Type III (PRD III)*
(formerly Generalized PRA)	(formerly Central PRA)	
Rod-cone dysplasia (Irish Setter, Miniature Poodle, Collie)	Pigment epithelial dystrophy (predominantly working breeds)	Hemeralopia (Alaskan Malamute)
Rod dysplasia (Norwegian Elkhound)		
Rod-cone degeneration (Miniature Poodle)		
Congenital night blindness (Appaloosa)		
Unclassified (PRD I) in many other breeds		

Breeds Affected

Type I	Type II	Types I and II	Type III
Afghan Hound	*Border Collie	Border Collie	Alaskan Malamute
Border Collie	Cardigan Corgi	Labrador Retriever	
Cardigan Corgi	English Springer Spaniel	Shetland Sheepdog	
*Cocker Spaniel (English & American)	*Golden Retriever		
Dachshund (Miniature & Long-haired)	*Labrador Retriever		
English Springer Spaniel	Red Bone Coon Hound		
Gordon Setter	Shetland Sheepdog		
Irish Setter			
Labrador Retriever			
Miniature Pinscher			
Norwegian Elkhound			
*Poodle			
Rough Collie			
Saluki			
Samoyed			
Shetland Sheepdog			
Tibetan Terrier			

*Most commonly affected breeds.

follows. In the early stages the pupils are dilated a bit and react sluggishly to light stimuli. Usually the fundi, including the optic discs, will appear normal. As loss of vision progresses, to include day vision as well, the dilatation of the pupils becomes more evident and eventually there will be no response to light stimuli at all. In addition, an increased tapetal reflectivity will be noted, the color of the tapetum appears to change, and the granular beading of the tapetum is lost. The tapetum often takes on an iridescent hue, in which the center of any field being examined appears hyperreflective, whereas the periphery of that field appears pinkish-grey.

11:57 Changes in the blood vessels then become marked. The large veins and arterioles remain at first, but are reduced in caliber and become paler. The smaller vessels, meanwhile, become fine and thread-like, and eventually disappear entirely. Meanwhile, the optic discs become paler, changing from pinkish grey to various shades of grey. Then the large vessels, too, become thread-like and the venous circles of the discs are lost. The nontapetal fundi lightens and the optic discs become pale white, and hardly any blood supply can be seen in the fundi.

11:58 The dogs are totally blind before these final stages, which may take from several months to several years to manifest themselves. In early cases the degeneration may be a little more advanced in one eye than in the other, but as the condition progresses both eyes become equally affected.

11:59 As Barnett[9] points out, "the rate of progression of the atrophy varies considerably from individual to individual, although all cases follow the same pattern. Some owners report a rapid deterioration in vision in a matter of a few weeks, whereas in other cases very little deterioration has been seen, even on ophthalmoscopic examination, in as much as 6 to 9 months. The degeneration seems more rapid early after its onset, the rate slowing down as the degeneration advances. It must be remembered, however, that the dog becomes so accustomed to its limited sight, that by using its other senses to an increasing extent, the true rate of degeneration may tend to be masked. It appears that in most cases dogs affected early in life progress to blindness more rapidly than do those which show the first signs of atrophy at a later age."

11:60 Often the owner will exclaim that his pet has gone blind "overnight." In these instances peripheral vision has been gradually lost (Fig. 11–7), but has gone unnoticed by the owners. Then when the central vision is affected, the dog's ability to see immediate objects is lost and the assumption is made that blindness was sudden. Although in the early stages of progressive retinal atrophy (PRD 1), the deterioration of rod cells, and hence ability to dark-adapt, starts centrally and progresses toward the periphery; in the late stage, the final atrophy and loss of sight progresses from the periphery toward the center. Sudden blindness is also sometimes reported by an owner who takes the dog into an unfamiliar environment, and suddenly realizes that the dog cannot see. Ophthalmoscopic examination will readily disclose the progressive changes that have ensued.

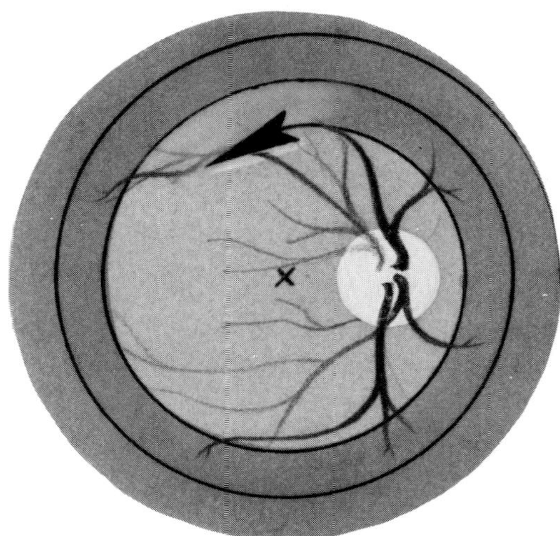

Fig. 11–7. Mode of progressive loss of vision. Arrow denotes loss from periphery toward the area centralis (X).

11:61 *Stages.* The changes in the fundi of the affected eyes have been described in stages.[61] For sake of convenience, the progressive findings can be divided into grades one through four.

11:62 *Grade 1.* Pupils semi-dilated and sluggish to response. Increased tapetal reflectivity, some loss of granular beading, small vessels diminished in caliber and peripheral circulation disappearing. Large venules and arterioles two-thirds normal size.

11:63 *Grade 2.* Pupils dilated, little response. Increased tapetal reflectivity, granular beading nearly gone, smaller vessels nearly all gone, major venules and arterioles one-half normal size, discs paler than normal, non-tapetal fundi lighter.

11:64 *Grade 3.* Pupils dilated, little to no response. Increased tapetal reflectivity, granular beading nearly gone or gone, small vessels completely gone, major venules and arterioles one-third normal size, discs pale, non-tapetal fundi lighter (ashen overcast).

11:65 *Grade 4.* Pupils in full dilatation and no response. Increased tapetal reflectivity, granular beading gone, all vessels gone except, possibly, at venous circle. Discs ashen white to white. (Total blindness.)

11:66 Cataract, secondary to retinal atrophy (Par. 10:37) (Plate 17E), will develop in a high percentage of the cases examined. The cataract may be slow or rapid in its development and may affect one eye before the other (Fig. 11–8). Its formation has been described (Par. 10:38).

11:67 *Histologically,* the main change is disappearance of the rods and cones together with reduction in width of the outer nuclear layer. Neither proliferation nor migration occurs from the pigment epithelium layer. The degenerative changes occur throughout the retina but are most severe at the periphery with a gradual change to less advanced degeneration in the area immediately surrounding the optic disc.[10]

11:68 The mode of inheritance of generalized PRA has been determined to be autosomal recessive in the Irish Setter, Miniature Poodle, Norwegian Elkhound and Collie. Clinical observations are consistent with an autosomal recessive mode of inheritance for PRA in other breeds as well. As mentioned previously (Par. 11:55), although PRA in several breeds appears similar, follows a similar clinical course, and is autosomal recessive, it is not inherited similarly in all breeds; and cross breeding of affected animals did not produce affected offspring in the 3 breeds studied.[1]

11:69 2. *Central progressive retinal atrophy* (CPRA) (Slatter PRD type II)[7,8,10] is also bilateral and progressive. Although CPRA still occurs rather commonly in the United Kingdom and continental Europe, it is much less common now in the U.S. The Labrador Retriever, Border Collie, English Springer Spaniel, Golden Retriever, Shetland Sheepdog and Red Bone Hound are among the breeds afflicted. Note that both PRA and

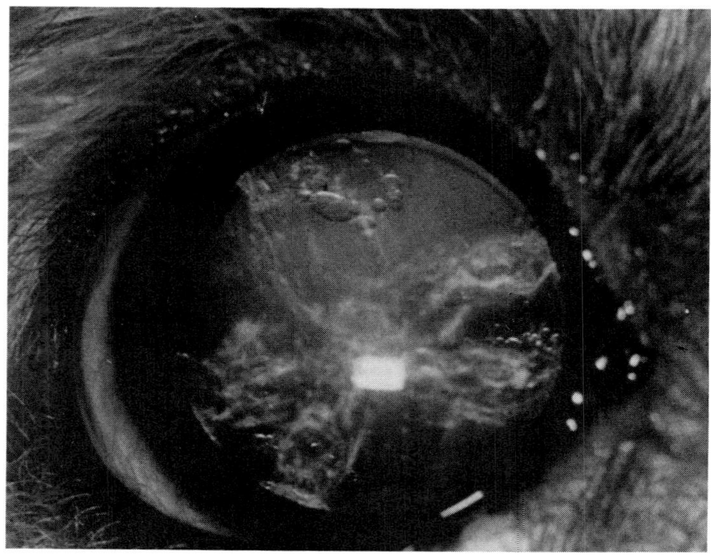

Fig. 11–8. Incipient cataract secondary to progressive retinal atrophy. Note vacuoles and streaks extending into the cortex, and dilatation of the pupil. (Courtesy of Keith C. Barnett, Cambridge, England.)

CPRA occur in the Border Collie, Labrador Retriever, Shetland Sheepdog and English Springer Spaniel (Table 11–2).

11:70 There is an early loss of central vision, with changes in the tapetal fundus, but peripheral vision may be retained for years. The pupil is normal in size and reaction early in the course, but as the retinal atrophy progresses the pupil becomes dilated and the light reflex is incomplete. Central vision loss is the main sign and dogs will often see moving objects until the atrophy is far advanced. A gun dog will see a shot bird fall but may be unable to mark it and may over-run it in the retrieve. Afflicted dogs will collide with objects directly in their path.

11:71 The electroretinogram is present until late in the course of central retinal atrophy. Unlike the generalized form an electroretinogram can be obtained when obvious ophthalmoscopic changes are present in the fundus.

11:72 *Ophthalmoscopically*, the optic disc is unchanged in the early stages but takes on a pallor in more advanced cases. In the beginning the blood vessels show no changes but later there is a narrowing. However, the narrowing of the retinal vessels in advanced cases is not the main fundus finding as it is in generalized progressive retinal atrophy. The tapetal or central fundus shows the first and main changes which take the form of brown pigment deposits scattered throughout the area (Plate 18O). The tapetum between this pigmented area increases in reflectivity. Eventually the deposits becomes less distinct and may even disappear in advanced cases.

11:73 The non-tapetal fundus is unchanged in the early course but as the atrophy progresses it assumes a "washed out" grey-brown color and sheen. Secondary cataract is less common in central retinal atrophy than in the generalized form (Par. 11:66).

11:74 *Histologically* the pigment epithelium in the central region shows the main change. This takes the form of hypertrophy with large cells, containing pale brown pigment granules, projecting into the inner retinal layers. These granules have been identified as lipofuscin.[5] The histopathologic changes are confined to the central retina in the early stages and the peripheral retina is unaffected until late in the course of the disease. There is a sharp line of demarcation between the affected and unaffected parts of the retina.

11:75 Although this type of retinal degeneration involves a significant number of breeds (Table 11–2) and a familial predisposition is indicated, the exact mode of inheritance is yet to be determined. It is thought by some to be dominant with incomplete penetrance.

11:76 *Treatment.* No treatment is of any value. Vitamin H was prescribed by some, in the past, but it has not been demonstrated to improve vision or retard progression of the disease.

Summation

11:77 Retinal atrophy in its two forms (PRA and CPRA) represents one of the most frequent intraocular diseases affecting many of the purebred and mixed breeds. Upon presentation the patient is invariably showing some degree of visual impairment, defective night vision in PRA and loss of central vision in CPRA. Secondary cataracts are commonly associated with PRA, less so with CPRA. The pupils may be somewhat dilated and sluggish in response to light stimuli. The age at which the clinical and ophthalmoscopic signs are first noted varies with the different breeds and the type of atrophy. The rate of progression also varies considerably from individual to individual. In general, the endstage is characterized ophthalmoscopically by retinal thinning and tapetal reflectivity, marked retinal vascular attenuation, and secondary atrophy of the optic disc. All treatments for retinal atrophy are invariably unsuccessful. Affected dogs, their parents and progeny must not be used for breeding.

11:78 *Hemeralopia*, a hereditary day blindness, has been reported in the Alaskan malamute.[54] The disease is classically seen in young dogs between 6 and 10 weeks of age when they are presented because of sudden and apparently complete blindness. The puppies have normal vision in dim light. Helpful diagnostic signs are a normal direct and consensual pupillary light response, normal appearing retinae, and absence of nystagmus. This disease is inherited as a simple recessive trait but selective breeding has resulted in the almost complete elimination of the disease from the breed. Diagnosis can be confirmed by electroretinography.

OPTIC NERVE

Anatomy

11:79 The optic nerve may be divided into (1) an *intraocular* portion, the head of the optic nerve; (2) an *orbital* portion extending from the eyeball to the optic foramen; and (3) an *intracranial* portion situated between the optic foramen and the chiasm.

11:80 The nerve varies from 1.2 to 2.4 mm in diameter including its sheaths until it enters the eye with the retinal vessels to form the nerve head or disc.[46] The disc (optic papilla) (Par. 2:58) measures about 1 mm in diameter, and is slightly below (about 2 mm) and lateral (about 1 mm) to the posterior pole of the globe. It varies in color as well as shape. It can be round, oval, triangular or quadrangular in appearance. As the optic nerve enters the myelin sheath may stop at the lamina cribrosa and the nerve becomes transparent (Plate 1D). However, the myelin may continue with the nerve fibers through the lamina cribrosa of the globe and out into the nerve fiber layer of the retina (Plate 1E). This myelin accounts for the variety of shapes and sizes of the optic disc (Par. 11:84).

11:81 The orbital portion of the optic nerve presents a curve, permitting free movement of the eyeball. It is enclosed within a dural sheath continuous with that of the brain, and therefore becomes a compact and enclosed pathway which has no connection with any other neural path until it reaches the cranial cavity. Once outside the orbits, the two optic nerves meet (chiasm) and decussate with each other before distributing to the lateral geniculate bodies (Fig. 1–3).

Diseases of the Optic Nerve

11:82 Affections of the optic nerve include: (1) congenital anomalies; (2) tumors; (3) atrophy; (4) papilledema (choked disc) and (5) optic neuritis.

11:83 *Congenital anomalies* include myelinated nerve fibers, coloboma, hypoplasia, and the "collie eye anomaly." Hypoplasia of the optic nerve and retina has been described (Par. 11:24).

11:84 Myelinated nerve fibers (Plate 1E) appear as white fiber bundles with featherlike margins or an actual flame-shaped enlargement of the fibers of the optic nerve stops at the disc margin. Occasionally, however, this myelinization overshoots and extends into the retina. This is a harmless anomaly which has little effect on vision. It is so common that it might be considered a variation of normal.

11:85 Typical colobomatous defects have been reported in the basenji breed in both the United States and England. It has been described as a colobomatous cupping into which the retinal vessels disappear. Colobomata of the peripapillary region have also been seen, as have small pits within the disc. There ordinarily is no effect on vision.

11:86 The most common anomaly involving the optic nerve head and surrounding structures was first[38] described as an excavation of the optic disc (Plate 19F). Since that time other researchers have employed the terms coloboma of the optic disc, congenital posterior ectasia of the sclera,[55] or simply the *collie eye anomaly.*

11:87 *Occurrence.* Different investigators[17,19,68] report the anomaly as occurring in from 75 to 90% of all purebred collie stock. The condition is bilateral but the clinical manifestations in paired eyes of one individual may be asymmetrical. This may range from one eye having only a slight pale area (choroidal hypoplasia) to a large colobomatous defect in the region of the optic nerve in the other. With or without retinal detachment, both sexes are involved and the condition is well distributed throughout this country and the world.[12,41] In addition to the smooth and rough collies, the anomaly is occasionally found in the Shetland Sheepdog and the Australian Shepherd.

11:88 *Significance.* This disease is important because of its hereditary aspect. Minor defects apparently produce little to no loss of vision, but ectasia of the posterior sclera may predispose to retinal detachment, intraocular hemorrhage (Plate 19G), and glaucoma. Although most detachments associated with collie eye anomaly occur in the first year or so, it is a complication that can occur after several or many years in an affected dog. Collies with large ectatic areas are predisposed to such detachment.

11:89 *Etiology.* The defect consists of arrest of mesodermal development which affects the sclera and the cribriform plate, and is probably related to abnormal differentiation of the optic cup.[55] It is now agreed that the most common manifestation of the collie eye anomaly, the choroidal hypoplasia, is inherited as a simple autosomal recessive characteristic. Evidence that staphyloma (coloboma), another manifestation of this anomaly, is inherited independently as a dominant characteristic is not generally accepted, however.[17] The idea that choroidal hyperplasia is an autosomal recessive trait, but that colobomas and retinal detachments are due to some additive factor, is now more generally accepted.

11:90 *Clinical signs.*[47] The signs depend upon the degree and duration of the involvement of the posterior structures of the eye. Collies may have vision ranging from normal to complete blindness. Most dogs involved will not be presented for examination by the singular pet collie owner unless there is a noticeable visual defect, or detachment of the retina with hyphema occurs. The age incidence in animals showing signs recognizable to the owner may vary from a few months to 5 or 6 years of age. Breeders, however, often present their litters for examination and evaluation because of their awareness of the problem within the breed.

11:91 The *ophthalmoscopic findings* vary from case to case. Wyman[69] described the following findings of collie eye anomaly that are now commonly referred to as *grades* by collie breeders:

(1) Increased tortuosity of retinal vessels.
(2) Chorioretinal change (now known as choroidal hypoplasia) (Plate 19D).
(3) Coloboma of the optic nerve with or without circumpapillary staphyloma (Plate 19E, F).
(4) Retinal detachment.
(5) Retinal hemorrhage.

It is now generally agreed that increased tortuosity of retinal vessels is not significant, so choroidal hypoplasia is the basic abnormality.

11:92 In those cases in which there is an enlargement (scleral ectasia) and excavation of the optic disc, the disc may appear to be from 2 to 5 times its normal size. The vessels drop off the edge of the excavation and may require a lens of minus 8 to minus 20 diopters to be brought into focus as they cross the floor of the disc. In others, a part of the disc will look normal while one edge will show a deep hole or a pale avascular area immediately adjacent to it. There may be a posterior bulging of the sclera at the inferonasal or temporal edge of the disc. Other eyes may take on a grey ground glass appearance in this same area and contain only a few retinal vessels with no sign of underlying choroid. The blood vessels usually show increased tortuosity as they approach the disc. Saunders[57] suggested that some of the tortuosity of the vessels is because the optic nerve enters the eye at a more acute angle than normal because the eyes are rotated away from the proper axis and getting too close to the midline.

11:93 Changes in the color of the tapetal portion of the fundus are frequently observed. The yellow-green reflex is replaced by an orange-red color, and the underlying choroidal vessels, which are normally invisible above the disc, can be seen. Some dogs show some degree of normal tapetal coloration, while others show none. Examination of many normal collies may prove this finding to have no significance other than it occurs in certain families of dogs.

11:94 Staphyloma (coloboma) was found in about 34% of collie eyes examined.[19] It was only seen in the presence of a chorioretinal hypoplasia. Large staphylomas were seen histologically as a cyst-like, thinned sclera, lined by an aberrant retinal membrane. Frequently retinal holes which lead to retinal detachment develop in this abnormal retinal lining.

11:95 Retinal detachments may be seen in a small percentage of affected animals. The most striking of these is the total detachment which prevents visualization of the disc and appears as a tremulous pink membrane which is thrown into folds which wave and change position as the eye moves (Par. 11:37). Donavan[19] reports a 4% incidence of rhegmatogenous retinal detachment in collies ranging from 4 weeks to 12 years of age.

11:96 The relationship of other abnormalities such as microphthalmia, excessive tortuosity of retinal vessels, vermiform streaks, and corneal opacities to other collie eye lesions seems inconclusive. Collies with normal-sized eyeballs are as frequently affected with defects as are collies with relatively small eyeballs.[17] It is interesting to note that many collies showing only slight chorioretinal hypoplasia when examined at an early age would be classified as normal some months later. By this time the "disputed" urea has become pigmented and does not differ ophthalmoscopically from the rest of the tapetum. These puppies are called "go normals" by breeders. Their exact genetic status is unclear.

11:97 At present, we are giving the following advice to collie breeders.

1. The optimal program for breeders who wish to eliminate collie eye defects from their stock involves breeding only those dogs found to have normal eyes. All progeny should be examined routinely, and affected pups should not be used as breeding animals.
2. As a first alternative to the optimal program, dogs with normal eyes would be bred to those with choroidal hypoplasia.
3. A least favored but still acceptable program would permit the breeding of dogs with choroidal hypoplasia to others with choroidal hypoplasia, recognizing no progress toward eliminating the anomaly.
4. All dogs with lesions worse than choroidal hypoplasia would be excluded from breeding.
5. The alternatives suggested in 2, 3, and 4 are valid only if colobomas and resulting detachments are caused by a genetic factor in addition to the autosomal recessive factor causing choroidal hypoplasia. My clinical impression is that this is the case.

11:98 In a retrospective study of the puppies of two breeders, we found that of 80 puppies from one breeder, about 80% had choroidal hypoplasia and 20% had colobomas and/or detachments. Of 90 puppies from the other breeder, 60% had choroidal hypoplasia, but *none* had colobomas or detachment. The only problem with the study was that, although the first breeder brought in all the puppies, the second, whose line of Collies did not have colobomas or detachments, only brought the show quality puppies and others she was interested in. One might suggest that she somehow was able to exclude all puppies with colobomas, but that seems unlikely. We concluded that the factor causing colobomas was not present in her line of dogs.

Tumors

11:99 Tumors of the optic nerve are rare, being derived from the nerve sheaths (meningioma[51]) and from the glial framework (glioma). Williams *et al.*[65] reported on a retrobulbar glioma of the optic nerve which developed along the course of the left optic nerve to the optic chiasm and then along the course of the right optic nerve. Magrane encountered a confirmed meningioma in a male, 11-year-old collie (Fig. 11–9A). The dog had been blind for 1 month and the left eye exhibited the classic findings of an advanced retrobulbar tumor (Par. 8:29). In addition, the retina appeared detached. The pupil of the right eye was dilated and responded slowly to light stimuli. On necropsy, a fairly round, firm tumor of the optic nerve was found tightly adhered to the posterior axis of the globe (Fig. 11–9B). It had started to necrotize.

11:100 Tumors of the optic nerve produce early loss of vision and exophthalmos (Par. 8:29). This condition is unilateral, and must be distinguished from other orbital inflammatory processes and causes of unilateral exophthalmos (Par. 8:17). Treatment consists in removal of the growth by exenteration of the orbit (Par. 8:51).

Atrophy

11:101 Atrophy is the end result of destructive disease involving the optic nerves.[32] Op-

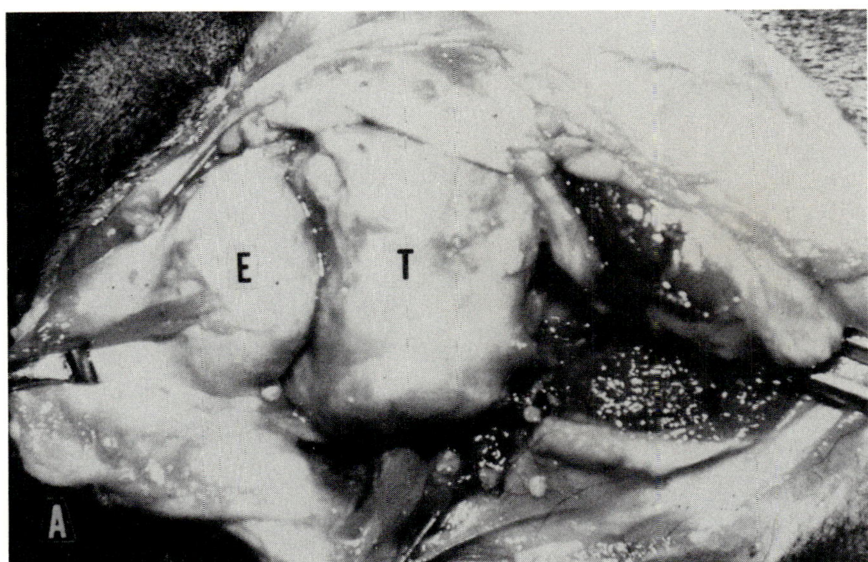

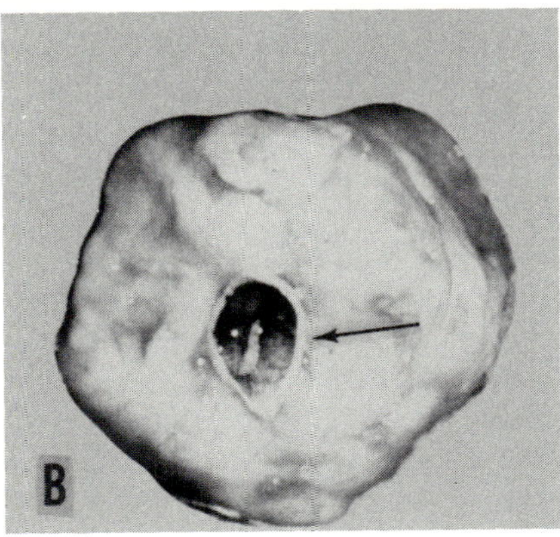

Fig. 11–9. *A.* Necropsy view of retrobulbar meningioma. E. Eyeball. T. Tumor. *B.* Tumor attached to a portion of the posterior sclera and to the optic nerve.

tic atrophy is caused by: direct pressure from neoplasia; glaucoma; chorioretinitis; intracranial hemorrhage; avitaminosis A; following optic neuritis; toxic conditions involving the optic pathway; and it is associated with progressive retinal atrophy (Fig. 11–10). Sometimes degenerative processes of unknown cause result in progressive atrophy.

11:102 McGrath[42] has observed unilateral optic atrophy in the dog in four cases, three in which a pathologic condition (a cyst or tumor) compressed the optic nerve within the orbital fossa (Fig. 11–11), and one case in which a middle fossa meningioma had compressed the right optic nerve within the cranial cavity.

11:103 Magrane[36] observed optic atrophy as an end result of all the aforementioned causes, including two cases of poisoning. In one, inhalation of exterminator gas was believed responsible and, in the second, dipping in a "lye" solution resulted in incoordination and loss of vision. Optic atrophy may also occur, following injury, caused by traumatic prolapse of the globe.

11:104 *Ophthalmoscopic signs* of optic atrophy vary and depend upon the cause and the stage. The disc is pale grey to chalk white or may be reduced in size and appear dark. Its margins may be sharply defined or irregular. The blood vessels normally present are few in number or gone altogether. Pigment migration from the surrounding structures may cause the outline to be blurred and indistinct.

11:105 *Prognosis.* Since atrophy of the

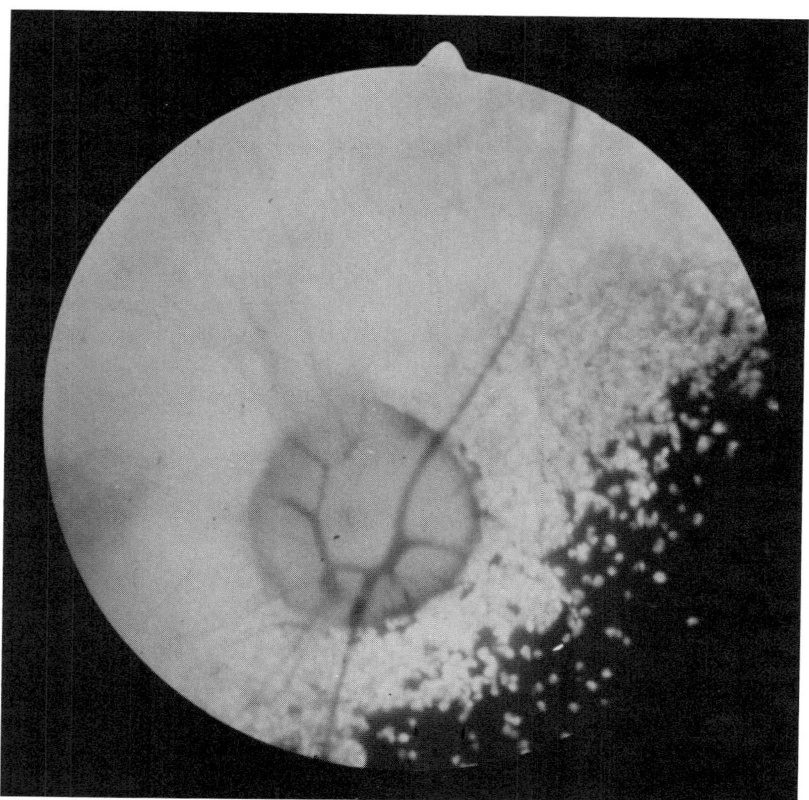

Fig. 11–10. Optic disc atrophy associated with progressive retinal atrophy. Note diminution in size and number of retinal vessels. (Courtesy of Keith C. Barnett, Cambridge, England.)

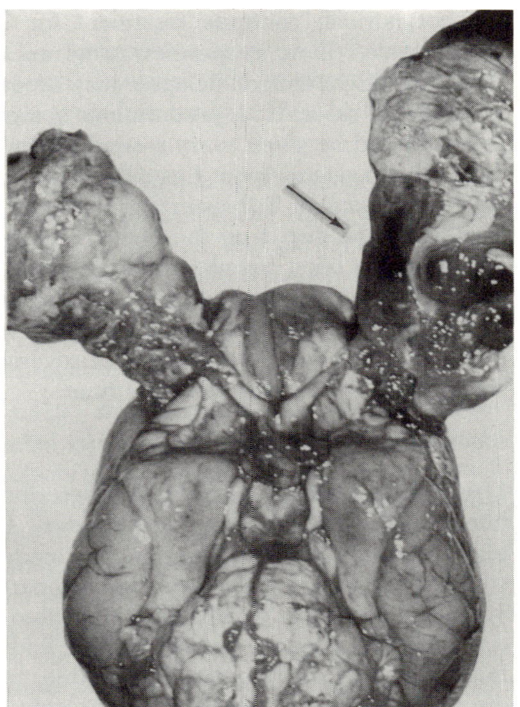

Fig. 11–11. Postorbital neurogenic sarcoma in a 9-year-old male boxer. The tumor produced unilateral atrophy by compression. Note exophthalmic deviation of the globe. (Courtesy of Dr. John T. McGrath, Philadelphia, Pa.)

nerve fibers has involved a great part of the optic nerve before a dog is presented and a diagnosis is made, the probability of restoration of function is poor. However, if some central vision remains, removal of the cause of the disease may preserve that vision.

11:106 *Treatment consists* in attempting to control the cause. Nothing can be done for the atrophy itself.

Papilledema

11:107 Papilledema (choked disc) has been defined as a swelling or edema of the optic nerve head resulting from increased intracranial pressure. In man, approximately 50% of patients with brain tumor exhibit this lesion. Routine fundic examinations have been carried out in many dogs with verified brain tumors, intracranial trauma, optic neuritis which occurred in association with viral encephalitis, and other lesions producing increased intracranial pressure. To date, true clinical examples of papilledema have been encountered seldom in the dog.[42]

11:108 One of the reasons for this relates to an anatomic difference from man. In man the presence of a central retinal artery and vein crossing the subarachnoid space makes those vessels subject to the effects of high intracranial pressure, and the stasis and subsequent congestion of the smaller vessels produce swelling of the optic nerve head.[51] In the dog there is no central retinal artery or vein, the retinal vessels piercing the sclera immediately around the optic nerve with no main vessels actually crossing the subarachnoid space. Thus, in most instances, papilledema in the dog is caused by disorders of the nerve itself. These can include tumors and the toxicities.

11:109 I encountered a pronounced papilledema in a boxer which later was euthanized and found to have a retrobulbar rhabdomyosarcoma (Par. 3:30). When initially presented, clinical signs included a moderate exophthalmos and conjunctival chemosis. The well-developed choked disc showed an elevation of 6 diopters over the surrounding area.

11:110 Papilledema and peripapillary retinal edema have been found in association with subacute and acute pancreatitis. The relationship between the ocular signs and pancreatitis is not clear.[51] Papilledema, itself, does not cause blindness, so diagnosis is often incidental. Papillitis, as a part of optic neuritis, may appear similar to papilledema, but causes blindness during the stage of active inflammation.

Optic Neuritis

11:111 Optic neuritis denotes inflammation of the optic nerve. It is often accompanied by demyelinization and degeneration. The term "optic neuritis" also includes *retrobulbar neuritis*, a form in which the nerve is affected posteriorly so that there are no visible oph-

7. Barnett, J.C.: Canine Retinopathies—III. The Other Breeds, J. Sm. Am. Pract., 6:185–196, 1965.
8. Barnett, K.C.: Canine Retinopathies—IV. Causes of Retinal Atrophy, J. Sm. An. Pract., 6,:229–242, 1965.
9. Barnett, K.C.: Hereditary Retinal Atrophy in the Poodle, Vet. Rec., *74*:672–675, 1962.
10. Barnett, K.C.: Primary Tapeto-retinal Degenerations in Dogs, Aspects of Comparative Ophthalmology, Pergamon Fress, Oxford and New York, 1966.
11. Barnett, K.C. and Grimes, T.D.: Unilateral Persistent and Hyperplasia of the Primary Vitreous in the Dog, J. Sm. An. Pract., *14*:561–565, 1973.
12. Blogg, J.R.: Collie Eye Anomaly, Aust. Vet. J., *46*:530–533, 1970.
13. Blogg, J.R.: *The Eye in Veterinary Practice*, North Melbourne, Victoria, V.S. Supplies, 1975.
14. Brightman, A.H., Brown, M., Johnson, B., et al.: Vitreous Centesis as a Diagnostic Procedure, Trans. ACVO/ISVO, pp. 82–87, 1986.
15. Carrig, C.B., MacMillan, A., Brundage, S., et al.: Retinal Dysplasia Associated with Skeletal Abnormalities in Labrador Retrievers, J.A.V.M.A., *170*:49, 1977.
16. Catcott, E.J.: Ophthalmoscopy in Canine Practice, J.A.V.M.A., *121*:35–37, 1952.
17. Catcott, E.J.: Summary and Conclusion—Collie Eye Panel, J.A.V.M.A., *155*:877, 1969.
18. Curtis, R., Barnett, K.C., and Leon, A.: Persistent Hyperplastic Primary Vitreous in the Staffordshire Bull Terrier, Vet. Rec., *115*:385, 1984.
19. Donavan, R.H., et al.: Anomaly of the Collie Eye, J.A.V.M.A., *155*:872, 1969.
20. Duke-Elder, Sir S.: *System of Ophthalmology*, Vol. II, St. Louis, C.V. Mosby Co., pp. 295–307, 1965.
21. Fine, B.S. and Tousimis, A.J.: The Structure of the Vitreous Body and the Suspensory Ligaments of the Lens, Arch. Ophth., *65*:95–110, 1961.
22. Fischer, C.: Optic Neuritis in Dogs, J.A.V.M.A., *160*:68–79, 1972.
23. Francois, J.: *Heredity in Ophthalmology*, St. Louis, The C.V. Mosby Co., 1961.
24. Gelatt, K.N., and Veith, L.A.: Hereditary Multiple Ocular Anomalies in Australian Shepherd Dogs, Vet. Med., *65*:39, 1970.
25. Grice, H.C. and Hutchison, J.A.: Retinoblastoma in a Dog, J.A.V.M.A., *136*:444–446, 1960.
26. Heywood, R. and Wells, G.H.: Retinal Dysplasia in the Beagle, Vet. Record, *87*:178–180, 1970.
27. Hodgman, F.S.J., Parry, H.B., Rasbridge, W.J. and Steel, J.D.: Progressive Retinal Atrophy in Dogs, Vet. Rec., *61*:185, 1949.
28. Jubb, K.U., Saunders, L.Z., and Coates, H.U.: The Intraocular Lesions of Canine Distemper, J. Comp. Path. & Ther., *67*:21–29, 1957.
29. Koch, S.A. and Rubin, L.F.: Distribution of Cones in the Retina of the Normal Dog, Am. J. Vet. Res., *33*:361–363, 1972.
30. Kock, Erik: Retinal Dysplasia—A Comparative Study in Human Beings and Dogs, Monograph, Dept. of Pathology, Karolinska Institute, Stockholm, and the Dept. of Surgery, Royal Vet. Coll., Stockholm, 1974.
31. Lavach, J.D., Murphy, J.M., and Severin, G.A.: Retinal Dysplasia in the English Springer Spaniel, J.A.A.H.A., *14*:192, 1978.
32. Leinfelder, P.J.: Outline of Neuro-ophthalmology. Home Study Course, Am. Ac. Ophth. & Otol., 1950.
33. Leinfelder, P.J.: Why is a Retinopathy?, Am. J. Ophth., *68*:427, 1969.
34. Leon, A.: PHPV in the Staffordshire Bull Terrier, Trans. ACVO/ISVO, pp. 31–39, 1986.
35. Magrane, W.G.: Personal observation, Radiobiology Lab., Atomic Energy Comm., University of California, Davis, Cal.
36. Magrane, W.: *Canine Ophthalmology*, 3rd ed., Philadelphia, Lea & Febiger, p. 256, 1977.
37. Magrane, W.G.: Progressive Retinal Atrophy and Associated Blindness: Breed Incidence, No. Am. Vet., *36*:743–746, 1955.
38. Magrane, W.G.: Congenital Anomaly of the Optic Disc in Collies, No. Am. Vet., *34*:646, 1953.
39. Magnusson, H.: Arch. Vergl. Ophth., *2*:147, 1911.
40. MacMillan, A.D., and Lipton, D.E.: Heritability of Multifocal Retinal Dysplasia in American Cocker Spaniels, J.A.V.M.A., *172*:568, 1978.
41. Mason, T.A. and Cox, K.: Collie Eye Anomaly, Aust. Vet. J., *47*:38–40, 1971.
42. McGrath, J.T.: *Neurologic Examination of the Dog*, 2nd Ed. Philadelphia, Lea & Febiger, p. 29, 1960.
43. Parry, H.B.: Degenerations of the Dog Retina, Brit. J. Ophth., *38*:295–309, 1954.
44. Parry, H.B.: Generalized Progressive Atrophy of Uncertain Etiology, Brit. J. Ophth., *38*:545, 1954.
45. Parry, H.B.: Vet. Rec., *63*:323, 1951.
46. Prince, J.H., Diesem, C.D., Eglitis,I., and Ruskill, G.L.: *Anatomy and Histology of the Eye and Orbit in Domestic Animals*, Springfield, Charles C Thomas, 1960.
47. Report—Comm. on Ophth. of the Am. An. Hosp. Assoc., 1960.
48. Rubin, L.F.: Asteroid Hyalosis in the Dog, Am. J. Vet. Res., *24*:1256–1262, 1963.
49. Rubin, L.F.: Atypical Coloboma of the Choroid in a Dog, J.A.V.M.A., *143*:841–842, 1963.
50. Rubin, L.F.: Heredity of Retinal Dysplasia in Bedlington Terriers, J.A.V.M.A., *152*:260, 1968.
51. Rubin, L.F.: *Atlas of Veterinary Ophthalmoscopy*, Philadelphia, Lea & Febiger, 1974.
52. Rubin, L.F.: *Ocular Manifestations of Arteriosclerosis and Hypertension in Dogs*, Proc. Am. Coll. Vet. Ophth., 1975.
53. Rubin, L.F.: Correction of Retinal Detachment in a Dog, J.A.V.M.A., *157*:461–466, 1970.
54. Rubin, L.F.: Clinical Features of Hemerolopia in the Alaskan Malamute, J.A.V.M.A., *158*:1696, 1971.
55. Roberts, S.R.: Congenital Posterior Ectasia of the Sclera in Collie Dogs, Am. J. Ophth., *50*:451–465, 1960.
56. Roberts, S.R.: The Collie Eye Anomaly, J.A.V.M.A., *155*:859, 1969.
57. Saunders, L.Z.: The Clinical Appearance and Pathology of Some Congenital Ocular Defects in Collie Dogs, Proc. Am. Soc. Vet. Ophth., 1960.
58. Saunders, L.Z.: Congenital Optic Nerve Hypoplasia in Collie Dogs, Cornell Vet., *62*:67–80, 1952.
59. Schnelle, G.B.: Progressive Retinal Atrophy in a Dog, J.A.V.M.A., *121*:177–178, 1952.
60. Slatter, B.H.: *Fundamentals of Veterinary Oph-*

thalmology, Philadelphia, W.B. Saunders Co., pp. 569–570, 1981.
61. Smythe, R.H.: *Veterinary Ophthalmology*, London, Baillière Tindall & Cox, p. 327, 1956.
62. Stades, F.C.: Persistent Hyperplastic Tunica Vasculosa Lentis and Persistent Hyperplastic Primary Vitreous (PHTVL/PHPV) in 90 Closely Related Doberman Pinschers: Clinical Aspects, J.A.A.H.A., *16*:739–751, 1980.
63. Vainisi, S.J., Font, R.L., Anderson, R., et al.: Idiopathic Photoreceptor Cell Degeneration in Dogs, Invest. Ophthalmol. Vis. Sci., 26:(3, suppl), 129, 1985.
64. Vainisi, S., Schmidt, G., West, C., et al.: Metabolic Toxic Retinopathy—A Preliminary Report, Trans. ACVO, pp 76–82, 1983.
65. Williams, J.O., Garlick, E.C. and Beard, D.C.: Glioma of the Optic Nerve, of a Dog, J.A.V.M.A., *138*:377–378, 1961.
66. Wolf, E.D., Vainisi, S.J., and Santos-Anderson, R.: Rod-Cone Dysplasia and Retinal Atrophy (letter), J.A.V.M.A., *174*:324–327, 1979.
67. Wolf, E.D., Vainisi, S.J., and Santos-Anderson, R.: Rod-Cone Dysplasia in the Collie, J.A.V.M.A., *173*:1331–1333, 1978.
68. Wyman, M., and Donavan, E.F.: Eye Anomaly of the Collie, J.A.V.M.A., *155*:866, 1969.
69. Wyman, M.: *Manual of Small Animal Ophthalmology*, New York, Churchill Livingstone, pp. 232–235, 245, 1986.

12

OCULAR MANIFESTATIONS OF SYSTEMIC DISEASE

"The eye is the lamp of the body."
MATTHEW 6:22

12:1 Ophthalmology should be considered as an integral part of internal medicine. The ocular condition often appears early in the course of a systemic disease and may be important to the diagnosis and prognosis. The ocular symptoms occurring with systemic affections are discussed more fully in the preceding chapters.

Diseases of the Blood and Cardiovascular System

12:2 *Anemia* gives rise to pale pink conjunctivae and a pearly white sclerae. The retinal vessels are more pale than normal and, depending upon the cause, retinal hemorrhages are occasionally found.

12:3 *Lipemia.* The anterior chambers are partially to fully filled with a very fluid milky exudate. When ophthalmoscopy is possible, the blood of the retinal vessels appears "creamy," *i.e.* like light tomato juice. The "silver wire" reflection (Par. 2:57) from the vessels in the non-tapetal fundus is absent. Lipemia retinalis may also occur with normal appearing aqueous. Thyroid and pancreatic function should be evaluated in such cases.

12:4 A paracentesis (Par. 6:163) will temporarily clear the anterior chamber, but the secondary aqueous which fills the chamber is also milky. Thyroid therapy and a low fat diet will result in permanent clearing within a week.

12:5 *Thrombocytopenic purpura* (Plate 20F) may be present as petechial or rather extensive hemorrhages beneath the conjunctiva, in the retina, and in the skin of the lids. A hyphema may be present and blindness may ensue. Systemic recovery can result in clearing of the eyes and restoration of vision.[12]

12:6 *Dysproteinemia.* Darraspen and Lescure[20] report a case of a dog with an endocular hemorrhage and a concurrent dysproteinemia.

12:7 *Arteriosclerosis* and *hypertension* may result in a severe and recurrent intraocular hemorrhage in older dogs.[45,46] When ophthalmoscopic examination is possible, retinal hemorrhages, localized or extensive, bullous detachment, and variation in the diameter of the retinal arterioles may be noted (Par. 11–29).

Diseases of the Digestive System

12:8 *Teeth.* A septic mouth from infected teeth may predispose to conjunctival congestion and iritis (Par. 7:34).

12:9 *Liver.* Diseases of the liver may cause jaundice, a yellowish discoloration of the sclera and of the conjunctiva. Retinal and subconjunctival hemorrhages are not uncommon in severe hepatic disorders.

12:10 *Pancreas.* In chronic pancreatitis interference with the digestion of fat may lead to a deficiency of vitamin A. This, in turn, can result in a loss of vision. Fortunately this type of blindness is reversible. If diagnosed in time, daily administration of vitamin A (Par. 3:69) will correct the condition. Papilledema and peripapillary retinal edema have been found in association with subacute and acute pancreatitis.[45]

Diseases of the Kidneys

12:11 *Nephritis* may present ocular manifestations in the late stages. In uremia, retinal hemorrhages are not uncommon (Par. 11:29) and are an indication of very serious illness. These hemorrhages vary in size and shape, are usually seen near the vessels, and may be large, keel-boat shaped (pre-retinal), flamed-shaped (nerve fiber layer) or small and round (deeper layers). Conjunctival congestion and discharges are also indicative of the toxic state of the animal.

Diseases of the Muscles

12:12 *Eosinophilic myositis* (Par. 8:23) produces striking ocular symptoms. Exophthalmos, edema of the lids, conjunctival chemosis, and hypertrophy and protrusion of the membrane nictitans can be expected in the acute form (Plate 13D).

12:13 *Atrophy* of the muscles around the eye and of the postorbital fat following an attack of eosinophilic myositis will result in an enophthalmos of the globe (Par. 8:41) (Plate 13H).

Diseases of the Endocrine Glands and Metabolic Disorders

12:14 *Pituitary.* Neoplasm of the pituitary gland causes impairment of vision of various degrees and an eventual partial or complete destruction of the optic nerve. This amaurosis (Par. 11:115) commonly remains unsolved until confirmed on necropsy. McGrath[37] has encountered pituitary adenocarcinomas in which amaurosis was initially noted.

12:15 *Diabetes.* The common ocular complication of diabetes in the dog is cataract (Par. 10:31). The retinopathy associated with diabetes in man has not been commonly observed in the dog. The characteristic diabetic retinopathy of man includes the findings of: capillary microaneurysms; dot and blot hemorrhages; retinal and vitreous hemorrhage; and retinal detachment. Sibay and Hausler[55] are of the opinion that a dog should have had diabetes for at least five years in order to show any significant retinal changes. The eyes of two diabetic dogs, father and son, were studied at necropsy. The father had been a known diabetic for 2 years and the son for 5 years. The father exhibited only dilatation of retinal arterioles, whereas the son showed retinopathy with typical capillary aneurysms. Blindness in dogs has not been reported as an effect of diabetic retinopathy.

12:16 Catcott[14] was unable to detect fundic changes in a series of dogs subjected to experimental diabetes. His observation period, however, was over a short period of time. Gross retinal lesions do not appear in diabetic humans until after a considerable time lapse. Recently capillary aneurysms have been clearly demonstrated by Patz and Maumenee[41] in a spontaneously diabetic dog. Engerman and Bloodworth[23] have produced experimental diabetic retinopathy in dogs. Retinas of ten dogs were studied histologically after 9 to 69 months of alloxan or metasomatropin diabetes. Either type of diabetes was found to result in a retinopathy comparable to that of human diabetes mellitus. The retinopathy occurred in each of three dogs that had been diabetic over 4 years. The evidence indicated that diabetic retinopathy is dependent to a lesser extent on the cause of diabetes than on its duration, and is a result not of a genetic disorder but of metabolic alterations initiated by deficiency of insulin.

12:17 The above and other reports agree that dogs may have the microaneurysms and exudative retinopathy reported in humans, but do not have the classical proliferation of blood vessels that is typical of diabetic retinopathy in the human.

Diseases of the Ear, Nose, Throat and Accessory Sinuses

12:18 *Ear.* Nystagmus is common in affections of the labyrinth and vestibular pathways. A chronic purulent conjunctivitis may be associated with purulent otitis (Par. 5:44).

12:19 *Nose and Throat.* The communication between the nose and the conjunctival sac by means of the lacrimal duct explains the occurrence of ocular symptoms as a result of nasal disease. Conjunctivitis may be a complication of chronic rhinitis. The lacrimal duct may be the means of conveying infective material from the nose to the conjunctival sac. In seasonal allergy there is often a conjunctival congestion or acute catarrhal conjunctivitis with marked lacrimation.

12:20 *Throat.* The tonsils merit consideration as a focus of infection in inflammations and infections of the eyes. Chronically infected tonsils must be regarded as a likely source for endogenous infection. Iritis and uveitis may occur as a manifestation of tonsillar infection (Par. 7:34).

12:21 *Sinus* disease may be responsible for ocular symptoms which include orbital cellulitis (Par. 8:19, 8:20) (Plate 13C); conjunctivitis; and iritis with deep keratitis in a small percentage of cases.

Diseases of the Nervous System

12:22 *Nystagmus.* Pendular nystagmus results from conditions present before or at the time of birth that cause great loss of vision in both eyes. In man, any of the ocular conditions such as congenital cataracts, anomalies of the retina or choroid, and congenital opacities on the cornea might produce pendular nystagmus.

12:23 Opacities of the cornea or lens that prevent central vision or retinal detachment interfere with the development of central fixation and may result in pendular nystagmus. In this type of nystagmus, there is no rhythm, but rather just wandering eye motion.[17] Pendular nystagmus in a young dog with cataracts is a clue that the cataracts are probably congenital.

12:24 *Horner's syndrome* is characterized by unilateral miosis, ptosis, and enophthalmos. The nictitating membrane usually covers about one half of the globe. It is caused most frequently by lesions producing paralysis of the cervical sympathetic portion of the autonomic nervous system and lesions of the hypothalamus. McGrath[36] has observed the syndrome with tumors of the anterior mediastinum, cervical cord lesions (especially tumors), and tumors of the hypothalamus.

12:25 Rubin[44] suggests the use of epinephrine (Par. 3:30) for the diagnosis and treatment of Horner's syndrome. We have been most satisfied by using the method proposed by Brightman, et al.[8] for diagnosis of Horner's syndrome. It is as follows:

> (In testing for Horner's syndrome, it is important that no other medication is applied to the eye concurrently or within 24 hours prior to testing)
>
> Instill 2 drops of 4% cocaine solution in each eye and repeat in 5 minutes. Measure and record pupil diameters every 5 minutes for 45 minutes. A normal eye should dilate in about 20 minutes, whereas in Horner's syndrome, the dilation will be absent or reduced throughout the 45-minute period. Cocaine dilates the pupil by blocking the reuptake of norepinephrine in the nerve endings in the iris, hence allowing continued action and pupil dilation. In Horner's syndrome no norepinephrine is being released, and therefore, the pupil does not dilate. Repeating the procedure after 24 hours or more using 1% hydroxyamphetamine will help delineate the location of the lesion. This drug causes release of norepinephrine from stores in sympathetic nerve endings. If the lesion is in the 3rd order neuron (above the superior cervical ganglion), there will be no stores to be released, hence the pupil will not dilate. If the lesion is in the 1st or 2nd order neurons, the pupil should dilate.

12:26 *Hemifacial spasm* in dogs is associated with a Horner's syndrome apparently resulting from interruption of sympathetic pathways which traverse the middle ear.[43] Ocular findings include blepharospasm, narrowing of the palpebral fissure, prolapse of the membrane nictitans, injection of conjunctival vessels and miosis. Associated signs are elevation and wrinkling of the lip with caudal displacement of the labial commissure and elevation of the ear. The nose deviates to the same side. The basic lesion in each case was a severe otitis media.

12:27 A variant of hemifacial spasm has been reported.[40] In this instance the eye appeared retracted and there was protrusion of the third eyelid. A Horner's syndrome was not diagnosed because of absence of a miosis. The character and site of the lesion found at necropsy confirmed the clinical diagnosis of an irritative lesion involving several cranial nerve nuclei. There was no associated otitis.

12:28 *Neuroparalytic* (neurotrophic) *keratitis* leads to corneal ulceration because of lack of sensation and tear film evaporation (Par. 6:108). The loss of sensation is due to denervation of the ophthalmic branch of the trigeminal nerve from varied causes.

12:29 *Primary reticulosis* of the central nervous system may lead to serious neuro-ophthalmologic manifestations.[25] Sudden blindness, pupils unresponsive to light, and bilateral inflammation of the optic discs were detected in a middle age poodle. In several cases, we have observed no ophthalmic lesions and normal ERGs. Treatment for optic neuritis (Par. 11:113) resulted in the return of sight, but deterioration of sight and other CNS signs occurred within several months.

Infectious Diseases

12:30 *Distemper.* A variable degree of conjunctivitis is to be expected in nearly every case of distemper. Corneal ulceration (Par. 6:109) and/or keratitis sicca (Par. 6:67) are less frequent manifestations.

12:31 Transient or permanent blindness occurs in still fewer instances (Par. 11:47). Intraocular lesions may be present concurrently with or in the absence of brain lesions.[31] Varying degrees of retinal atrophy have been found on histologic examination. Gross findings include dilatation of the pupil, but an essentially normal appearing fundus (Par. 11:47). Recovered animals will often exhibit areas of quiescent chorioretinitis (Plate 18H) upon ophthalmoscopic examination. This is probably due to an optic neuritis, retinitis focal encephalitis syndrome.

12:32 Fischer[24] describes a specific pattern of retinal and retinochoroidal lesions in dogs with early neuropathic distemper. The majority of the lesions were seen in the peripheral and midperipheral nontapetal fundus. Fewer and less easily observed lesions were seen in the tapetal fundus. There was no noticeable visual deficit.

12:33 *Hepatitis.* A serious conjunctivitis may be present, but in the mild form, ocular manifestations are seldom apparent. A corneal opacity due to endothelial cell damage of one or both eyes may appear 5 to 10 days after the acute illness (Par. 7:35). These opacities are usually transitory.

12:34 *Leptospirosis.* Inflammation of the conjunctiva and a catarrhal to crusty discharge can be expected. In the icterohemorrhagiae form, a jaundiced sclera and petechial hemorrhages beneath the conjunctiva are the usual findings. Acute anterior or posterior unveitis occurs and can produce secondary retinal detachments.

12:35 *Toxoplasmosis* of man is known to be responsible for uveitis and chorioretinitis. Sufficient evidence has been accumulated to indicate that some relationship may exist between animal and human toxoplasmosis, although evidence of communicability is lacking.[19] Heeley[29] believes that this organism may be involved in some of our more obscure clinical problems (Par. 7:60). Barron and Saunders[4] have found toxoplasma organisms in the enucleated eye of a dog. The associated pathologic changes were retinitis, iridocyclitis, and optic neuritis. The ocular lesions of experimental and naturally occurring toxoplasmosis in 60 dogs has been described.[42]

Lesions were found most frequently in the iris, ciliary body, and retina. Focal necrosis, especially of the retina, was frequently observed. Masses of organisms, severe necrosis, and suppurative myositis occurred in the extraocular muscles.

12:36 Undoubtedly an occasional case of uveitis with a subsequent chorioretinitis in the dog can be attributed to toxoplasmosis. In general, however, fewer ocular manifestations will be found in dogs infected with toxoplasma than in a like number in man.[18] In cases of recurrent uveitis it has been my practice to confirm or eliminate toxoplasma as a source through use of the Sabin-Feldman dye test.

12:37 *Rabies.* Possible findings in this disease include: reddened conjunctiva; mucopurulent exudate; anisocoria (uneven pupils); divergent or convergent strabismus; and a membrane nictitans protruding over the globe.

12:38 *Tetanus.* The membrane nictitans is usually prominent and is seen to flick over the eyes. The pupils are miotic.

12:39 *Septicemia* alone may produce manifestations in almost any of the structures of the eye. The more common are those of the conjunctiva (discharge, petechial hemorrhages). A generalized septicemia can lead to involvement of the uveal tract (iridocyclitis with hypopyon) or an endophthalmitis and ultimate loss of the eyeball (Par. 7:62).

12:40 *Coccidioidomycosis* can produce severe corneal and conjunctival involvement. Cello[15] has demonstrated the natural occurrence of a granulomatous uveitis in dogs with disseminated coccidioidomycosis and points out that a true evaluation of the incidence of this condition can only be obtained from careful examination of the eye by veterinarians practicing in areas where the disease is endemic. Shively and Whiteman[54] reported granulomatous uveitis, retinitis, keratitis, and occasional focal scleritis as unilateral ocular lesions in two cases of coccidioidomycosis in dogs. Armstrong[2] provides a good literature review of canine coccidioidomycosis and a report of 8 cases. No lesions were reported in these cases. Angell and Meredith[1] reported on ocular lesions associated with coccidioidomycosis in 35 dogs. The eye lesions in order of frequency were keratitis, 17 eyes, iritis, 15 eyes, and glaucoma, 11 eyes. Other lesions include retinal separation, conjunctivitis, hyalitis, hyphema, cataracts, and retinitis. The lesions were unilateral in 28 dogs, and 15 dogs did not have clinical signs other than those of ocular disease. Diagnosis was confirmed by serologic testing and/or histologic examination. They recommend ketoconazole administered orally, 5 to 10 mg/kg, q 12h for a minimum of 8 months in dogs with disseminated disease. If one eye appears to be the only site of active infection, is sensitive and/or nonresponsive to medication, they recommend enucleation and ketoconazole treatment until there is no active titer for C. immitis.

12:41 *Blastomycosis* may produce eye discharges, severe uveitis, granulomatous choroiditis and retinitis, secondary glaucoma, detached retina and panophthalmitis.[24,53,56,59,61] Blindness has been reported in 25% of dogs with ocular manifestations of the disease.[39,45] The ocular form has a sudden onset and the acute form must be treated immediately if any hope can be given for survival or preservation of vision. Ausherman[13] reports good results with amphotericin B, systemically and subconjunctivally, along with supportive therapy. Our long-term results have generally been unsatisfactory, especially if chorioretinitis is present. Even when the general systemic infection and ocular infection are controlled with systemic amphotericin, reactivation of the ocular lesions is common. Diagnosis can best be established by vitriocentesis (Par. 11:16) (Fig. 11–3) if chorioretinitis lesions are present.

12:42 *Cryptococcosis* (Plate 20G) has been reported as being the cause of blindness in the dog.[10,58] Full pupil dilatation was observed in those cases reported. In other dogs with cryptococcosis of the central nervous system, ocular findings included optic neuritis, nonsuppurative granulomas in the retina, choroid, around both optic nerves and an occasional retinal detachment.[7,27,32,34,47]

12:43 *Histoplasmosis.* Salfelder[50] demonstrated that, in dogs, histoplasmosis can be a cause of granulomatous uveitis and ophthalmitis and that histologic examination aids in establishing the causative agent. A case of confirmed histoplasmosis had a loss of vision associated with a granulomatous uveitis.[13] Treatment was initiated with intravenous amphotericin B, topical atropine and systemic chloramphenicol. Subconjunctival and systemic steroids were used when recovery seemed apparent. Partial recovery of vision was attained.

12:44 *Canine Ehrlichiosis* (tropical canine pancytopenia) has been known to cause conjunctival hemorrhage, retinal hemorrhage and hyphema. In experimentally infected dogs these hemorrhages were not noted.[22] Rather, these induced dogs went through a stage of retinal vascular engorgement coincident with an initial febrile response. Regression of the vascular engorgement was followed by generalized tapetal reflectivity. Histologically, a mild nongranulomatous uveitis was usually found. In experimental cases, at the University of Illinois, chronic, low-grade, anterior uveitis with corneal edema was observed in some dogs.

12:45 *Rocky Mountain Spotted Fever* can cause thrombocytopenia and ocular lesions similar to those of Ehrlichiosis. Rutgers, et al.[63] reported on five cases. Ocular lesions included retinal hemorrhage, chorioretinitis, and anterior uveitis. Three dogs died despite tetracycline therapy. It is of interest to note that Rocky Mountain Spotted Fever is now more common in the Carolinas and surrounding states than in the Rocky Mountains.

Malignancies

12:46 *Malignant Lymphoma* (lymphosarcoma) (Plate 8H and Fig. 12–1). The ocular changes in malignant lymphoma of dogs are striking. These changes are significant in that they occur more frequently than has been supposed, and they may, on occasion, precede the actual systemic symptoms of the disease.

12:47 Cello and Hutcherson[16] summarize the most important changes found in the various parts of the globe. Conjunctivitis ranges in severity from a mild inflammation with hyperemia, chemosis, and scanty mucous discharge to a severe purulent discharge with thickening and induration of the tissue. Changes in the cornea include edema, vascularization, keratic precipitates, and intrastromal hemorrhage. Ulcerative keratitis is a common finding in the final stages of the disease and usually appears after the cornea has undergone one or more of the other corneal changes. A dense white band around the limbal margin of the cornea may be noted. This infiltrate is an invasion of tumor cells.

12:48 Spontaneous hemorrhage into the anterior chamber (hyphema) is a frequent gross sign of tumor involvement. Uveitis and a hazy ocular media are part of the picture. This makes ophthalmoscopy difficult, if not impossible, in some cases. When the fundus can be viewed, a retinopathy with superficial flame-shaped and deep round hemorrhages may be evident.

12:49 Glaucoma is to be expected as a secondary complication of the later stages.[52] Tumor involvement of the iris, ciliary body and retina will, in turn, produce the rise in tension.

12:50 In general, examination of the eye will not be helpful in detecting early cases of malignant lymphoma, since by the time the ocular changes occur, the more common systemic symptoms are evident. This is not always true, however. In some eyes, the neoplastic infiltration of the cornea has been mistaken clinically for an obscure keratitis, and in others the tumor tissue had partially filled the anterior chamber. Further examination of the patient then revealed the beginning lymph node enlargement.

12:51 *Intracranial Tumors.* Interruption of

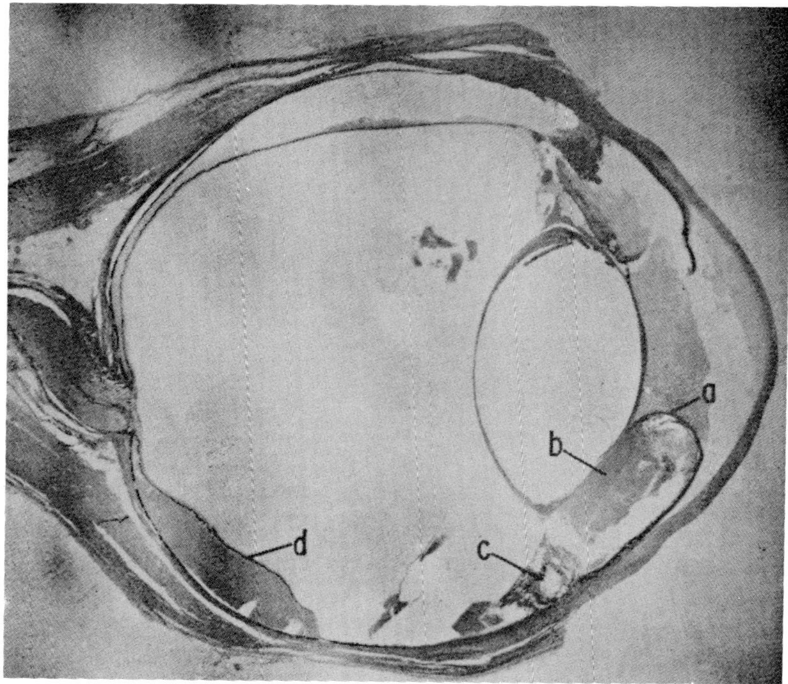

Fig. 12–1. Canine malignant lymphoma. Section of eye showing iris bombé and atrophic iris *(a)*, hemorrhage in posterior chamber *(b)*, atrophy of ciliary body *(c)*, subretinal hemorrhage *(d)*. (Cello and Hutcherson, courtesy of Cornell Veterinarian.)

the optic pathways in association with neoplasia will produce partial to total loss of vision of one or both eyes. This amaurosis (Par. 11:115) may precede certain specific neurologic signs and symptoms which are then suggestive of an intracranial malignancy. According to Hoerlein,[30] tumors in the pyriform and parietal lobes of the mid-brain are characterized by blindness, convulsions and incoordination.

12:52 *Retrobulbar Tumors* (Par. 8:28) (Plate 13E, F and G). Depending upon the stage of development, one or all of these ocular manifestations are present: exophthalmos; globe deviation; diminished movement; prominent hypertrophied membrane nictitans; pupil dilated and/or eccentric; exposure keratitis; and blindness.

12:53 *Secondary Intraocular Tumors.* These tumors occur by hematogenous metastasis from the internal organs. They also occur from the orbit, conjunctiva, or cornea via the optic nerve or cornea.[5] Metastatic tumor infiltration of the iridocorneal angle, iris, ciliary body and anterior choroid has been reported as arising from canine mammary adenocarcinoma.[6,33,51] Records of the Armed Forces Institute of Pathology show adenocarcinoma and malignant lymphoma to be the most common secondary intraocular tumors. Other less frequent include hemangiosarcoma, fibrosarcoma, meningioma, rhabdomyosarcoma, and malignant melanoma. Symanski[57] records an unusual intraocular metastasis of a widely disseminated systemic hemangiosarcoma. The ophthalmic signs were exophthalmos, episcleral congestion, a firm subconjunctival mass at the superior limbus, edematous cornea, miotic pupil, consolidated hyphema and a tension increase. It is believed that the examination of the eye in cases of generalized neoplasia in animals will reveal that intraocular metastasis is far from rare.[51]

12:54 *Metastasis.* A visual deficit from metastatic neoplasms of the brain may result from adenocarcinoma of the mammary glands, carcinoma of the lung[21] and transitional cell carcinoma of the urinary bladder.[26]

Parasitism

12:55 *Hookworm.* A severe hookworm infestation will give rise to a pale conjunctivae and pearly white sclera (anemia). An accompanying mucopurulent conjunctival discharge can be expected.

12:56 *Toxocara.* The clinical and histologic features are described in four cases of intraocular larva migrans in dogs.[48] Clinically, a small, raised, greyish nodule about one-fourth to one-sixth the diameter of the optic disc was visible on the surface of the retina. In three of the cases the lesion was recognized during ophthalmoscopic examination, and in one it was discovered histologically. The lesion is a granuloma resembling those seen in other organs of dogs affected by visceral larva migrans, and contains nematode larvae of the genus Toxocara.

12:57 Dubielzig[29a] reported a generalized retinal degeneration and blindness in sheep herding dogs in New Zealand, associated with severe intraocular larvae migrans. We[30a] have reported a similar retinal degeneration and blindness, associated with severe Toxocara infestation, in a kennel of Border collies in Illinois used for herding pigs and sheep.

12:58 *Heartworm.* The filarial worm has been observed in the anterior chamber on a number of occasions. An increase in lacrimation and corneal hazing can be expected. When the parasite has been present for some time an iritis and interstitial keratitis results. Removal is performed through a small limbal incision and "snaring" the worm with a dull iris hook. Heartworm disease, even without visible filaria in the eye, may cause mild to severe anterior uveitis and chorioretinitis. In my experience, the uveitis may become more severe during treatment.

12:59 *Leishmaniasis.* The ocular effects of visceral leishmaniasis have been recorded in dogs imported into the United States from Greece.[28,35] Ocular manifestations of the disease included a severe bilateral endophthalmitis and associated blepharitis. *Leishmania donovani* was cultured from conjunctival swab, eyelid, anterior chamber and vitreous body, and found, histologically, in reticuloendothelial cells of the eye.

12:60 *Protothecosis* with ocular involvement has been reported.[9] Signs included blindness; a dilated, unresponsive pupil of one eye; lowered tension; a bilateral chorioretinitis, and eventual retinal detachment.

12:61 *Pseumonyssus* mites in the nasal and paranasal sinuses have been incriminated as a cause of chronic orbital cellulitis (Par. 8:20).

12:62 *Cysticercosis* infection of the brain was reported to be associated with retinal abnormalities.[60] Ocular signs consisted of mydriasis, retinal hemorrhage, retinal vascular attenuation and detachment.

13:63 *Thelazia californiensis* infestation of the conjunctival cul-de-sac will cause lacrimation and exudation with a possible associated keratopathy (Par. 5:53).

12:64 *Mange.* Demodex or sarcoptic mange can produce a blepharitis (Par. 4:79).

Deficiencies

12:65 *Vitamin A.* The principal ocular manifestations of an avitaminosis A are erosion of corneal tissue (keratomalacia) (Par. 6:110) (Plate 7D), xerosis (dryness) of the conjunctiva and cornea (Par. 6:70), and loss of vision. Vitamin A deficiency continues to be one of the most widely prevalent and devastating nutritional diseases of man.[38] In the dog the symptom of night blindness should always suggest the possibility of vitamin A deficiency although it more often results from generalized progressive retinal atrophy (Par. 11:54). Diminution in the supply of vitamin A in the form of the aldehyde (retinene) to the rod cells of the retina results in impairment of the function of dark adaptation.

12:66 I have examined blind puppies and

adult dogs that were being fed diets deficient in vitamin A. In some instances the pupil response was good and, from all appearances, the fundi was still unaffected. In others, pupillary response was sluggish and retinal degeneration was in evidence. Correction of the diet and a therapeutic regimen of vitamin A resulted in return of vision (Par. 3:67). A case in point involved a 6-year-old Chihuahua that had whelped 6 weeks before. She had bloody, foul-smelling stools, was on an "odd-and-end" diet and was seeing poorly in subdued light. Examination of the ocular structures disclosed a corneal haze and an overall stain visible with magnification. The pupils were moderately dilated with a sluggish response to light stimuli. The fundi appeared normal. Correction of the diet and an additional vitamin A supplement resulted in return of normal vision and clearing of the cornea within a few days.

12:67 *Riboflavin* (B_2) deficiency is characterized by superficial vascularization with a possible ulceration and subsequent opacity of the cornea.

Poisonings and Intoxications

12:68 Drug and chemical poisonings may produce eye manifestations. These may develop as the direct result of an acute or chronic intoxication and include contraction or dilatation of the pupils, retinal hemorrhages, amblyopia (Par. 11:115) and cataract.

REFERENCES

1. Angell, J.A., Meredith, R.E., Shively, J.N., et al.: Ocular Lesions Associated with Coccidioidomycosis in Dogs: 35 Cases (1980–1985), J.A.V.M.A., *190*:1319–1322, 1987.
2. Armstrong, P.J., DiBartola, S.P.: Canine Coccidioidomycosis: A Literature Review and Report of Eight Cases, J.A.A.H.A., *19*:937–946, Nov/Dec 1983.
3. Ausherman, R.J.: Treatment of Blastomycosis and Histoplasmosis in the Dog, J.A.V.M.A., *163*:1048–1049, 1973.
4. Barron, Von C.N. and Saunders, L.Z.: Ein Fall von intraokulärer Toxoplasmose beim Hund, Schweizer Archiv für Tierheilkunde, *101*:7, 1959.
5. Barron, Von C.N., Saunders, L.Z. and Jebb, K.V.: Intraocular Tumors in Animals. III. Secondary Intraocular Tumors, Am. J. Vet. Res., *24*:835–853, 1963.
6. Bellhorn, R.W.: Secondary Ocular Adenocarcinoma in Three Dogs and a Cat, J.A.V.M.A., *160*:302–307, 1972.
7. Bistner, S., deLaHunta, A., and Lorenz, M.: Generalized Cryptococcosis in a dog, Cornell Vet., *61*:440–457, 1971.
8. Brightman, A.H., Helper, L.C., and Parker, A.J.: Congenital Horner's Syndrome—A Case Report, J. Canine Practice, pp. 19–23, Oct. 1977.
9. Buyukmihci, N., Rubin, L.F., and De Paoli, A.: Protothecosis with Ocular Involvement in a Dog, J.A.V.M.A., *167*:158–160, 1975.
10. *Canine Medicine*, 2nd ed., Santa Barbara, American Veterinary Publications, Inc., p. 636, 1959.
11. Carlton, W.W.: A Case of Blastomycosis in Dog with Pulmonary, Cutaneous and Ocular Lesions, J.A.A.H.A., *10*:586–590, 1974.
12. Carter, J.D., et al.: Ocular and Clinical Features of Thrombocytopenic Purpura, VM/SAC, *66*:125–128, 1972.
13. Case Records, personal and Univ. of Ill. College of Vet. Med.
14. Catcott, E.J.: Ophthalmoscopy in Canine Practice, J.A.V.M.A., *121*:37, 1952.
15. Cello, R.M.: Ocular Manifestations of Coccidioidomycosis in a Dog, Arch. Ophth., *64*:897–903, 1960.
16. Cello, R.M. and Hutcherson, B.: Ocular Changes in Malignant Lymphoma, Cornell Vet., *52*:492–523, 1962.
17. Cogan, David G.: *Neurology of the Ocular Muscles, 2nd Ed.*, Springfield, Charles C Thomas, pp. 189–193, 1956.
18. Cole, C.R.: Personal Communication, 1954.
19. Cole, C.R., et al.: Toxoplasmosis III. Study of Families Exposed to Their Toxoplasma-Infected Pet Dogs, A.M.A. Arch. Int. Med., *92*:308–313, 1953.
20. Darraspen, E. and Lescure, F.: A Propos d'un cas d'hémorrhagie endoculaire Relation possible avec une dysprotéinémie, Revue de Medecine Veterinaire, *111*:275, 1960.
21. de Lahunta, A. and Cummings, J.F.: Neuro-Ophthalmologic Lesions as a Cause of Visual Deficit in Dogs and Horses, J.A.V.M.A., *150*:994, 1967.
22. Ellett, E.W., Playter, R.F., and Pierce, K.R.: Retinal Lesions Associated with Induced Canine Ehrlichiosis, J.A.A.H.A., *9*:4–7, 1973.
23. Engerman, R.L. and Bloodworth, J.M.B.: Experimental Diabetic Retinopathy in Dogs, Arch. Ophth., *73*:205–210, 1965.
24. Fischer, C.A.: Retinal and Retinochoroidal Lesions in Early Neuropathic Canine Distemper, J.A.V.M.A., *6*:740–752, 1971.
25. Fischer, C.A. and Liv, S.K.: Neuro-Ophthalmologic Manifestations of Primary Reticulosis of the Central Nervous System in a Dog, J.A.V.M.A., *7*:1240–1248, 1971.
26. Geib, L.W., et al.: Transitional Cell Carcinoma of the Urinary Bladder in the Dog with Unusual Clinical Signs, Am. Hosp., *3*:22–27, 1967.
27. Gelatt, K.N., McGill, L.D., and Perman, V.: Ocular and Systemic Cryptococcosis in a Dog, J.A.V.M.A., *162*:370–375, 1973.
28. Giles, R.C., et al.: Visceral Leishmaniasis in a Dog

with Bilateral Endophthalmitis, J.A.A.H.A., *11*:155–159, 1975.

29. Heeley, D.M.: Toxoplasmosis, J. Sm. An. Pract., *4*:435–446, 1963.

29a. Hughes, P.L., Dubielzig, R.R., and Kazacos, K.R.: Multifocal Retinalis in New Zealand Sheepdogs, Vet. Path., *24*:22–27, 1987.

30. Hoerlein, B.F.: *Canine Neurology*, Philadelphia, W.B. Saunders Co., p. 255, 1965.

30a. Johnson, B.W., Kirkpatrick, C.E., Morton, D.B., et al.: Ocular Larval Migrans in a Border Collie, Trans. ACVO, p. 300, 1987.

31. Jubb, K.V., Saunders, L.Z. and Coates, H.V.: The Intraocular Lesions of Canine Distemper, J. Comp. Path. & Ther., *67*:21–29, 1957.

32. Kurtz, H.J., and Finco, D.R.: Granulomatous Chorioretinites Caused by Cryptococcus Neoformans in a Dog, J.A.V.M.A., *157*:934–937, 1970.

33. Ladds, P.W., et al.: Canine Ocular Adenocarcinoma of Mammary Origin, J.A.V.M.A., *156*:63, 1970.

34. Lipton, D.: Intraocular Cryptococcosis in a Dog, VM/SAC, *68*:357–358, 1973.

35. McConnell, E.E., et al.: Visceral Leishmaniasis with Ocular Involvement in a Dog, J.A.V.M.A., *156*:197, 1970.

36. McGrath, J.T.: *Neurologic Examination of the Dog*, Philadelphia, Lea & Febiger, p. 26, 1956.

37. McGrath, J.T.: Personal Communication, 1954.

38. McLaren, D.S., et al.: Ocular Manifestations of Vitamin A Deficiency in Man, Bull. World Health Org., *34*:357–361, 1966.

39. Menges, R.W.: Blastomycosis in Animals. A Review of an Analysis of 116 Canine Cases. Vet. Med., *55*:45–54, 1960.

40. Parker, A.J., et al.: Hemifacial Spasms in a Dog, Vet. Record, *93*:514–516, 1973.

41. Patz, A. and Maumenee, A.E.: Studies on Diabetic Retinopathy, 1. Retinopathy in Dog with Spontaneous Diabetes Mellitus, Am. J. Ophth., *54*:532–541, 1962.

42. Piper, R.C., et al.: Natural and Experimental Ocular Toxoplasmosis in Animals, A.J.O., *69*:662–668, 1970.

43. Roberts, S.R. and Vainisi, S.J.: Hemifacial Spasm in Dogs, J.A.V.M.A., *150*:381, 1967.

44. Rubin, L.F.: Applications of Adrenergic Drugs in Ophthalmology J. Am. An. Hosp. Assoc., *4*:251, 1968.

45. Rubin, L.F.: *Atlas of Veterinary Ophthalmoscopy*, Philadelphia, Lea & Febiger, 1974.

46. Rubin, L.F.: *Ocular Manifestations of Arteriosclerosis and Hypertension in Dogs*, Proc. Am. Coll. Vet. Ophth., 1975.

47. Rubin, L.F. and Craig, P.H.: Intraocular Cryptococcosis in a Dog, J.A.V.M.A., *147*:27, 1965.

48. Rubin, L.F. and Saunders, L.Z.: Intraocular Larva Migrans in Dogs, Path. Vet., *2*:566–573, 1965.

49. Rutgers, C., Kowolski, J., Cole, C.R., et al.: Severe Rocky Mountain Spotted Fever in 5 Dogs, J.A.A.H.A., 2[illegible]:361–369, (May–June) 1985.

50. Salfelder, K., et al.: Experimental Ocular Histoplasmosis in Dogs, Am. J. Ophth., *59*:290, 1965.

51. Saunders, L.Z.: *Pathology of the Eye*, edited by Ernst Joest, Berlin, Verlag Paul Pary, 1968.

52. Saunders, L.Z. and Barron, Von C.N.: Intraocular Tumors in Animals: IV. Lymphosarcoma, Brit. Vet. J., *120*:25–35, 1964.

53. Selby, L.A., et al.: Canine Blastomycosis, Sm. An. Clinician, *59*:1221–1228, 1964.

54. Shively, J.N. and Whiteman, C.E.: Ocular Lesions in Disseminated Coccidioidomycosis in Two Dogs, Path. Vet., *7*:1–6, 1970.

55. Sibay, T.M. and Hausler, H.R.: Eye Findings in Two Spontaneously Diabetic Related Dogs, Am. J. Ophth., *63*:289, 1967.

56. Simon, J. and Helper, L.C.: Ocular Disease Associated with Blastomycosis in Dogs, J.A.V.M.A., *157*:922–925, 1970.

57. Symanski, C.M.: Bilateral Metastatic Intraocular Hemangiosarcoma in a Dog, J.A.V.M.A., *161*:803–805, 1972.

58. Trautwein, G. and Nielsen, S.W.: Cryptococcosis in 2 Cats, a Dog and a Mink, J.A.V.M.A., *140*:438, 1962.

59. Trevino, G.S.: Canine Blastomycosis with Ocular Involvement, Path. Vet., *3*(6):653–658, 1966.

60. Wilson, F.D.: Cytophlegia due to Cysticercus Cellulosae in the Brain of a Dog, Indian Vet. J., *39*:393–396, 1962.

61. Wolf, G.F., et al.: Blastomycosis in the Dog. Two Cases with Ocular Manifestations, Vet. Med., *53*:595, 1958.

62. Wyman, M., and McKissick, G.E.: Lipemia Retinalis in a Dog and Cat: Case Reports, J.A.A.H.A., 9:288–291, 1973.

Appendix 1
BREED PREDISPOSITION TO CONDITIONS OF THE EYE

Afghan Hound
Juvenile cataract
Akita
Progressive retinal atrophy
Australian Shepherd
Microphthalmia
Persistent pupillary membrane
Retinal dysplasia
Scleral ectasia
Basenji
Persistent pupillary membrane
Basset Hound
Ectropion
Primary glaucoma (mesodermal dysgenesis of the iridocorneal angle) (goniodysgenesis)
Secondary glaucoma ? (subluxation of the lens)
Beagle
Glaucoma (primary open-angle glaucoma or primary angle closure glaucoma)
Hypoplasia (or aplasia) of the optic nerve
Progressive retinal atrophy
Prolapse of the gland of the third eyelid
Retinal dysplasia
Bedlington Terrier
Atresia of lacrimal puncta or canaliculi
Distichiasis
Retinal dysplasia (detachment)
Bloodhound
Chronic keratoconjunctivitis
Ectropion
Border Collie
Central retinal atrophy
Boston Terrier
Entropion (medial canthus)
Juvenile cataract
Prolapse of the gland of the third eyelid
Boxer
Superficial corneal erosion (Boxer ulcer)
Briard
Central retinal atrophy
Bulldog (English)
Distichiasis
Ectropion
Entropion (lower lid, medial canthus, lateral canthus)
Bull Mastiff
Entropion
Eversion of the cartilage of the third eyelid
Cairn Terrier
Scleral pigment hyperplasia syndrome
Secondary glaucoma (subluxation of lens)
Chesapeake Bay Retriever
Entropion
Progressive retinal atrophy
Chihuahua
Keratoconjunctivitis sicca
Prolapse of the gland of the third eyelid
Secondary glaucoma (subluxation of lens)
Chow Chow
Entropion (lateral canthus)
Narrow palpebral fissure

Cocker Spaniel
Chronic blepharoconjunctivitis and KCS
Corneal dystrophy
Distichiasis
Ectropion
Glaucoma (acute primary narrow-angle glaucoma)
Juvenile cataract
Oversized upper eyelashes
Progressive retinal atrophy
Prolapse of the gland of the third eyelid
Retinal dysplasia
Secondary glaucoma ? (subluxation of lens)

Collie
Collie eye anomaly
Corneal dystrophy
Hypoplasia of the optic nerve
Microphthalmia
Persistent pupillary membrane
Progressive retinal atrophy and central retinal atrophy
Proliferative keratoconjunctivitis

Dachshund
Chronic superficial keratitis (pannus)
Superficial corneal erosion
Punctate keratitis

Doberman Pinscher
Persistent hyperplastic primary vitreous (PHPV)

Fox Terrier (Smooth and Wire-haired)
Corneal dystrophy—both epithelial (superficial) and endothelial (Wire-haired Terriers)
Superficial corneal erosion (Wire-haired Terriers)
Juvenile cataract
Secondary glaucoma (subluxation of lens)

German Shepherd
Chronic superficial keratitis (pannus)
Plasma cell infiltration of the third eyelid

Golden Retriever
Cataract (Congenital and juvenile)
Central retinal atrophy
Distichiasis
Entropion (lower lid and lateral canthus)
Retinal dysplasia

Gordon Setter
Progressive retinal atrophy

Great Dane
Ectropion
Entropion
Eversion or inversion of the third eyelid
Microphthalmia

Irish Setter
Progressive retinal atrophy

Labrador Retriever
Progressive retinal atrophy and central retinal atrophy
Entropion
Juvenile cataract
Retinal dysplasia and detachment

Manchester Terrier
Secondary glaucoma (subluxation of lens)

Norwegian Elkhound
Glaucoma (primary open-angle glaucoma)
Progressive retinal atrophy

Old English Sheepdog
Cataract (congenital)

Pekingese
Atresia of lacrimal drainage apparatus
Corneal ulceration
Distichiasis
Entropion (medial canthus)
Keratoconjunctivitis sicca
Pigmentary keratitis
Trichiasis

Pinscher (Miniature)
Keratoconjunctivitis sicca

Pointer
Progressive retinal atrophy

Pomeranian
Distichiasis
Epiphora
Trichiasis

Poodle (Miniature and Toy)
Chronic superficial keratitis (Miniature Poodles)
Distichiasis
Entropion (medial canthus)
Epiphora
Hypoplasia (or aplasia) of the optic nerve (Miniature Poodles)
Iridal atrophy
Juvenile cataract
Microphthalmia
Progressive retinal atrophy

Pug
Entropion (medial canthus)
Exposure keratitis and corneal ulcers
Keratoconjunctivitis sicca
Pigmentary keratitis
Trichiasis

Rottweiler
Entropion
Retinal dysplasia

Saint Bernard
Dermoid
Distichiasis
Ectropion
Entropion
Eversion or inversion of the third eyelid

Samoyed
Progressive retinal atrophy

Schnauzer (Miniature)
Atresia of lacrimal drainage apparatus
Congenital cataract
Juvenile cataract
Microphthalmia

Sealyham Terrier
Atresia of the nasolacrimal duct
Cataract
Retinal dysplasia (detachment)
Secondary glaucoma (subluxation of lens)

Shetland Sheepdog
Central retinal atrophy
Collie eye anomaly

Siberian Husky
Corneal dystrophy—both epithelial (superficial) and endothelial
Juvenile cataract

Springer Spaniel
Central retinal atrophy
Progressive retinal atrophy
Retinal dysplasia

Staffordshire Bull Terrier
Persistent hyperplastic primary vitreous (PHPV)

Tibetan Terrier
Progressive retinal atrophy
Stationary night blindness ?

Toy Terrier
Secondary glaucoma (subluxation of lens)

Weimaraner
Eversion or inversion of the third eyelid

Welsh Corgi
Superficial corneal erosion
Secondary glaucoma (subluxation of lens)

West Highland White Terrier
Keratoconjunctivitis sicca

Yorkshire Terrier
Keratoconjunctivitis sicca
Retinal dysplasia